OKANAGAN UNIVERSITY COLLEGE
LIBRARY
BRITISH COLUMBIA

Neurological, Psychiatric, and Developmental Disorders

Meeting the Challenge in the Developing World

Committee on Nervous System Disorders in
Developing Countries

Board on Global Health

INSTITUTE OF MEDICINE

NATIONAL ACADEMY PRESS
Washington, D.C.

NATIONAL ACADEMY PRESS ● 2101 Constitution Avenue, N.W. ● Washington, DC 20418

NOTICE: The project that is the subject of this report was approved by the Governing Board of the National Research Council, whose members are drawn from the councils of the National Academy of Sciences, the National Academy of Engineering, and the Institute of Medicine. The members of the committee responsible for the report were chosen for their special competences and with regard for appropriate balance.

Support for this project was provided by Centers for Disease Control and Prevention, Global Forum for Health Research, National Institute for Child Health and Human Development, National Institute for Mental Health, National Institute for Neurological Disorders and Stroke, and the Fogarty International Center of the National Institutes of Health. The views presented in this report are those of the Institute of Medicine Committee on Nervous System Disorders in Developing Countries and are not necessarily those of the funding agencies.

Library of Congress Control Number: 2001090472
International Standard Book Number: 0-309-07192-5

Additional copies of this report are available for sale from the National Academy Press, 2101 Constitution Avenue, N.W., Box 285, Washington, D.C. 20055. Call (800) 624-6242 or (202) 334-3313 (in the Washington metropolitan area), or visit the NAP's home page at www.nap.edu. The full text of this report is available at www.nap.edu.

For more information about the Institute of Medicine, visit the IOM home page at: www.iom.edu.

Copyright 2001 by the National Academy of Sciences. All rights reserved.

Printed in the United States of America.

Cover: Mbangu mask, Central Pende, Bandundu, Zaire, registered in 1959. One of the great masterworks of Pende art in Western collections, this Mbangu mask represents the bewitched him. It dances to the song, "We look on (unable to help), the sorcerers have bewitched him." The masker wears a humpback from which an arrow extends. The arrow refers to the popular image of sorcerers "shooting" their prey with invisible arrows when they cast their spell. The metaphor communicates the perception of sudden onslaught in illness or misfortune, just as we might say, "It came out of the blue."

Mbangu is "bewitched"; however, since the Pende worldview attributes almost all illness and personal misfortune to the malice of others, what is really at issue is chronic illness or disability and our response to it. If he does not carry a bow and arrows, the dancer usually avails himself of a cane to indicate his physical weakness. The black-and-white division of his face refers to the scars of someone who fell into the fire due to epilepsy or some other medical condition. This sculptor has also depicted traces of smallpox on the black eyelid, and the face is pulled down on one side due to a paralysis of the facial nerve. Sculptor and performer collaborate to make Mbangu a composite sign of illness and disability, of all the misfortunes that can befall someone.

What then is to be our response to Mbangu? Some sculptors render the mask comedic, but this work conveys an extraordinary delicacy and sympathy by contrasting the gentle perfection of the features on one side with the systematic distortion on the other. This sculptor responds to the widespread version of Mbangu's song: "Do not mock your neighbor, do not laugh at your brother, the sorcerers have bewitched him." In other words, anyone can fall prey to misfortune; it could happen to you. Our brother, our neighbor, deserves our support.

Permission to use this image was kindly granted by the Royal Museum of Central Africa. ©AFRICA-MUSEUM TERVUREN(BELGIUM)

The serpent has been a symbol of long life, healing, and knowledge among almost all cultures and religions since the beginning of recorded history. The serpent adopted as a logotype by the Institute of Medicine is a relief carving from ancient Greece, now held by the Staatliche Museen in Berlin.

"Knowing is not enough; we must apply.
Willing is not enough; we must do.
—Goethe

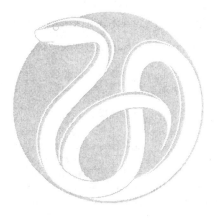

INSTITUTE OF MEDICINE

Shaping the Future for Health

THE NATIONAL ACADEMIES

National Academy of Sciences
National Academy of Engineering
Institute of Medicine
National Research Council

The **National Academy of Sciences** is a private, nonprofit, self-perpetuating society of distinguished scholars engaged in scientific and engineering research, dedicated to the furtherance of science and technology and to their use for the general welfare. Upon the authority of the charter granted to it by the Congress in 1863, the Academy has a mandate that requires it to advise the federal government on scientific and technical matters. Dr. Bruce M. Alberts is president of the National Academy of Sciences.

The **National Academy of Engineering** was established in 1964, under the charter of the National Academy of Sciences, as a parallel organization of outstanding engineers. It is autonomous in its administration and in the selection of its members, sharing with the National Academy of Sciences the responsibility for advising the federal government. The National Academy of Engineering also sponsors engineering programs aimed at meeting national needs, encourages education and research, and recognizes the superior achievements of engineers. Dr. William A. Wulf is president of the National Academy of Engineering.

The **Institute of Medicine** was established in 1970 by the National Academy of Sciences to secure the services of eminent members of appropriate professions in the examination of policy matters pertaining to the health of the public. The Institute acts under the responsibility given to the National Academy of Sciences by its congressional charter to be an adviser to the federal government and, upon its own initiative, to identify issues of medical care, research, and education. Dr. Kenneth I. Shine is president of the Institute of Medicine.

The **National Research Council** was organized by the National Academy of Sciences in 1916 to associate the broad community of science and technology with the Academy's purposes of furthering knowledge and advising the federal government. Functioning in accordance with general policies determined by the Academy, the Council has become the principal operating agency of both the National Academy of Sciences and the National Academy of Engineering in providing services to the government, the public, and the scientific and engineering communities. The Council is administered jointly by both Academies and the Institute of Medicine. Dr. Bruce M. Alberts and Dr. William A. Wulf are chairman and vice chairman, respectively, of the National Research Council.

COMMITTEE ON NERVOUS SYSTEM DISORDERS IN DEVELOPING COUNTRIES

ASSEN JABLENSKY (*Co-chair*), Professor, Department of Psychiatry, University of Western Australia, Perth

RICHARD JOHNSON (*Co-chair*), Professor, Department of Neurology, Co-Chair of Department of Microbiology and Neurosciences, John Hopkins University School of Medicine, Baltimore, Maryland

WILLIAM BUNNEY, JR., Professor and Della Martin Chair, Department of Psychiatry and Human Behavior, University of California at Irvine

MARCELO CRUZ, Professor, Neurosciences Institute, Central University of Ecuador, Quito

MAUREEN DURKIN, Professor, Sergievsky Center, Joseph L. Mailman School of Public Health, Columbia University, New York, New York

JULIUS FAMILUSI, Professor, Department of Pediatrics, University College Hospital, Ibadan, Nigeria

M. GOURIE-DEVI, Director-Vice Chancellor, and Professor of Neurology, National Institute of Mental Health and Neurosciences, Bangalore, India

DEAN JAMISON, (Board on Global Health Liaison), Director, Program on International Health, Education, and Environment, University of California at Los Angeles

RACHEL JENKINS, Director, World Health Organization Collaborating Centre, Institute of Psychiatry, London, United Kingdom

SYLVIA KAAYA, Professor, Department of Psychiatry, Muhimbili University College of Health Science, Dar es Salaam, Tanzania

ARTHUR KLEINMAN, Presley Professor of Anthropology and Psychiatry, Departments of Anthropology and Social Medicine, Harvard University, Boston, Massachusetts

THOMAS MCGUIRE, Professor, Department of Economics, Boston University, Massachusetts

R. SRINIVASA MURTHY, Dean, and Professor of Psychiatry, National Institute of Mental Health and Neurosciences, Bangalore, India

DONALD SILBERBERG, Professor of Neurology, Director of International Medical Programs, University of Pennsylvania School of Medicine, Philadelphia

BEDIRHAN ÜSTÜN, Group Leader of Assessment, Classification, and Epidemiology Group, World Health Organization, Geneva, Switzerland

Study Staff

STACEY KNOBLER, Study Director (from February 2000 to May 2001)

JUDITH BALE, Director, Board on Global Health and Study Director

PAMELA MANGU, Study Director (from September 1999 to February 2000)

CHRISTINE COUSSENS, Research Associate

ALISON MACK, Consultant Writer

LAURIE SPINELLI, Project Assistant

KEVIN CROSBY, The National Academies Christine Mirzayan Internship Program

CARLA HANASH, The National Academies Christine Mirzayan Internship Program

BOARD ON GLOBAL HEALTH

DEAN JAMISON, *(Chair)*, Director, Program on International Health, Education, and Environment, University of California at Los Angeles

YVES BERGEVIN, Senior Health Specialist, Canadian International Development Agency

HARVEY FINEBERG, Provost, Harvard University, Boston, Massachusetts

EILEEN KENNEDY, Deputy Under Secretary for Research, Education, and Economics, U. S. Department of Agriculture, Washington, D.C.

ARTHUR KLEINMAN, Presley Professor of Medical Anthropology and Psychiatry, Harvard Medical School, Boston, Massachusetts

PATRICIA DANZON, Professor of Health Care Systems Development, Wharton School, University of Pennsylvania, Philadelphia

NOREEN GOLDMAN, Professor, Woodrow Wilson School of Public and International Affairs, Princeton University, Princeton, New Jersey

ALLAN ROSENFIELD, Dean, Mailman School of Public Health, Columbia University, New York, New York

ADEL MAHMOUD, President, Merck Vaccines, Whitehouse Station, New Jersey

SUSAN SCRIMSHAW, Dean, School of Public Health, University of Illinois at Chicago

JOHN WYN OWEN, Secretary, Nuffield Trust, London, United Kingdom

GERALD KEUSCH, *(Liaison)*, Director, Fogarty International Center, National Institutes of Health, Bethesda, Maryland

DAVID CHALLONER, *(IOM Foreign Secretary)*, Vice President for Health Affairs, University of Florida, Gainesville

Staff
JUDITH BALE, Director
JONATHAN DAVIS, Study Director
STACEY KNOBLER, Study Director
KATHERINE OBERHOLTZER, Project Assistant
LAURIE SPINELLI, Project Assistant

REVIEWERS

This report has been reviewed in draft form by individuals chosen for their diverse perspectives and technical expertise, in accordance with procedures approved by the National Research Council's Report Review Committee. The purpose of this independent review is to provide candid and critical comments that will assist the institution in making the published report as sound as possible and to ensure that the report meets institutional standards for objectivity, evidence, and responsiveness to the study charge. The review comments and the draft manuscript remain confidential to protect the integrity of the deliberative process. We wish to thank the following individuals for their review of this report:

Naomar Almeida-Filho, Campus Universitario-Canela, Salvador-Bahia, Brazil
Nancy Andreasen, University of Iowa Hospitals and Clinics, Iowa City
Gretchen Birbeck, Michigan State University, East Lansing
Daniel Chisholm, World Health Organization, Geneva, Switzerland
Sir David Goldberg, King's College, United Kingdom, London
Nora Groce, Yale University, New Haven, Connecticut
Vladimir Hachinski, University of Western Ontario, Canada
William Harlan, National Institutes of Health, Bethesda, Maryland
Guy Mckhann, John Hopkins University School of Medicine, Baltimore, Maryland
Alberto Minoletti, Ministry of Health, Santiago, Chile
Malik Mubbashar, WHO Collaborating Centre for Research Training in Mental Health, Rawalpindi, Pakistan
Elena Nightingale, Institute of Medicine, Washington, D.C.
Nimal Senanayake, University of Peradeniya, Sri Lanka
Rune Simeonsson, University of North Carolina, Chapel Hill
R. Thara, Schizophrenia Research Foundation, Chennai, India
Myrna Weissman, Columbia University College of Physicians and Surgeons, New York

Although the reviewers listed above have provided many constructive comments and suggestions, they were not asked to endorse the conclusions or recommendations nor did they see the final draft of the report before its release. The review of this report was overseen by Arthur Asbury, University of Pennsylvania School of Medicine, Philadelphia, and Floyd Bloom, The Scripps Research Institute, La Jolla, California, who were responsible for making certain that an independent examination of this report was carried out in accordance with institutional procedures and that all review comments were carefully considered. Responsibility for the final content of this report rests entirely with the authoring committee and the institution.

Preface

The continuing existence of gross disparities in health between affluent and poorer countries is becoming a major challenge for policy makers in the new millennium. While the link between poverty and disease is well established and has been recognized by public health leaders and social reformers for a century and a half, the complexity of this relationship has become apparent only in the last several decades as national governments and international organizations have accorded health increasing priority in development programs. It is now widely accepted that socioeconomic development and population health must advance together to be sustainable in the long term. Improvements in population health are not merely or even necessarily a by-product of economic growth. They are a prerequisite and a driving force of economic and social productivity. Reductions in maternal and infant mortality, improvements in nutrition and environmental sanitation, and control of communicable diseases have made important contributions to economic growth. Conversely, high levels of preventable morbidity and mortality, survival with chronic disability, reduced quality of life, and widespread demoralization are a drain on society's resources and impede overall development.

For several decades, investments in health in the context of national and international development strategies have targeted primarily the major communicable diseases, malnutrition, and poor sanitation in low-income countries. A number of such programs have successfully lowered infant mortality rates and, as a result, increased life expectancy at birth. However, the net effect of such gains has been largely offset by the epidemiological transition from a morbidity and mortality pattern dominated by acute and often fatal communicable diseases to one characterized by a rapid rise in chronic and potentially disabling diseases such as cardiovascular disorders, diabetes, and neoplasms. As a consequence, middle- and low-income countries are increasingly facing an epidemic of chronic diseases along with the unfinished agenda of infectious disease and malnutrition.

This complex epidemiological situation is further complicated by the widespread incidence of neurological, psychiatric, and developmental disorders, all involving a congenital or acquired brain dysfunction and affecting the behavior and quality of life of some 250 million people in the developing world. Their global importance was highlighted in the *Global Burden of Disease* study published in 1996 by the World Health Organization (WHO), the World Bank, and the Harvard School of Public Health. Although brain disorders account for only 12 percent of all deaths in these estimates, they are responsible for at least 27 percent of all years of life lived with disability, and this combined share of the total global burden of disease was estimated at nearly 15 percent in 1990 and projected to rise significantly by 2020. Negative attitudes, prejudice, and stigma are associated with many of the neurological, psychiatric, and developmental conditions. As a result, the majority of people affected by these disorders in developing countries remain virtually untreated, while for many others the conditions remain undiagnosed. Since many of these disorders run a continuous or recurrent course that is often lifelong, they profoundly affect an individual's capacity to relate to others and perform culturally expected roles, and result in significant distress and dysfunction among family members and the community. Therefore, their socioeconomic impact is likely to be greater than their prevalence would suggest.

Despite negative attitudes, prejudice, and neglect, many brain disorders can be successfully addressed: some can be prevented from occurring, and all the disabling sequelae of others can be mitigated. Treatment, prevention, and reduction of disability for this group of disorders could therefore have a major impact on the total burden of disease and disability in developing countries.

Indeed, the timeliness of initiatives to raise global public awareness of brain disorders in developing countries is underscored by major advances in scientific understanding of the neurobiology of brain development and function, epitomized by the Decade of the Brain, 1990–2000. Echoing the farsighted aphorism of one of the founders of modern psychiatry that "mental diseases are brain diseases" (Griesinger, 1845), current neuroscience research now recognizes mental disorders as arising from brain dysfunctions that interact with environmental triggers at different stages of neurodevelopment. The mapping and cloning of specific genes that contribute to vulnerability to psychiatric disorders will be greatly accelerated by the complete sequencing of the human genome and by powerful new technologies for gene tracking and functional analysis. Such knowledge will inevitably provide new insights into the pathophysiology of these disorders and lead to novel treatments. Similarly, the diagnosis and treatment of many neurological disorders are likely to be revolutionized as a result of advances in molecular neuroscience. An increasing number of such disorders may become preventable in the not-too-distant future.

It is important at the same time to recognize that, regardless of the promise of future developments, many of the brain disorders accounting for a major share of the burden of disease and disability in the developing world can be treated effectively with means that are currently available and, in principle, affordable. To highlight these opportunities and the prerequisites for implementing appropriate interventions, was the principal task of the Committee on Nervous System Disorders in Developing Countries, convened by the U.S. Institute of Medicine.

This study was sponsored and supported by the U.S. Centers for Disease Control and Prevention, the Fogarty International Center of the National Institutes of Health, the Global Forum for Health Research, the National Institute of Child Health and Human Development, the National Institute of Mental Health, and the National Institute of Neurological Disease and Stroke.

The charge to the committee was first to address the broad burden of neurological, psychiatric, and developmental disorders and then to focus on six groups of conditions: developmental disabilities affecting the central nervous system in early life, epilepsy, unipolar depression, bipolar disorder, schizophrenia, and stroke. These conditions share the following characteristics:

- highly prevalent;
- potentially disabling;
- often subject to stigma and neglect; and
- amenable to interventions that are effective and relatively low cost.

The specific focus on six groups of disorders does not imply future exclusion from consideration of other conditions that meet the same criteria, fully or in part. Peripheral neuropathies, alcohol and drug dependence, dementia, and disorders resulting from trauma and interpersonal violence are examples of conditions that merit commensurate attention and it is hoped that they will be the subject of future studies.

The membership of the committee reflects both the multidisciplinary nature of the problems to be addressed and the need for first-hand familiarity with and expertise in their socioeconomic and cultural context in various regions of the world. Thus, the committee comprised 15 members with expertise in fields as diverse as clinical neurology and psychiatry, developmental neuroscience, epidemiology, cultural anthropology, and health economics. In addition, the committee had the benefit of access to consultants and advisers with expertise in primary health care, health statistics, and public policy. A complete list of contributors is included in Appendix A. Invaluable technical and administrative support throughout the study, including compilation of an extensive bibliography, literature research, technical writing, and editing, was provided by the staff of the Institute of Medicine. We thank each of these individuals and organizations for their assistance and support over the course of this study.

Assen Jablensky, M.D.   Richard Johnson, M.D.

Acknowledgments

The breadth and scope of the issues considered within this report are extensive. The committee is grateful for the many individuals who contributed their time and expertise toward the committee's understanding of these complex issues and the development of the report. Particular thanks are in order to the authors of the background papers, whose efforts provided important information bearing on the topic of this report and the development of draft chapters: Eduardo Castilla, Eclamc/Genetica, Fiocruz, Brazil; Oyewusi Gureje, University College Hospital, Nigeria; Nalia Khan, Bangladesh Institute of Child Health; Kwame McKenzie, Institute of Psychiatry, University College, London; Vikram Patel, London School of Tropical Hygiene and Sangath Centre, Goa, India; Gregory Powell, University of Zimbabwe; and Marigold (Molly) Thorburn, 3D Projects of Jamaica and the Jamaica Coalition on Disabilities.

The committee thanks Marcelo Cruz, Maureen Durkin, Assen Jablensky, Rachel Jenkins, Tom McGuire, and Donald Silberberg for their chapter drafts; and William Bunney, Julius Familusi, M. Gourie-Devi, Dean Jamison, Dick Johnson, Sylvia Kaaya, Arthur Kleinman, Srinivasa Murthy, and Bedirhan Üstün for their substantive contributions to the committee deliberations and draft chapter reviews.

Special thanks is expressed to the following workshop participants for advising and informing the committee's efforts: Alex Cohen, Harvard Medical School; Beugre Kouassi, University of Abidjan-Cocody, Ivory Coast; Thomas Langfitt, University of Pennsylvania; Jessie Mbwambo, Muhimbili University College of Health Science, Tanzania; Norman Sartorius, University of Geneva,

Switzerland; Peter Schantz, Centers for Disease Control and Prevention; and Harvey Whiteford, the World Bank.

The committee is particularly grateful for those who provided technical review of and substantive contributions to draft chapters: Gretchen Birbeck of Michigan State University, East Lansing; Jose Biller of Indiana University School of Medicine; Ellis D'Arrigo Busnello of the Universidade Federal do Rio Grande do Sul, Brazil; Robert Edgerton and Jerome Engel of University of California, Los Angeles; Joop T. V. M. de Jong of the Transcultural Psychosocial Organisation, Amsterdam; Matthew Menken of the World Federation of Neurology Research Group on Medical Education; Pierre-Marie Preux and Michel Dumas of the Institut de Neurologie Tropicale, Limoges, France; Leonid Prilipko of the Department of Mental Health and Substance Dependence, World Health Organization; Niphon Poungvarin of Mahidol University, Thailand; Ralph Sacco of Columbia University; Josemir W. A. S. Sander and Robert Scott of the Institute of Neurology, University College, London; and Rune Simeonsson of the University of North Carolina, Chapel Hill.

The committee gratefully acknowledges those who provided data, information, and guidance critical to the committee's deliberations: Gallo Diop of the Centre Hospitalier Universitaire De Fam, Dakar, Senegal; Ronald Kessler of Harvard Medical School; Robert Kohn of Brown University; Itzhak Levav, Charles Godue, and Felix Rigoli of the Pan American Health Organization; Beverly Long of the World Federation for Mental Health; Ronald Manderscheid of the Substance Abuse and Mental Health Services Administration, U.S. Department of Health and Human Services; Benedetto Saraceno of the World Health Organization; Hisao Sato of the Japan College of Social Work; Koon Sik Min of the Sam Yook Rehabilitation Center, Korea; B.S. Singhal of the Bombay Hospital Institute of Medical Sciences, India; James Toole of the Wake Forest University School of Medicine and the World Federation of Neurology; and the African Medical and Research Foundation.

Finally, and in particular, the committee would like to express its deep appreciation of the Institute of Medicine (IOM) staff who facilitated the work of this committee. We especially thank Judith Bale, Stacey Knobler, and Alison Mack for translating and transforming the discussions and draft chapters of the committee and technical review comments into final prose; Laurie Spinelli for her tireless efforts in research verification and preparation of the manuscript for publication; and Christine Coussens, Stephanie Baxter-Parrott, Kevin Crosby, Carla Hanash, Amber Johnson, Witney McKiernan, Katherine Oberholtzer, and Tara Rao for their valuable research and logistical support of the committee's efforts. The committee is grateful for the contributions of Pamela Mangu during the initial stages of the project. Others within the IOM and the National Academies who were instrumental in seeing the project to completion were Paige Baldwin, Clyde Behney, Andrea Cohen, Mike Edington, Janice Mehler,

Jennifer Otten, Sarah Schlosser, and Curt Taylor. Thanks are also due to editorial consultants Rona Briere, Phillip Sawicki, and Beth Gyorgy.

This project was funded by the Centers for Disease Control and Prevention (CDC), Global Forum for Health Research (GFHR), Fogarty International Center of the National Institutes of Health (FIC), National Institute of Child Health and Human Development (NICHD), National Institute of Mental Health (NIMH), and the National Institute of Neurological Disorders and Stroke (NINDS). The committee is appreciative of their support and of the commitment and productive efforts of Duane Alexander (NICHD), Coleen Boyle (CDC), Robert Eiss (FIC), Gerald Fischbach (NINDS), Walter Gulbinat (GFHR), Gray Handley (NICHD), Steven Hyman (NIMH), Gerald Keusch (FIC), Grayson Norquist (NIMH), Mary Lou Oster-Granite (NICHD), Darrel Regier (NIMH), Joana Rosario (NINDS), and Agnes Rupp (NIMH).

Contents

Neurological, Psychiatric, And Developmental Disorders

Meeting the Challenge in the Developing World

Part I

Executive Summary

Neurological, psychiatric, and developmental disorders exact a profound economic and personal toll worldwide, yet public and private health care systems, particularly in developing countries, have paid little attention to them. Today, growing recognition of the prevalence of these disorders and the availability of prevention strategies and cost-effective treatment make it both important and possible to substantially reduce their impact, even where resources are limited.

Neurological, psychiatric, and developmental disorders encompass a wide range of disabling conditions, including epilepsy, stroke, schizophrenia, unipolar depression, bipolar disorder, mental retardation, cerebral palsy, and autism. Although diverse, these conditions are increasingly recognized as disorders of the brain and its neural connections interacting with the environment; accordingly, in this report they are often referred to in the aggregate as *brain disorders*.

Brain disorders are currently estimated to affect as many as 1.5 billion people worldwide—a number that is expected to grow as life expectancy increases. Since most disorders affecting the brain and its neural connections result in long-term disability and many have an early age of onset, measures of prevalence and mortality vastly understate the disability they cause. Social isolation and stigma often add to the medical and financial burden borne by patients and their families.

The breadth and diversity of brain disorders present a complex task to researchers attempting to measure their impact. Health care economists have widely adopted the term *burden of disease* to express a combination of the frequency and distribution of a disorder or group of disorders, the death and disabil-

1

ity they cause, and the resulting economic impact. Brain disorders are responsible for at least 27 percent of all years lived with disability in developing countries. The collective impact of brain disorders is partially captured by disability-adjusted life years (DALYs), a measure of the burden of disease that combines years lost as a result of death and disability, the latter being weighted according to severity. When disability is taken into consideration along with death, brain disorders comprise nearly 15 percent of the burden of disease in developing countries. Current figures are seriously underestimated, however, since many patients with these conditions in developing countries, particularly children, are not diagnosed and do not receive medical care. In the United States, 12 to 18 percent of children are estimated to be disabled in some way. The numbers are likely to be substantially higher in developing countries, where children are also more frequently exposed to infectious diseases and nutritional deficiencies. As improvements in health care and sanitation enable more children in the developing world to survive, the number of children with developmental disabilities is very likely to rise without concomitant efforts to reduce their occurrence.

Today's rapidly changing global economy poses a significant challenge to the developing world. To meet it, developing countries must foster healthy, educated workers, a process that begins with prenatal care and continues to adulthood. Since many brain disorders interfere with education as well as health, they present a threat to economic development. For low-income countries, the social and economic consequences of ignoring the burden of brain disorders are large and will continue to grow.

BACKGROUND

Responding to growing awareness of the impact of brain disorders and initiatives undertaken to address them, the Committee on Neurological, Psychiatric, and Developmental Disorders in Developing Countries, convened by the U.S. Institute of Medicine, was charged to prepare a consensus report that would define the increasing burden caused by neurological, psychiatric, and developmental disorders in developing countries, and to identify opportunities for effectively reducing that burden with cost-effective strategies for prevention, diagnosis, and treatment. The committee was also asked to identify areas for research, development, and capacity strengthening that would contribute most significantly to reducing the overall burden of these disorders in developing countries (Part I of the report) and to focus on several major groups of conditions: developmental disabilities, epilepsy, schizophrenia, bipolar disorder, unipolar depression, and stroke (Part II of the report).

The study was sponsored by the Global Forum for Health Research, U.S. National Institutes of Health's Fogarty International Center, U.S. National Institute of Child Health and Human Development, U.S. National Institute of

Mental Health, U.S. National Institute of Neurological Disorders and Stroke, and U.S. Centers for Disease Control and Prevention.

The U.S. Institute of Medicine assembled a study committee with broad international expertise in neurology, psychiatry, pediatrics, microbiology, epidemiology, public health, economics, and clinical and basic research. Members of the committee were chosen for their first-hand experience with these disorders in a wide range of middle- and low- income countries.[*]

SCOPE

In its 1997 report, *America's Vital Interest in Global Health,* the Institute of Medicine's Board on Global Health presented the long-term benefits that would accrue to the developed countries from improvements in global health. Building on the findings of that report and in conjunction with initiatives supported by this report's sponsors, international development agencies, development banks, and developing country communities, this report provides an evidence base to inform steps needed to address brain disorders in developing countries. The report committee considered a wide base of scientific evidence on these disorders in order to:

- define the burden of morbidity and disability due to brain disorders;
- describe the causes and risk factors associated with these disorders;
- identify effective, affordable strategies for their prevention and treatment, and rehabilitation of the afflicted;
- identify mechanisms for incorporating care for brain disorders into existing health care systems in developing countries.

The data for this study were identified by the committee and other experts from several disciplines through bibliographic references on related topics, and through databases such as Medline, university libraries, and Internet sites of organizations associated with research and services for neurological and psychiatric disorders. Although much of the published information on neurological and psychiatric disorders in developing countries was found in international and national journals and reports, some of the evidence is from regional journals, the proceedings of meetings, and unpublished reports prepared for the World Health Organization (WHO) and other international organizations. To review this knowledge base, the committee enlisted experts with recent research or service experience in developing countries. Data and supportive evidence were provided by these experts in workshop presentations, commissioned papers, and technical consultation. The framework for the committee's deliberations included an

---

[*] The countries addressed in this report have per capita incomes of $9266 or less. Low-income countries have per capita incomes of less than $766. The poorest people live on less than $2 a day.

overview of epidemiological parameters, a review of the evidence that supports interventions, and projections of the feasibility, cost, and expected impact of proposed interventions.

The combined weight of such evidence, the committee believes, provides an accurate account of the epidemiology of the six disorders covered in this report, their treatment and management in developing countries, and the capacity of local health care systems to treat them. Evaluation of the available evidence enabled the committee to identify areas where gaps in knowledge exist and to propose strategies for a research agenda that would inform these areas. The findings, strategies, and recommendations of this report have been developed from this broad base of evidence. The report also specifies where the data are inadequate to support additional conclusions.

This report is intended to engage a broad spectrum of individuals, including policy makers at the international level, such as WHO, the World Bank, and UNICEF; at the national level, such as ministries of health, finance, education, and social welfare; and at regional and local levels. It is also addressed to health care providers and professionals, researchers in relevant fields and the funding agencies that support them, health care advocates, and interested members of the public.

MAGNITUDE OF THE PROBLEM

Disease control efforts in the developing world have been effective in increasing life expectancy and reducing fertility. The result has been a demographic transition from predominantly youthful populations to older and aging ones. This transition has been accompanied by increases in the health problems associated with older people who are particularly vulnerable to chronic diseases, including a number of brain disorders. As a consequence, many low-income countries now face the double burden of increases in these noninfectious diseases and continuing high levels of infectious ones, including some that result in brain disorders (e.g., AIDS and cerebral malaria).

Each of the six classes of brain disorders examined in Part II of this report has a range of personal, social, and economic impacts:

Developmental disabilities include such conditions as mental retardation, behavioral disorders, and cerebral palsy that result from abnormal development or injury to the brain and central nervous system during infancy or childhood. These disorders often impose enormous personal, social, and economic costs as a result of early onset and lifetime disability. Many of the causes of developmental disabilities—including genetic and nutritional factors, infectious diseases, and traumatic events—are particularly common in low-income countries.

Epilepsy affects an estimated 40 million people in developing countries, roughly 85 percent of the total number affected worldwide. The disorder commonly attacks young adults in the most productive years of their lives and frequently leads to their being unemployed. Because of stigmatization and false beliefs, epilepsy is frequently untreated and even unrecognized in the developing world.

Schizophrenia causes severe and chronic disability, due in part to its connotations of "insanity." The disorder is estimated to affect 33 million people in developing countries. Schizophrenia, however, can be controlled with a variety of treatments that offer patients significant improvements in productivity and quality of life.

Bipolar disorder accounts for about 11 percent of the neuropsychiatric disease burden in developing countries. The disorder is characterized by alternating episodes of extreme elation (mania) and severe depression. Between 25 and 50 percent of patients in developed countries with bipolar disorder attempt suicide, and as many as 15 percent are successful. Treatments that significantly reduce the debilitating symptoms of the disease are available, yet few of these treatments are being used in developing countries.

Depression is estimated to be the leading cause of disability worldwide. Its risk factors include family history of the disease, chronic social adversity, and poverty. Because depression typically results from a combination of causes, prevention and treatment require a multifaceted approach. In developing countries this approach may involve a combination of health care, public health awareness, community care, and socioeconomic development.

Stroke and its associated disability are increasing in developing countries, where the disorder is projected to become the fifth leading condition contributing to the disease burden by 2020. Because of the high risk of death, long-term disability, and recurrence after a first stroke, prevention is key to reducing the public health impact of cerebrovascular disease.

Statistics alone do not express the social and economic losses suffered by patients, their families, and the community because of brain disorders. The social and economic demands of care, treatment, and rehabilitation strain entire families, seriously diminishing their productivity and quality of life. The stigma often associated with these disorders adds to the burden; indeed, in some communities the stigma leads to denial of basic human rights.

Despite the burden of disease represented by brain disorders, these conditions are largely absent from the international health agenda. The need for attention is particularly urgent in the developing world, where poverty and brain disorders tend to reinforce each other, and where the vicious cycle is frequently exacerbated by gender inequalities. Yet there is some hope in the fact that in some developing country settings, people have drawn on their strong family and community relationships to develop programs that provide cost-effective health care for those afflicted.

FINDINGS AND FUTURE STRATEGIES

Where resources are scarce, policy makers face difficult choices in allocating limited funds for health care. Such decisions are best made on the basis of rigorous evaluation of the efficacy of proposed interventions and, for those interventions that prove efficacious, their cost-effectiveness. Since most brain disorders impair cognitive function, the determination of cost-effectiveness must encompass the costs associated with prevention, detection, treatment, rehabilitation, chronic care, and lost wages as well as the impact on family members. Because only preliminary and limited evidence is available, more research will be required to refine the calculations of these costs and apply them in developing countries. Since health care interventions are only as good as their implementation, research on cost-effectiveness must also address health care management as well as prevention and treatment outcomes. Thus, the expansion of health care systems in developing countries to include cost-effective care for brain disorders requires not only increased capacity for delivery of services but also increased capacity for operational research to evaluate the quality and effectiveness of care. The findings of such research would guide an iterative process of improving clinical care at affordable costs.

Review of prevention, treatment, and rehabilitation programs in developing countries and of cost-effective treatments in both developed and developing countries reveals several effective interventions for brain disorders. Some developing countries have successfully integrated low-cost prevention, screening, and treatment methods for developmental disabilities, epilepsy, and depression into primary health care programs. Similarly, some have created affordable, community-based rehabilitation programs that help people disabled by brain disorders live as normally as possible. Where these programs provide good care, they serve as a starting point for addressing the burden of brain disorders in the developing world. However, the existence of effective treatments alone does not ensure programmatic success. Programs need to be designed and implemented according to the needs and resources of each location. A one-size-fits-all approach is not likely to succeed.

Determination of the appropriate level of effective, affordable care for brain disorders depends on cost-effectiveness analyses for a range of treatments in different systems of health care. Variability among communities in their recognition of neurological and psychiatric illness, their expectations for medical care, and ability to pay for drugs and other services complicates choices. Optimal approaches will reflect local costs and benefits.

Once care for brain disorders has been incorporated into a system of health care, maintaining a cost-effective program will require monitoring, evaluation, and investigation of alternatives. Moreover, research on the cost-effectiveness of treating brain disorders is a key element in educating governments, missions, and nongovernmental organizations on the affordability of these services.

The strategies presented below and discussed in Chapters 1 through 4 are aimed at reducing the overall burden of brain disorders. Recommendations appear in Part II of the report: Chapters 5 through 10. Each of these chapters presents a description of a disorder; its prevalence, incidence, and other epidemiological parameters in developing countries; the risk factors for the disorder; an analysis of interventions and capacity-building strategies; and recommendations on policies, interventions, capacity building, and future research needs.

To Reduce the Burden of Brain Disorders Now

Strategy 1. Increase public and professional awareness and understanding of brain disorders in developing countries, and intervene to reduce stigma and ease the burden of discrimination often associated with these disorders.

Both the public and health professionals may be unaware that effective, affordable treatments are available. Educational programs should be tailored to the needs of local communities, and messages adapted to local cultural beliefs. Advocacy groups, educators, religious leaders, and traditional healers can be effective at delivering this information. Governments can reinforce these efforts with laws that protect people with brain disorders from abusive practices, ensure access to health care, and prevent discrimination in education, employment, housing, and other opportunities.

Strategy 2. Extend and strengthen existing systems of primary care to deliver health services for brain disorders. Secondary and tertiary centers should train and oversee primary care staff, provide referral capacity, and provide ongoing supervision and support for primary care systems in developing countries.

Many countries have specific disease-control and primary care programs for infectious diseases and maternal and child health. These programs can be expanded to include effective services for prevention, identification, treatment, rehabilitation, and surveillance of brain disorders. Integration of care for brain disorders into the primary health care system should occur as part of national policy. Because diagnosis and treatment of these disorders often requires specialized skills and training, primary care programs must be closely linked with secondary and tertiary facilities, such as district and regional hospitals. Cooperative funding for this additional care should come from national and local governments, international nongovernmental organizations, and development agencies.

Strategy 3. Make cost-effective interventions for brain disorders available to patients who will benefit. Financial and institutional constraints require selectivity and sequencing in setting goals and

priorities. The continued implementation of these interventions should also be informed by ongoing research to reveal the applicability and sustainability of such programs.

Cost-effective interventions are available now to address much of the disease burden (see Table 1). To the extent possible, treatment programs for brain disorders should follow best-practice guidelines. Where this is not possible because of capacity or resource limitations, however, implementation of component practices is likely to be more cost-effective than inaction. Adapting existing interventions to local levels of resource availability is feasible, and standard approaches for assessing the cost-effectiveness of health care delivery should be used to this end. Once care for brain disorders has been incorporated into a system of health care, maintaining a cost-effective program will require monitoring, evaluation, and comparison with alternatives.

TABLE 1 Cost-Effective Interventions for Management of Brain Disorders*

Condition(s)	Primary and secondary prevention goals	Treatment and management modalities
Developmental Disabilities	• Provision of folic acid and iodine supplements to women of child bearing age • Expansion of vaccination programs and other proven methods of infectious disease control	• Early detection and treatment of infections that threaten the nervous system • Implementation of prenatal, newborn, and developmental screenings
Epilepsy	• Public education to destigmatize the disorder and to create awareness of available treatments • Prevention and treatment of cysticercosis • Reduce incidence of head injury, brain infection, and parasitosis	• Phenobarbital and phenytoin • Low-cost carbamazepine and valproate
Schizophrenia	• Public education to destigmatize the disorder • Suicide prevention • Relapse prevention	• Low-cost antipsychotic drugs, such as chlorpromazine and haloperidol • Community rehabilitation programs for patients to improve social and occupational skills • Psychosocial interventions to reintegrate patients into family and community life
Major Depression	• Public education to destigmatize the disorder and to create awareness of available treatments • Early identification and counseling of high-risk individuals • Suicide prevention • Relapse prevention	• Tricyclic antidepressants and, where available, low-cost SSRIs • Adjunctive problem-solving and interpersonal psychotherapy
Bipolar Disorder	• Early identification and counseling against substance abuse among high-risk individuals • Relapse prevention	• Long-term treatment with lithium, carbamazepine, valproate, or other agents • Adjunctive psychosocial treatments
Stroke (Cerebrovascular Disorders)	• Use of public health and education strategies for lowering stroke-related risk factors (e.g., hypertension, smoking, diet, and exercise)	• Control of hypertension with low-dose thiazide, beta-blockers, and low-cost statins and ACE inhibitors • Sulphonylureas with metformin if needed for diabetes

* Supporting evidence for these recommended interventions is derived from research in both developed and developing countries. Specific discussion of the evidence base for each of these interventions appears in Part II of the report.

To Create Options for the Future

Strategy 4. Conduct operational research to assess the cost-effectiveness of specific treatments and health services in local settings, along with epidemiological research to monitor the incidence, prevalence, and disease burden of brain disorders in developing countries.

Because of limited knowledge about the delivery of appropriate interventions in developing countries, there is a need for continuing research to identify local risk factors and their prevalence, to estimate the economic costs associated with these disorders, to assess cost-effective modes of prevention and treatment, and to develop and evaluate approaches for overcoming nonfinancial barriers to implementation.

Strategy 5. Create national centers for training and research on brain disorders in developing countries. Link these centers with institutions in high-income countries through multicenter research projects, staff exchanges and training, and Internet communication.

National centers for training and research can conduct applied research that is tailored to local needs and resources while simultaneously developing the technical capacity of professional and community health care providers. Such centers can also provide leadership to establish priorities and develop planning strategies. These centers should establish and coordinate professional information networks as repositories of knowledge on effective prevention and intervention strategies, training programs, and research findings.

Strategy 6. Create a program to facilitate competitive funding for research and for the development of new or enhanced institutions devoted to brain disorders in developing countries. This effort should be global, and spearheaded by the Global Forum for Health Research, the World Health Organization, and well-funded research centers, such as the U.S. National Institutes of Health and the Centers for Disease Control and Prevention. To ensure the sustainability of the program, major donors—such as the World Bank, foundations, and governmental and non-governmental aid organizations—must commit initial investments to this effort, and longer-term annual budgets must be established.

The integration of brain disorders into primary care, with monitoring and assistance from secondary and tertiary centers in developing countries, will require broad international support and multiple funding sources. This support should include collaborative research with institutions in developed countries as well as opportunities for training of professionals from developing countries in operational research and surveillance. Substantial long-term funding will be required to develop a worldwide network of national training and research centers, and to enable the participation of researchers in developing countries.

CONCLUSION

A growing body of evidence indicates that the social and economic impact of neurological, psychiatric, and developmental disorders is large and increasing. Present figures almost certainly underestimate the impact of brain disorders, particularly in the developing world, yet these disorders have largely been ignored by the health systems of those countries.

Immediate and long-term remedies exist that could significantly reduce the burden of brain disorders in the developing world. These include low-cost preventive and diagnostic measures, medicines, and therapeutic and rehabilitative techniques. The benefits of these remedies could be maximized if they were implemented through a comprehensive health care system, with operational research being carried out on needs and cost-effectiveness in local settings. The identification and testing of interventions for brain disorders in developing countries should eventually yield more and better strategies. Research on incidence, prevalence, and socioeconomic impact will provide the information needed to set goals and priorities.

A sustained, comprehensive, and integrated effort to reduce brain disorders in developing countries will require broad institutional support. This support could be achieved through cooperative links among the full spectrum of organizations associated with brain disorders, spearheaded by the sponsors of this report: the Global Forum for Health Research, the U.S. National Institutes of Health (National Institute of Mental Health, National Institute of Neurological Disorders and Stroke, National Institute of Child Health and Human Development, and the Fogarty International Center), and the U.S. Centers for Disease Control and Prevention.

1

Introduction

During the last century, impressive improvements in health care have decreased maternal and infant mortality, malnutrition, and infectious disease while raising life expectancy in most countries. Together with associated declines in fertility, increased life expectancy has generated a demographic transition; developing countries,[1] which customarily had youthful populations, now have older and aging ones. This transition has in turn created an emerging set of health problems resulting from the fact that older populations are more vulnerable to chronic diseases, including neurological and psychiatric disorders. This is a particularly challenging situation for countries still struggling with high levels of poverty and communicable disease. Additionally, improvements in health care and sanitation are enabling more children in developing countries to survive infancy, but without concomitant efforts to reduce the occurrence of developmental disabilities, the number of disabled children is likely to increase.

Neurological, psychiatric, and developmental disorders are estimated to affect as many as 1.5 billion people worldwide—a number that is expected to grow as life expectancy increases around the globe. Most disorders affecting the brain and its neural connections result in long-term disability, and many have an early age of onset. Measures of the mortality associated with these disorders miss the major burden of disease, while measures of associated disability vastly

---

[1] In this report, the term developing countries includes those countries with economies classified as middle- and low-income in the 1999/2000 *World Development Report* (for additional information, see Appendix A).

understate the burden. Social isolation and stigma often add to the medical and financial burden borne by patients and their families.

NEUROLOGICAL, PSYCHIATRIC, AND DEVELOPMENTAL DISORDERS

Although numerous and diverse, the neurological, psychiatric, and developmental disorders addressed by this report share several important features. First, they are increasingly recognized as disorders of the brain and its neural connections that are precipitated by injury, psychological trauma, chronic adversity, or genetic vulnerability. Several psychiatric disorders, including schizophrenia, are now understood to have a strong biological component, while disabling psychiatric symptoms are known to result from neurological diseases, as when depression follows stroke.[2] Indeed, integrated knowledge of psychiatry and neurology now holds promise for greatly improving medical care for illnesses affecting the brain.[1,2] Thus, throughout this report, neurological, psychiatric, and developmental disorders are collectively referred to as *brain disorders*. The aggregate examination of these disorders not only reflects their common systemic origins, but also represents a strategy that can leverage the limited resources available to provide the widest possible benefit in developing countries.

Many of these disorders are chronic, debilitating conditions. Programs and research show that much of the disability associated with these disorders can be prevented or reduced through effective, affordable measures. As discussed in Chapter 2, poverty frequently accompanies and exacerbates the proximal causes of brain disorders. Thus people in low-income countries face increased risk of developing these disorders. This report is therefore intended to call attention not only to the serious toll exacted by brain disorders in low- and middle-income countries, but also to the significant potential for reducing that impact through cost-effective measures.

While recognition of common features among brain disorders should inform efforts to reduce their impact, it will also be necessary to develop targeted strategies for the prevention and treatment of specific illnesses and rehabilitation for those who suffer from them. The committee's contribution to this endeavor appears in Part II of this report, whose chapters focus on six classes of brain disorders: developmental disabilities, epilepsy, schizophrenia, bipolar disorder, unipolar depression, and stroke. Other brain disorders contributing to the burden of disease in developing countries but not among the disorders discussed in Part II include Alzheimer's disease, addictive disorders, HIV encephalopathy, meningitis, peripheral neuropathies, autism, posttraumatic stress disorder, cerebral palsy, dementia, and Parkinson's disease.

---

[2] See chapters 7 and 10.

CHALLENGES FOR THE CARE OF
BRAIN DISORDERS

Despite their profound consequences, brain disorders have received little attention in the developing world. The reason for this neglect is that health planning and priority setting have been based mainly on mortality data, which do not reflect the long-term disabilities commonly associated with these and other chronic disorders. As a result of the 1996 publication of the *Global Burden of Disease Study*,[3] policy makers have begun to recognize the social and economic impact of brain disorders. That landmark study compared the total cost of various diseases on the basis of disability-adjusted life years (DALYs), a measure that accounts for the overall burden of a disease by combining years of potential life lost as a result of premature death with years of productive life lost because of disability.[3] Projections based on this method indicate that brain disorders will account for an increasing proportion of the future disease burden in both developing and developed countries.

Brain disorders frequently present different challenges in the developing than in the developed world. Differences in incidence and prevalence, in social and economic factors, and in timely access to adequate health care may cause a disorder such as epilepsy, which is largely controlled in industrialized countries, to go unrecognized or untreated in low- and middle-income countries. In the latter countries, medications and other treatments are often unavailable, adherence to available treatment is poor, records of care and health statistics are often incomplete, and research on effective treatments and methods of delivery are lacking.

In some communities, traditional beliefs lead to stigmatization of patients with brain disorders and their families, or to the use of treatments that exacerbate the disorder or harm the patient. The problem is further complicated because many of the mentally ill in developing countries have been homeless or housed in asylums for a large part of their adult lives. On the other hand, the strong family and community ties often found in developing countries can form the core of cost-effective prevention, care, and rehabilitation (see Chapter 3). Overcoming discrimination against those who suffer from brain disorders requires the educating of communities to gain their active collaboration in respecting and caring for patients.

Medical care for the majority of the world's population living in developing countries is provided through community health care centers organized and financed by national governments or by religious and other nongovernmental organizations. These health care centers often focus on the prevention and treatment of acute conditions to the exclusion of brain disorders and other chronic illnesses.

---

[3]The indicator *burden of disease* measured in disability-adjusted life years (DALYs) reflects the burden due to both death and disability. It does not attempt to measure the suffering and loss of the affected individuals and their families.

During the past several decades, basic care for brain disorders has become available in a small number of developing countries through nationally sponsored public health programs and community primary care centers. In many developing countries, however, care for the vast majority of patients with these disorders— poor people who live in rural communities or urban shantytowns—is limited by a general lack of physicians (and an even greater lack of specialists), as well as unavailability of resources for treatment. The physician:patient ratio in rural areas of the developing world can be 1:20,000, and is much greater for psychiatrists and neurologists. Given current resource limitations and development trends,[4] it is unlikely that health care centers can be adequately staffed by physicians or specialist nurses in the foreseeable future. The most feasible approach to filling the staffing gap will be by providing trained health care workers with protocols for the prevention, diagnosis, and treatment of common disorders along with es- sential medications and guidelines for their use (see Chapter 3).

This report does not attempt to define a system that will work in every situation. It does describe a general approach that needs to be supported by training of staff at all levels. Implementation of this approach will depend on the adaptation of effective, affordable treatments from developed countries, even if they are not state of the art; referral of cases by primary care workers, rather than dependence on traditional healers or the chance of being hospitalized later; diagnosis and provision of treatment by general physicians with some training in neurological and psychiatric care; supervised follow-up and maintenance ther- apy by primary care workers (nurses in some settings, health care workers in others); continued consultation on and referral of patients as needed; govern- ment support through policy and law; national centers guided by specialists; and increased capacity for operational research.

GOALS OF THE STUDY

The committee was charged to prepare a consensus report that would define the increasing burden caused by brain disorders and identify opportunities for ef- fectively reducing that burden with cost-effective strategies for prevention, diag- nosis, and treatment. The committee was also asked to identify areas of research, development, and capacity strengthening that would contribute most significantly to reducing the overall burden of these disorders in developing countries.

In its 1997 report, *America's Vital Interest in Global Health,* the Institute of Medicine's Board on Global Health [4] examined the long-term benefits to the developed world of improving global health. Building on the findings of that report and in conjunction with recent initiatives supported by the sponsors of the

---

[4] The countries addressed in this report have per capita incomes of $9266 or less. Low-income countries have per capita incomes of less than $766. The poorest people live on less than $2 a day.

present study, international development agencies, development banks, and developing-country communities, this report provides an evidence base to inform the next steps in addressing brain disorders in the developing world. The committee analyzed the scientific evidence available on these disorders to:

- define the overall disease;
- describe the causes and risk factors associated with brain disorders;
- identify effective and affordable strategies for prevention, treatment, and rehabilitation; and
- identify mechanisms for incorporating care for brain disorders into existing health systems in developing countries.

This report does not examine a number of significant brain disorders, such as Alzheimer's disease, HIV encephalopathy, meningitis, addictive disorders, peripheral neuropathies, posttraumatic stress disorder, and injuries of the brain and central nervous system. We emphasize that their exclusion here is not intended to imply that these disorders and others meeting the criteria listed above are unworthy of future study. On the contrary, the committee hopes that future efforts focusing on those other disorders will also advance the goals of the present report.

The findings, strategies, and recommendations of this report are intended to engage a broad spectrum of individuals and organizations that have the potential to play vital roles in addressing the global impact of brain disorders. They include, but are not limited to, policy makers worldwide, United Nations agencies, multilateral development banks, international donor agencies, foundations, nongovernmental organizations, professional societies, the pharmaceutical industry and medical device companies, advocacy groups, health care professionals, researchers, consumer and patient advocacy groups, and interested members of the public. This diverse and influential audience holds the key to raising public awareness and generating the commitment and resources necessary to reduce the burden of brain disorders in developing countries.

STUDY APPROACH

The Institute of Medicine assembled a study committee with broad international expertise in clinical and basic research, economics, epidemiology, microbiology, neurology, pediatrics, psychiatry, and public health. The members of the committee were also chosen for their first-hand experience with these disorders in a wide range of middle- and low-income countries. The committee members are listed at the beginning of the report, and brief biographies are given in Appendix E.

The data for this study were identified by the committee and other experts representing various disciplines through bibliographic references on related topics and through databases, such as Medline, university libraries, and Internet sites of organizations associated with research and services for brain disorders.

Although much of the published information on these disorders in developing countries was found in international and national journals and reports, some of the evidence has appeared in local journals, the proceedings of meetings, and unpublished reports prepared for the World Health Organization (WHO) and other international organizations. To tap this knowledge base, the committee enlisted a broad range of experts with recent research or service experience in developing countries. Data and supportive evidence were provided by these experts through workshop presentations, commissioned papers, and technical consultation on report chapters (for additional information see Appendix A). The framework for the committee's deliberations and examination of each of the selected disorder groups included an overview of the available epidemiological parameters, a review of the existing knowledge base on interventions, and projections of the feasibility, cost, and impact of proposed interventions.

The combined weight of such evidence, the committee believes, has produced an accurate account of the state of knowledge concerning the epidemiology of the six groups of disorders covered in this report, their treatment and management in developing countries, and the capacity of local health care systems to provide such treatment. Evaluation of the available evidence enabled the committee to identify gaps in knowledge and to propose strategies for a research agenda that would fill these gaps. The findings, strategies, and recommendations included in the report were developed from this broad base of evidence; we also indicate where the data are inadequate to support additional conclusions.

ORGANIZATION OF THE REPORT

Part I of this report reviews challenges and opportunities for the prevention, treatment, and rehabilitation of the broad range of brain disorders in developing countries. Chapter 2 describes the magnitude of the problem caused by these disorders and reviews the various factors—including poverty and gender inequalities—that serve to magnify their effects. Chapter 3 explores the process of designing and maintaining health systems capable of addressing brain disorders in developing countries. Chapter 4 summarizes the committee's findings and proposes strategies for addressing core issues of policy, intervention, research, and capacity building.

Part II examines the six groups of brain disorders cited earlier: developmental disabilities (Chapter 5); epilepsy (Chapter 6); schizophrenia (Chapter 7); bipolar disorder (Chapter 8); unipolar depression (Chapter 9); and stroke (Chapter 10). Each chapter presents a description of the disorder; its prevalence, incidence, and other relevant epidemiological parameters; associated risk factors; an analysis of interventions and capacity-building strategies from the point of view of cost-effectiveness and applicability in developing countries; and recommendations for policies, interventions, capacity building, and future research.

REFERENCES

1. B.H. Price. D. Adams, and J.T. Coyle. Neurology and Psychiatry: closing the great divide. *Neurology* 54:8–14, 2000.
2. S.E. Hyman. The milennium of mind. brain, and behavior. *Archives of General Psychiatry* Jan 57:88–89, 2000.
3. C.L. Murray and A.L. Lopez, eds. *The Global Burden of Disease*. Boston: The Harvard Press. 1996.
4. Institute of Medicine (IOM). *America's Vital Interest in Global Health*. National Academy Press. Washington. D.C., 1997.

Summary of Findings:
The Magnitude of the Problem

- Brain disorders—neurological, psychiatric, and developmental—are a leading cause of death and disability worldwide and are responsible for a large proportion of the burden of disease in developing countries.

- Brain disorders are projected to increase in the coming decades as a result of large-scale demographic and epidemiological shifts. By 2020, for example, depression is projected to be the second and stroke the leading cause of disability-adjusted life years (DALYs) lost worldwide.

- The stigma associated with epilepsy, schizophrenia, and mental retardation often prevents people with these disorders from seeking and getting medical attention. It also results in the denial of social, educational, and employment opportunities to affected individuals and their families.

- The relationship between poverty and illness is complex and circular; poverty can be both a cause and a result of ill health.

- Poverty is associated with specific risk factors for brain disorders, including poor nutrition, unhygienic living conditions, inadequate access to health care, lack of educational and employment opportunities, and debt.

- These disorders can substantially worsen people's economic circumstances because of the cost of medical or traditional treatments; the limits they impose on educational opportunities; and interference with effective functioning at home, work, and school.

- Considerable research in developing countries indicates that poverty and several psychiatric disorders, such as depression, exacerbate each other.

- Poverty is more common and more severe for women than for men. Women also have a more severe health burden from psychiatric disorders. Depression affects women disproportionately.

- Specialist and physician care for brain disorders is extremely limited in most developing countries. Health care services in many countries lack the capacity, in terms of physicians, nurses, and trained health care workers, to provide care for these disorders to the majority of their populations.

2

The Magnitude of the Problem

Neurological, psychiatric, and developmental disorders exact a profound economic and personal toll in developing countries. Brain disorders affect the highest human faculties and, left untreated, can destroy a person's dignity, productivity, and autonomy. Yet despite their importance, these disorders have been largely ignored by public and private health systems in developing countries as compared with diseases that are better understood.[1]

Health policy on brain disorders has long been limited by the following misperceptions:

- The illnesses are a problem in the developed but not the developing world.
- They do not cause mortality.
- They are not amenable to treatment.
- They are too expensive to manage in developing countries.

This report seeks to counter each of these notions, the first of which is addressed in this chapter. The impact of brain disorders in developing countries is reviewed from several perspectives: the impact on nations and communities in terms of the overall disease burden due to death and disability, the impact on individuals and families due to lost time, lost productivity, stigmatization and discrimination, the reinforcing roles of poverty and gender inequality, and the lack of capacity to address these problems.

EFFECTS ON COMMUNITIES AND NATIONS

The Disease Burden

Prompted by estimates of the disease burden first published in 1993, health leaders have begun to recognize the major role of brain disorders in the overall burden of disease.[1–3] Governments and public health policy makers are starting to investigate the impact of this burden on communities and nations (see, for example, Box 2-1 on the 1999 report of the U.S. Surgeon General). Previous comparisons of the contribution of various disorders to the overall burden of disease were based most commonly on the cause of death alone, or sometimes years of life lost (YLLs) by cause. These comparisons dramatically underestimated the importance of brain disorders because these conditions tend to be chronic (not an acute cause of death) and therefore are rarely listed as the immediate cause of death in official records.[2,4] Yet depression, epilepsy, and other brain disorders often cause many years of serious disability. Brain disorders are responsible for at least 27 percent of all years lived with disability (YLDs) in developing countries.[1][5] With the exception of Sub-Saharan Africa, brain disorders are the leading contributors to YLDs in all regions of the world (see Table 2-1).[5]

In these calculations, the disability-adjusted life year, or DALY (a variant of the better known quality-adjusted life years, or QALY), assesses both disability and premature mortality in a single measure. In combining assessments of YLLs and YLDs, current DALY estimates highlight the significant contribution of brain disorders to the overall disease burden in developing countries (see Table 2-2).[5]

Absent data on most developmental disabilities and many adult neurological diseases,[2] 1998 estimates for brain disorders still show these conditions responsible for nearly 34 percent of all noncommunicable disease DALYs in developing countries (see Figure 2-1). Table 2-2 and Figure 2-2 show the contribution of brain disorders to all DALYs and mortality in developing countries. These conditions account for nearly 15 percent of DALYs and 12 percent of mortality among all disease categories.[3][6]

Current DALY calculations for developing countries, however, reflect only a portion of the disease burden imposed by brain disorders. These sizable cal-

---

[1] The percentage distribution of YLDs attributed to brain disorders is estimated using the 1990 data for neuropsychiatric conditions (25.5 percent), the cerebrovascular disease component of cardiovascular disease (approximately one percent), and the self-inflicted injury component of intentional injuries (approximately .5 percent).

[2] Data on such developmental disorders as mental retardation, cerebral palsy, and autism along with adult neurological conditions such as peripheral nerve disease and severe migraine were not accounted for in the estimates of the 1996 *Global Burden of Disease* study.

[3] Category I: Communicable disease, maternal and perinatal conditions and nutritional deficiencies; Category II: Non-communicable disease; and Category III: Injuries.

BOX 2-1 Mental Health: A Report of the U.S. Surgeon General

In 1999, the U.S. Department of Health and Human Services issued its first Surgeon General's report on the topic of mental health. The report describes recent defining trends in research, treatments, care provision, and public opinion; reviews current knowledge on mental health care for children, adults, and the elderly; and charts a course for improving access to mental health services and effective treatment for mental disorders. About 10 percent of the U.S. adult population uses mental health services in the health sector in any given year, with another 5 percent seeking such services from social service agencies, schools, or religious or self-help groups. Yet despite the relative abundance of mental health care in the United States, as compared with most developing countries, critical gaps exist between those who need mental health care and those who receive service, as well as between optimally effective treatment and the care many people actually receive.

Many of the findings in the Surgeon General's report concur with those in this volume. In the United States, as well as in much of the developing world, the stigma of having a mental illness represents a major barrier to treatment. A lack of awareness of the range of treatments for mental illness also hinders access to effective care. Financial barriers prevent many people from seeking mental health care, and capacity is limited by personnel shortages in several key fields.

The two main findings of the Surgeon General's report are equally applicable in the developing world and in the United States:

- The efficacy of mental health treatments is well documented, and
- A range of treatments exists for most mental disorders.

Accordingly, several recommended courses of action based on these findings are also relevant in a broader context: to fight stigmatization by dispelling myths about mental illness and by increasing public awareness of the effectiveness of existing treatments; to establish effective, evidence-based community mental health services; to facilitate access to mental health care by increasing potential points of entry and reducing financial barriers; and to provide "culturally competent" treatment that recognizes individual differences.

While focusing on a subset of the brain disorders discussed in this volume, the Surgeon General's report emphasizes the central importance of the brain. "We recognize that the brain is the integrator of thought, emotion, behavior, and health," states Surgeon General David Satcher, M.D., Ph.D, in his preface to the report. "Indeed, one of the foremost contributions of contemporary mental health research is the extent to which it has mended the destructive split between 'physical' and 'mental' health."

Source: [7]

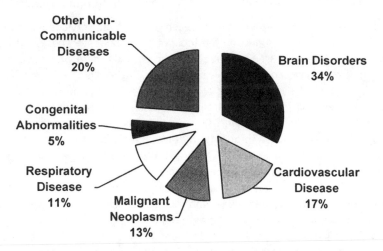

FIGURE 2-1 Non-communicable disease DALYs attributable to brain disorder, estimates for 1998.

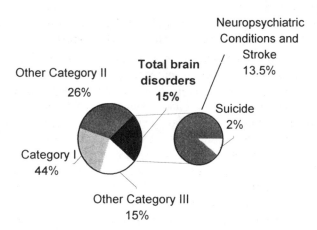

FIGURE 2-2 Burden of brain disorders as a percentage of total disease burden in low- and middle-income countries, estimates for 1998.

Source:[6]

culations are surely lower-bound estimates of the true impact of brain disorders because they do not fully incorporate many of the known neurological and psychiatric sequelae of infectious, nutritional, genetic, and perinatal disorders, as well as environmental exposures.[4] Current data estimating the prevalence of brain disorders is considered inadequate because many patients in developing countries, particularly children with developmental disorders, do not receive medical care. In the United States, 12 to 18 percent of children are estimated to be disabled in some way.[8] Comparable measures would be expected to be substantially higher in developing countries, where children are exposed more frequently to infectious diseases and nutritional deficiencies. While improvements in health care and sanitation are enabling more children to survive infancy in developing countries, concomitant efforts to reduce the occurrence of the number of disabled children is very likely to rise.[5]

Brain disorders in general are expected to play an increasingly important role in the disease burden of developing countries during the next two decades. Data for 1990 on the burden of disease in developing countries have been projected to 2020,[5] based on trends in cause-specific mortality rates, life expectancy, income per capita, human capital, smoking intensity, and HIV and tuberculosis infection rates. One projected calculation is that unipolar depression (the fourth leading cause of DALYs in 1990 for all age groups and the leading cause of DALYs among those aged 15 to 44) will become the leading cause among all age groups combined in 2020 (see Tables 2-3 through 2-5). This projected increase in DALYs attributable to depression reflects not only an aging population, but also recent increases in the rate of depression among younger people. Stroke, ranked as the tenth leading cause of DALYs in developing countries in 1990 (see Table 2-3), is projected to be the fifth leading cause in 2020 (see Table 2-5). Improvements in the reliability and validity of data and collection methods for brain disorders in developing countries may well reveal an even greater contribution to disease burden estimates.

It should be noted that in calculating disease burden estimates (e.g., YLDs and DALYs), the years of productive life lost as a result of disability are weighted according to expert opinion regarding the severity of a given disability. For example, the disability caused by major depression is estimated by panels of experts as approximately equivalent to that caused by blindness or paraplegia, while the disability caused by schizophrenia lies between that caused by paraplegia and quadriplegia.[4] The assumptions and judgments underlying DALY

---

[4] Neurological and psychiatric sequelae not fully expressed in current DALY estimates include those caused by infectious disease (e.g., cerebral malaria, HIV encephalopathy, and congenital rubella), nutritional deficiencies (e.g., iodine-deficiency syndrome and vitamin A blindness), perinatal conditions (e.g., birth trauma), genetic conditions (e.g., phenylketonuria and Duchenne's muscular dystrophy), and environmental exposures (e.g., fetal alcohol syndrome and lead poisoning).

estimates are complex and have been controversial. Some of the problems involve the relative value of living assigned to each age group, the comparative severity of different disabilities at different ages, diagnoses of diseases and their classifications, the presumption of disability weights as universal, and the accuracy and completeness of data sets for each country (see Appendix B for additional information on measurement limitations). The estimates will continue to be refined as stronger data and more widely tested assumptions become available. Meanwhile, current estimates using this indicator have provided the public health community with a valuable way to rank the impact of various diseases on health and to recognize the major role of diseases that cause a high level of disability.

TABLE 2-1 Percentage distribution of years lived with disability (YLDs) for specific causes, 1990

Condition Group	Region										
	EME	FSE	IND	CHN	OAI	SSA	LAC	MEC	Developed	Developing	World
All Causes	100.0	100.0	100.0	100.0	100.0	100.0	100.0	100.0	100.0	100.0	100.0
I. Communicable, maternal, perinatal and nutritional conditions	5.5	7.8	33.6	18.9	28.5	39.3	19.0	24.6	6.3	27.8	24.4
A. Infectious and parasitic diseases	2.6	3.0	14.3	6.4	12.6	22.4	9.7	6.4	2.7	12.3	10.7
B. Respiratory infections	0.3	0.4	1.4	1.4	1.4	1.3	1.0	1.8	0.4	1.4	1.2
C. Maternal conditions	0.6	1.9	4.7	1.9	4.0	5.8	2.7	5.0	1.1	4.0	3.5
D. Conditions arising during the perinatal period	0.5	0.5	3.5	1.1	1.7	3.2	1.6	2.9	0.5	2.3	2.0
E. Nutritional deficiencies	1.5	2.0	9.8	8.2	8.7	6.6	4.1	8.6	1.7	7.9	6.9
II. Noncommunicable diseases	86.7	79.5	43.7	66.9	56.1	39.8	67.3	61.5	84.2	54.8	59.5
A. Malignant neoplasms	3.8	2.5	0.6	1.2	0.9	0.5	0.8	0.5	3.3	0.8	1.2
B. Other neoplasms	1.2	1.1	0.2	0.6	0.4	0.4	0.8	0.4	1.2	0.4	0.5
C. Diabetes mellitus	3.2	1.5	1.0	0.5	1.0	0.3	1.3	1.5	2.6	0.9	1.1
D. Endocrine disorders	1.7	0.7	0.1	0.4	0.4	0.9	2.1	1.2	1.4	0.7	0.8

E. Neuro-psychiatric conditions	47.2	37.6	20.9	30.7	28.5	16.3	34.6	25.4	43.9	25.5	28.5
F. Sense organ diseases	0.2	0.2	3.4	2.0	2.7	2.9	1.4	2.0	0.2	2.5	2.1
G. Cardiovascular diseases	6.2	7.1	3.6	3.5	2.9	1.6	2.4	3.8	6.5	3.0	3.6
H. Respiratory diseases	6.1	7.1	5.0	14.0	4.7	6.6	6.1	7.8	6.5	7.7	7.5
I. Digestive diseases	4.1	5.5	2.4	5.1	5.8	3.6	4.3	7.1	4.6	4.5	4.5
J. Genito-urinary diseases	1.1	2.0	0.5	0.8	0.8	0.9	1.3	3.4	1.4	1.1	1.2
K. Musculo-skeletal diseases	8.0	10.2	1.6	3.6	3.1	1.5	6.9	1.8	8.8	2.9	3.8
L. Congenital anomalies	2.0	14.8	3.2	3.0	2.6	3.1	2.8	3.6	1.9	3.0	2.9
M. Oral conditions	1.8	1.8	1.2	1.1	2.0	0.6	2.4	3.0	1.8	1.5	1.6
III. Injuries	7.9	12.7	22.8	14.2	15.4	20.9	13.6	13.9	9.5	17.4	16.1
A. Unintentional injuries	7.1	10.7	22.4	12.9	14.6	16.3	12.3	10.0	8.3	15.4	14.3
B. Intentional injuries	0.8	2.0	0.4	1.3	0.8	4.6	1.4	3.9	1.2	1.9	1.8

Note: EME = Established Market Economies; FSE = Formerly Socialist Economies of Europe; IND = India; CHN = China; OAI = Other Asia and Islands; SSA = Sub-Saharan Africa; LAC = Latin America and the Caribbean; MEC = Middle Eastern Crescent

Source: [5]

TABLE 2-2 Contribution of brain disorders to disability-adjusted life years (DALYs) and Mortality in low- and middle-income countries, estimates for 1998.

Condition	DALYs (1,000s)	% of Total DALYs	Deaths (1,000s)	% of Total Deaths
All Disease	1,274,259		45,897	
Brain Disorders				
Unipolar major depression	51,217	4.02	0	0
Stroke	36,407	2.86	4,213	9.20
Self-inflicted injuries	19,095	1.50	818	1.80
Bipolar affective disorder	14,421	1.13	15	0.03
Alcohol dependence	13,553	1.06	42	0.09
Psychoses	11,984	0.94	40	0.08
Obsessive compulsive disorders	10,062	0.79	0	0
Alzheimer's disease and other dementias	5,527	0.43	111	0.24
Drug dependency	4,782	0.38	7	0.02
Panic disorders	4,710	0.37	0	0
Epilepsy	4,659	0.37	60	0.13
Post traumatic stress disorders	1,896	0.15	0	0
Multiple sclerosis	1308	0.10	20	0.04
Parkinson's disease	621	0.05	30	0.07
Other neuropsychiatric disorders	9,308	0.73	170	0.37
Total Brain Disorders	189,550	14.90	5,526	12.00

Source: [6]

TABLE 2-3 Causes of DALYs (percentage total) in descending order, 1990

		Developing Regions	
Rank	Disease or Injury	DALYs (1,000s)	% of Total
	All causes	1,218,244	
1	Lower respiratory infections	110,506	9.1
2	Diarrheal diseases	99,168	8.1
3	Conditions arising during the perinatal period	89,193	7.3
4	Unipolar major depression	41,031	3.4
5	Tuberculosis	37,930	3.1
6	Measles	36,498	3.0
7	Malaria	31,705	2.6
8	Ischemic heart disease	30,749	2.5
9	Congenital anomalies	29,441	2.4
10	Cerebrovascular	29,099	2.4
11	Road traffic accidents	27,253	2.2
12	Chronic obstructive pulmonary disease	25,771	2.1
13	Falls	24,232	2.0
14	Iron-deficiency anaemia	23,465	1.9
15	Protein-energy malnutrition	20,758	1.7
16	War	18,868	1.6
17	Tetanus	17,513	1.4
18	Violence	15,632	1.3
19	Self-inflicted injuries	15,199	1.3
20	Drownings	14,819	1.2

Source: [5]

TABLE 2-4 Ten leading causes of DALYs at ages 15–44 years in developing regions, 1990

		Both Sexes		Males			Females		
Rank	Disease or Injury	DALYs (1,000s)	Cumulative %	Disease or Injury	DALYs (1,000s)	Cumulative %	Disease or Injury	DALYs (1,000s)	Cumulative %
Developing Regions									
	All causes	357,437		All causes	180,211		All causes	177,277	
1	Unipolar major depression	35,398	9.9	Unipolar major depression	12,658	7.0	Unipolar major depression	22,740	12.8
2	Tuberculosis	19,451	15.3	Road traffic accidents	11,387	13.3	Tuberculosis	8,703	17.7
3	Road traffic accidents	14,321	19.4	Tuberculosis	10,747	19.3	Iron-deficiency anemia	7,135	21.8
4	War	12,382	22.8	Violence	9,844	19.3	Self-inflicted injuries	6,526	25.5
5	Iron-deficiency anemia	12,033	26.2	Alcohol use	8,420	24.8	Obstructed labor	6,033	28.9
6	Self-inflicted injuries	12,004	29.5	War	7,448	29.4	Chlamydia	5,364	31.9
7	Violence	11,448	32.7	Bipolar disorder	5,601	36.7	Bipolar disorder	5,347	34.9
8	Bipolar disorder	10,948	35.8	Self-inflicted injuries	5,478	39.7	Maternal sepsis	5,226	37.8
9	Schizophrenia	9,514	38.5	Schizophrenia	5,068	42.5	War	4,934	40.6
10	Alcohol use	9,371	41.1	Iron-deficiency anemia	4,898	45.3	Abortion	4,856	43.4

Source: [5]

TABLE 2-5 Ten leading causes of DALYs in developing regions in 2020 (baseline scenario)

Both Sexes				Males				Females			
Rank	Disease or Injury	DALYs (1,000s)	Cumulative %	Disease or Injury	DALYs (1,000s)	Cumulative %	Disease or Injury	DALYs (1,000s)	Cumulative %
Developing Regions									
	All causes	1,228,302		All causes	701,018		All causes	527,284	
1	Unipolar major depression	68,037	5.6	Road traffic accidents	44,907	6.4	Unipolar major depression	44,652	8.5
2	Road traffic accidents	64,388	10.8	Ischemic heart disease	40,922	12.2	Ischemic heart disease	23,406	12.9
3	Ischemic heart disease	64,328	16.1	Cerebro-vascular disease	31,252	16.7	Chronic obstructive pulmonary disease	22,817	17.2
4	Chronic obstructive pulmonary disease	52,677	20.4	Chronic obstructive pulmonary disease	29,859	21.0	Road traffic accidents	20,266	21.1
5	Cerebrovascular disease	51,518	24.6	Unipolar major depression	24,185	24.4	Tuberculosis	19,481	24.8
6	Tuberculosis	42,364	28.0	Violence	23,911	27.8	Lower respiratory infections	19,382	28.4
7	Lower respiratory infections	41,107	31.4	War	23,285	31.1	War	18,766	32.0
8	War	40,190	34.6	Tuberculosis	22,982	34.4	Diarrheal diseases	16,379	35.2
9	Diarrheal diseases	36,960	37.6	Lower respiratory	22,341	37.6	HIV	15,605	38.3
10	HIV	33,962	40.4	Diarrheal disease	20,581	40.5	Abortion	4,856	41.3

Source:[5]

EFFECTS ON INDIVIDUALS AND FAMILIES
Lost Productivity

Brain disorders interfere with the highest level of human functioning, greatly reducing productivity and social interaction.[9,10] Since these disabilities usually last for many years, they have profound emotional and financial effects on individuals and families.[11–14] These consequences are increased where treatment and support are not available.[15–17] A large economic cost is the lost productivity of workers whose disability prevents them from working at full capacity, if at all and those who die accidentally or by suicide as a result of brain disorders.[15,17–26] Additional economic costs result from the time and other resources required to care for a dependent family member.[11,15,19,20] Social costs of these disorders include the emotional burden of suffering a chronic disorder or caring for an affected family member, learning and developmental problems in children whose parents have brain disorders, and (in some cases) lifelong dependency.[18,21,22,27–30]

Stigma and Discrimination

The stigma and discrimination associated with disorders such as epilepsy, schizophrenia, and mental retardation increase the toll of illness for many people with brain disorders and their families. These individuals are often rejected by neighbors and the community, and as a result suffer loneliness and depression. The psychological effect of stigma is a general feeling of unease or of "not fitting in," loss of confidence, increasing self-doubt leading to depreciated self-esteem, and a general alienation from society.[31] Moreover, the stigma is frequently irreversible,[32,33] so that even when the behavior or physical attributes disappear, an individual continues to be stigmatized by others and by their own self-perception.[34]

People with brain disorders and their families may also be subjected to other forms of social sanction, such as being excluded from community activities. One of the most damaging results of stigmatization is that affected individuals or those responsible for their care may not seek treatment, hoping to avoid the negative social consequences of diagnosis. This leads in turn to delayed or lost opportunities for treatment and recovery; underreporting of these conditions can also reduce efforts to develop appropriate strategies for prevention and treatment.[35]

Because the symptoms of brain disorders can be frightening to others or embarrassing to the afflicted, the social rejection of affected individuals takes several forms. Most frequently, rejection is manifested as lost opportunity for employment and a normal social life, sometimes for family members as well as for patients. Many individuals affected by schizophrenia, for example, experience a vastly diminished quality of life because they are excluded from social events and social networks.[36] They often become homeless and spend years on the streets, in the criminal justice system, or in psychiatric hospitals. In all these situations they are exposed to abuse.[37,38]

Epilepsy carries a particularly severe stigma that is sustained by misconceptions, myths, and stereotypes.[9,39,40] In some communities, children who do not receive effective treatment for this disorder are removed from school; lacking a basic education, they may not be able to support themselves.[36,41] People in some African countries believe that saliva can spread epilepsy or that the "epileptic spirit" can be to transferred to anyone who witnesses a seizure. These misconceptions cause people to retreat in fear from someone having a seizure, leaving that person unprotected from open fires and other dangers they might encounter in cramped living conditions.[42–44]

Stigmatization and rejection can be reduced by providing factual information on the causes and treatment of brain disorders; by talking openly and respectfully about the disorder and its effects; and by providing and protecting access to appropriate health care.[45] Governments can reinforce these efforts with laws that protect people with brain disorders and their families from abusive practices and prevent discrimination in education, employment, housing, and other opportunities.

THE ROLES OF POVERTY AND GENDER INEQUALITY

Poverty and gender inequality underlie many key risk factors for disease generally; neurological, psychiatric, and developmental disorders are no exception. Indeed, these are the two risk factors of greatest salience for brain disorders in the developing world.

The Role of Poverty

A growing body of economic and epidemiological research suggests a reciprocal relationship between poverty and illness.[25,46] Rather than simply pointing to poverty as the root cause of ill health, decision makers—particularly in developing countries, where most people remain poor throughout their lives—should also begin to recognize illness as a major cause of poverty, and one that is amenable to public intervention.[46] The linkages between poverty and illness are likely to be as complex and variable as poverty itself. For example, in addition to suffering physical adversity and high mortality and morbidity resulting from poverty, many poor people in developing countries face the emotional hardship of living with gross income inequalities.[47–49]

Poverty-Associated Risk Factors for Brain Disorders

Several poverty-associated causes of ill health stand out as risk factors for brain disorders.

Unsafe and Unhygienic Living Conditions

Many of the world's poorest people live in extreme poverty in shantytowns and urban slums where they face squalor, corruption, drugs, violence, and predation. The relationship between such unhealthy physical environments and somatic disease is well established.[50–53] Given inadequate shelter, no control of sewage, limited access to potable water, and crowding, the poor are constantly exposed to infectious agents and environmental toxins that can cause epilepsy and developmental disabilities.[9,54–56] In unprotected living conditions, individuals suffering an epileptic seizure have a high mortality rate due, for example, to falling into an open fire or becoming lost in the bush.[9,39]

Hunger and Malnutrition

Several micronutrient deficiencies in mothers, when severe, can cause developmental disabilities in their infants (see Chapter 5).[57] Folic acid deficiency has been shown to cause spina bifida;[58] iodine deficiency can lead to cognitive deficits;[59] vitamin A deficiency can cause blindness [60] and increase a child's vulnerability to severe infections.[61] Anxiety and depression have also been associated with chronic hunger,[62] while high infant and child mortality among families living in extreme poverty can have significant psychosocial effects on parents and other family members.[63]

Inadequate Access to Health Care

Poor people in the developing world rarely receive preventive care or effective treatment for brain disorders. In Brazil, for example, poverty and lack of education have been shown to reduce access to prevention and treatment of stroke.[64] In Zambia, risk factors for stroke, such as hypertension and diabetes, frequently go undetected and therefore untreated because caregivers lack basic diagnostic technology.[34] Similarly, untreated substance abuse, epilepsy, schizophrenia, and depression can lead to chronic disability or death. In India, patients with psychiatric disorders may receive a combination of vitamin injections, herbal medicines, and benzodiazepines from tradtional healers,[65] the total cost of which can exceed that of effective biomedical care.[66–69]

Lack of Educational and Employment Opportunities

Poverty is commonly associated with a substandard education. It is also associated with decreased cognitive potential,[70,71] poor nutrition, and lack of home support for educational achievement. The all-too-frequent result is inadequate achievement and outcomes in school, and lifelong limitations of employment opportunities.[72–75]

Each of these poverty-related factors tends to exacerbate the impact of the others.[70] The illnesses—including brain disorders—to which these factors predispose people can in turn lead to depressed economic circumstances, thus creating a vicious cycle of illness and economic deprivation.[14] Brain disorders interfere with effective functioning at school, work, and home, causing social and economic hardship. Substance abuse, learning disabilities, and schizophrenia, for example, can prevent students from completing their education, thereby limiting their ability to find employment and support themselves.[72–73]

Beyond the aforementioned general threats to brain health, poverty has been shown to pose specific risks. Poverty can profoundly affect early development, beginning with the prenatal period and continuing through early childhood. Poverty-related factors are associated with increased neonatal and postneonatal mortality rates; developmental disorders; and injuries from accidents, abuse, or neglect.[76] When health and housing are inadequate, infection and malnutrition often limit a child's growth and development.[77] Living in a poor family has been shown to be the single strongest predictor for developmental disabilities in preschoolers, outweighing the role of maternal age and educational attainment.[71]

Malnutrition, physical illness, exposure to toxins such as alcohol and lead, perinatal injury, and lack of educational and social stimulation have been shown to adversely affect the cerebral mechanism of attention, which has been identified as a major source of cognitive deficits in school children.[71] Similar observations have been made in the United States, where perinatal complications, exposure to lead, and lack of cognitive stimulation have been found to account for diminished cognitive function in children of low socioeconomic status.[73] Malnutrition, along with perinatal complications and infection, has been associated with increased risk for epilepsy among Indian children.[78] Food deprivation leading to low birth weight or slow weight gains during the first year has been suggested as contributing to stroke risk during adulthood if food later becomes plentiful.[79,80]

Schizophrenia and other severe mental illness can lead to unemployment, family breakdown, and homelessness in a wide range of settings.[81–83] Research in the developed world indicates that people with schizophrenia experience a downward socioeconomic drift,[82] a trend that is probably echoed in developing countries.

Depression, alcohol dependence, stroke, and epilepsy rank among the leading causes of disability worldwide and share disabling consequences, such as stigmatization, suicide, violence, family disruption, and long-term disability.[84,85] A combined analysis of five recent surveys from Brazil, Zimbabwe, India, and Chile reveals a consistent and significant association between low income and risk of one of these disorders.[48,64] The data also suggest associations between indicators of impoverishment, such as hunger or indebtedness, and these disorders. In Indonesia, lower rates of depression and other common mental disorders were observed in individuals with higher levels of education, access to amenities such as electricity, and television ownership. This association applied to entire communities as well as to individuals: the least-developed villages surveyed had common mental disorder rates of 28 percent, compared with 13 percent in the most-developed villages.[86] Similar findings have been made in other countries.[83] Other studies have demonstrated a higher risk for common mental disorders and suicide among unemployed persons,[15,84,87] those with lower incomes,[87,88] and those with a lower standard of living.[81,89]

The Role of Gender Inequality

For many years, public health has equated women's health with reproductive and child health, and rarely considered women's well-being for its own sake.[48] This lack of attention appears particularly egregious in the case of brain disorders, given that women make up a disproportionate share of those living in poverty and also face gender inequalities—both of which, as noted earlier, are exacerbating factors in the development of these disorders.

Studies of psychiatric disorders across cultures reveal that depression is more prevalent in women (see Figure 2-3).[90,91] One large epidemiological study in China showed that depression was nine times higher in women than in men.[92] In addition to the higher risks to their health, women have in the past also received inferior care and, as a result, suffered more severe consequences than men with similar disorders. Although schizophrenia is diagnosed more frequently in women than in men in China, Chinese women occupy fewer psychiatric hospital beds and generally receive less assistance than men.[93] A few studies conducted in developing countries indicate that the situation is improving.[94–96]

Similarly, the consequences of having epilepsy appear to be more severe for African women than for African men. They are less likely to receive treatment for their illness, are less likely to marry, and are often rejected by their families. To support themselves, many African females with epilepsy become prostitutes and thereby become vulnerable to sexually transmitted disease.[39]

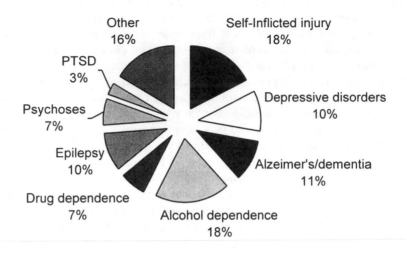

Males

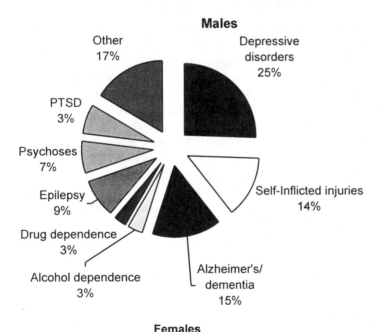

Females

FIGURE 2-3: Mental Health Problems of Males and Females Worldwide Percentages of DALYs Lost

Note: DALY = disability-adjusted life years; PTSD = posttraumatic stress disorder
Source: [1]

The conclusions of several studies describing the disproportionately severe effects of depression and other psychiatric disorders on women in the developing world enumerate the factors found to contribute to women's vulnerability: unequal status, not being valued by husbands or society, dependence on husbands, marital stress, low education, social isolation, economic deprivation, multiple family responsibilities, hard physical labor, lack of employment, and employment in a low-income job.[88,90,97–99] The evidence points in particular to a link between the latter two factors and psychiatric disorders. A classic study in London, for example, found depression to be more severe for working-class than middle-class women.[98] In low-income societies, a woman's workday is an exhausting dawn-to-dusk routine that causes frustration, chronic fatigue, and demoralization, and leads to feelings of powerlessness and lack of opportunity.[1,88] Considerable evidence links these stressful feelings, experienced by many more women than men, with the onset of depression.[89,98,100–103] Additional stresses arise for rural women in developing countries when men migrate to urban areas and leave wives to do the farming as well as other chores; in rural China this practice has led to high suicide rates among overburdened young wives.[104] Biological differences between men and women may also contribute to differences in the prevalence of depression among the sexes.[99,105,106] This issue is separate from gender inequality, though biology may serve to reinforce societal causes of high depression rates among women.

Many of women's reproductive health issues also have significant implications for mental health. These issues, which include childbirth, adverse maternal outcomes (stillbirths and abortions), premarital pregnancies in adolescents, menopause, and infertility, challenge women's emotions and coping abilities.[107] For example, when couples fail to conceive, women tend to take the brunt of the disappointment and blame.[108] In India, infertility and failure to produce a male child have been linked to wife battering and female suicide.[108,109] The effects of women's reproductive health on their mental health include the following.

Postnatal Depression

Many women suffer depression during the period immediately following childbirth.[99,109–111] Although limited, the literature on postnatal depression (PND) in developing countries suggests that it can be detected in 10 to 36 percent of new mothers.[112–115] The detection of PND is of great public health interest because of its profound impact on maternal and child health. Compelling evidence implicates PND in a range of adverse cognitive and emotional outcomes in children.[95] One recent study recorded a high prevalence of postnatal depression and demonstrated its adverse impact on the relationship between mother and infant.[96] Although the majority of cases of PND are self-limiting, the untreated disorder may take up to a year to resolve.[109] Interventions such as nondirective counseling can prevent the adverse outcomes associated with PND.[97]

Rape and Sexual Violence

The consequences of rape and sexual violence can include emotional trauma, depression, physical injury, pregnancy, sexually transmitted diseases such as AIDS, and death.[116–119] Involuntary prostitution has occurred more frequently in recent years through the luring of women into sexual slavery with promises of marriage or work. Female genital mutilation, forced sterilization or involuntary abortion, and partners who demand unprotected sex also contribute to dire mental health consequences.[120–122]

HIV/AIDS

People with HIV are at increased risk for depression for a variety of reasons: the stigma and discrimination associated with the disorder, the knowledge that they are likely to die prematurely of AIDS, the discovery that other family members may also have the disease, and the direct and indirect effects of HIV on the brain, as well as the effects of secondary neoplastic and infectious diseases.[123,124] Evidence also suggests that caregivers for people with HIV/AIDS, who tend to be women, suffer mental and physical health problems, particularly depression.[125] The impact of HIV/AIDS on women's mental health is likely to be enormous in countries such as Zimbabwe, where 30 percent of pregnant women attending antenatal health clinics were found to be HIV-positive.[126] In such situations, women must cope not only with illness in their male partners but also with their own failing health and that of their children.

Domestic Violence

Women are overwhelmingly the targets of domestic violence. This is a largely hidden problem, but routine battering is estimated to affect 25 to 65 percent of women across diverse cultures, including India,[88] Sri Lanka,[127] Bangladesh, Papua New Guinea,[128] Thailand, and Mexico.[129] South American countries have a particularly high rate of alcohol-related spouse abuse.[1] Domestic violence resulting in death occurs increasingly through dowry deaths of brides in India and female infanticide in India and China. Female victims of violence are likely to suffer disabling and long-lasting health effects, such as depression and posttraumatic stress disorder, as well as dissociation disorders, somatization, sexual dysfunction, and self-harm behavior.[116,130–132] Elderly women in poor societies are often vulnerable to personal abuse, isolation, suicide, and the stigma associated with accusations of witchcraft, particularly when issues of land ownership are disputed.[133,134]

While the associations between gender and mental health justifiably focus on the substantial vulnerability of women in the developing world, men are more commonly dependent on alcohol and drugs than are women (see Figure 2-3). Substance abuse and dependence have been linked to premature mortality (from cirrhosis, accidents, lung cancer, and other associated causes), risky behavior (with consequences such as hepatitis B and HIV infection), and greater exposure to violence and injuries.[130,135,136] Although depression occurs more frequently in women, men complete a greater proportion of suicides,[5] a statistic that appears to reflect the higher rates of substance abuse among men and perhaps also wider access to the most effective means of suicide, such as guns.[138–140] Men are also at higher risk than women for stroke.[141,142]

CAPACITY TO ADDRESS BRAIN DISORDERS

In many developing countries, health care for brain disorders is in even shorter supply than health care for other important diseases. Figures 2-4 through 2-7 compare the numbers of neurologists, psychiatrists, general physicians, and nurses per capita for several developing countries. In India, for example, there are about 3,000 psychiatrists and 565 neurologists to serve a billion people,[143,144] while in Zimbabwe there are 10 psychiatrists and 29 neurologists to serve 11 million people.[145,146] Specialists in the prevention and management of pediatric brain disorders are even more scarce, especially as compared with the large pediatric population in developing countries. In addition, most of these specialists are located in cities, leaving rural populations unserved. Among the larger number of general physicians in the developing world, only a minority are experienced in the care of brain disorders, and they tend to be more familiar with hospital than with primary care presentation of cases.

With human resources being so limited, policy makers in the developing world face difficult choices on how to allocate these and equally limited financial resources to best meet health care needs. Since many brain disorders impair cognitive function, an attempt must be made to estimate the costs and benefits associated with all aspects of care, as well as lost wages and the time and financial commitments borne by family members (see Chapter 4). Cost-effectiveness data from developed countries, along with limited evidence from developing countries, reveal certain cost-effective interventions (see Chapters 5 through 10). Demonstration projects and operational research should be conducted to measure their sustainability and impact on brain disorders in a range of low-income communities.

---

[5] Except in China, where women commit suicide more often than men.[137]

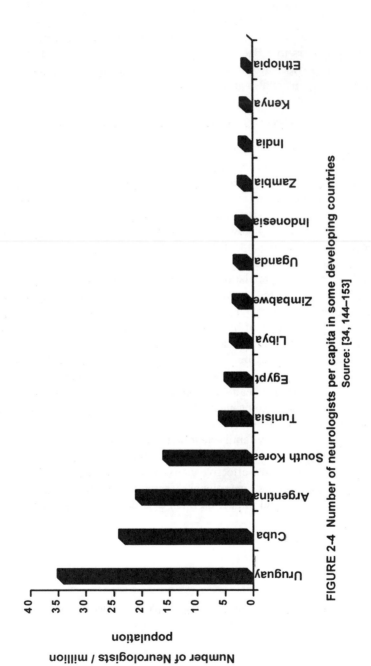

FIGURE 2-4 Number of neurologists per capita in some developing countries
Source: [34, 144–153]

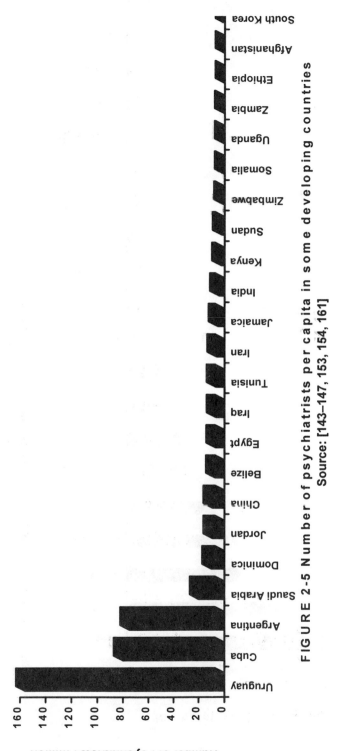

FIGURE 2-5 Number of psychiatrists per capita in some developing countries
Source: [143–147, 153, 154, 161]

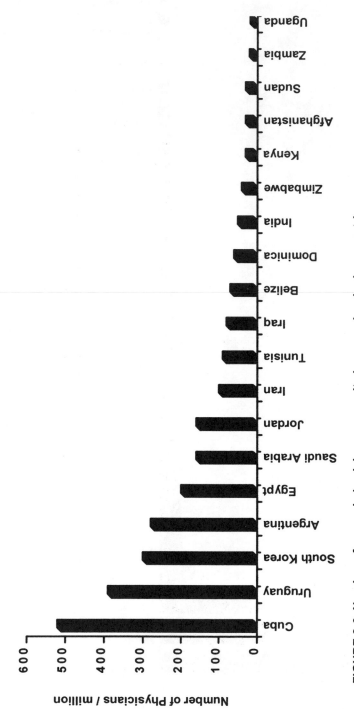

FIGURE 2-6 Number of general physicians per capita in some developing countries
Source: [153,157,162]

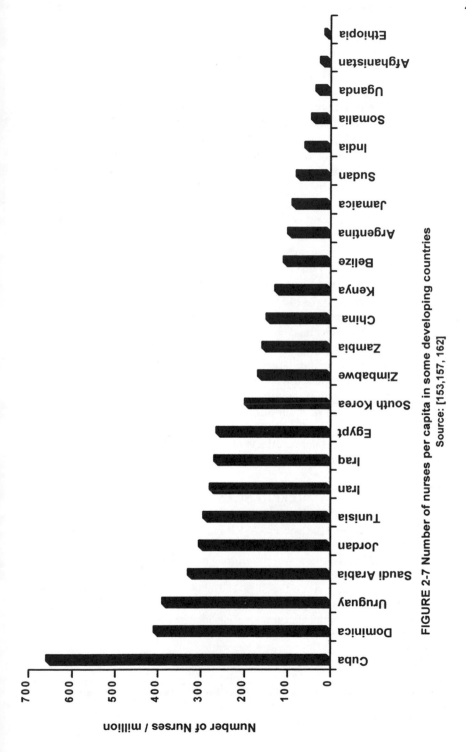

FIGURE 2-7 Number of nurses per capita in some developing countries
Source: [153,157, 162]

CONCLUSION

To compete in international markets and to build stronger national and local infrastructures, developing countries must produce well-educated workers, a process that begins with prenatal care and continues through the adult years of employment. Since many brain disorders interfere not only with health but also with education, they present an especially insidious limitation to developing economies. The consequences for a country's development of ignoring the burden imposed by these disorders are clearly large, and growing larger.

These disorders create special problems for developing countries not only because of the scarcity of resources available to address them but also because of their mutually reinforcing relationship with poverty. Poor women bear an even heavier burden than poor men as a result of several gender-specific risk factors, many of which are preventable. The implementation of cost-effective interventions can help to reduce the impact of these disorders and break this debilitating cycle. Thus, poverty and gender inequality, which contribute greatly to the burden of brain disorders in developing countries, should be viewed as a target of the recommendations made in this report.

Despite the increasingly significant contribution of brain disorders to disease burden, these conditions are largely missing from the international health agenda.[1] Stigma, discrimination, economic and gender inequalities, and lack of capacity for addressing these add to their burden in developing countries. Recognizing the importance of brain disorders is the first step toward reducing this burden. The process can be further advanced through increased understanding of the social and economic effects of brain disorders as well as through provision of cost-effective care.

REFERENCES

1. R. Desjarlais, L. Eisenberg, B. Good, and A. Kleinman. *World Mental Health.* Oxford University Press: New York, 1995.
2. World Bank. *World Development Report: Investing in Health Research Development.* World Bank: Geneva, 1993.
3. N. Sartorius, T. B. Ustun, J. A. Costa e Silva, D. Goldberg, Y. Lecrubier, J. Ormel, et al. An international study of psychological problems in primary care. Preliminary report from the World Health Organization Collaborative Project on "Psychological Problems in General Health Care." *Archives of General Psychiatry* Oct,50(10):819–824, 1993.
4. T. B. Ustun. The Global Burden of Mental Disorders. *American Journal of Public Health* Sept. 89(9), 1999.
5. C. Murray and A. Lopez, eds. *The Global Burden of Disease.* The Harvard Press: Boston, 1996.

6. WHO (World Health Organization). *The World Heath Report.* World Health Organization: Geneva, 1999.
7. U.S. Department of Health and Human Services. *Mental Health: A Report of the Surgeon General-Executive Summary.* U.S. Department of Health and Human Services Administration, Center for Mental Health Services, National Institutes of Health, National Institute of Mental Health: Rockville, MD, 1999.
8. T.W. Langfitt. Presentation to IOM Committee on Neurological, Psychiatric, and Developmental Disorders in the Developing World, 2000.
9. K. Kahn and S.M. Tollman. Stroke in rural south Africa: Contributing to the little known about a big problem. *South Africa Medicine Journal* 89,63–65, 1999.
10. D. Kebede, A. Alem, T. Shibre, A. Fekadu, D. Fekadu, A. Negash et al. The Bitajira-Ethiopia study of the course and outcome of schizophrenia and bipolar disorders. I. Description of study settings, methods and cases. Unpublished manuscript, 1999.
11. R. Goeree, B.J. O'Brien, P. Goering, G. Blackhouse, K. Agro, A. Rhodes, et al. The economic burden of schizophrenia in Canada. *Canadian Journal of Psychiatry* Jun;44(5),464–472, 1999.
12. M. Zhang, K.M. Rost, J.C. Fortney, and G. R. Smith. A community study of depression treatment and employment earnings. *Psychiatric Service* Sep;50(9),1209–1213, 1999.
13. L.L. Judd, M.P. Paulus, K.B. Wells, and M.H. Rapaport. Socioeconomic burden of subsyndromal depressive symptom and major depression in a sample of the general population. *American Journal of Psychiatry* Nov;153(11),1411–1417, 1996.
14. J. Westermeyer. Economic losses associated with chronic mental disorder in a developing country. *British Journal of Psychiatry* 144,475–481, 1984.
15. S.V. Thomas. Money matters in epilepsy. *Neurology India* Dec;48(4),322–329, 2000.
16. G.E. Simon, D. Revicki, J. Heiligenstein, L. Grothaus, M. Von Korff, W.J. Katon, and T.R. Hylan. Recovery from depression, work productivity, and health care costs among primary care patients. *General Hospital Psychiatry* May-Jun;22(3),153–162, 2000.
17. W. Mak, J.K. Fong, R. T. Cheung, and S. L. Ho. Cost of epilepsy in Hong Kong: Experience from a regional hospital. *Seizure* Dec;8(8),456–464, 1999.
18. Health-related quality of life among persons with epilepsy—Texas, 1998. *Morbidity Mortality Weekly Report* Jan 19;50(2),24–26, 35, 2001.
19. L.M. Brass. The impact of cerebrovascular disease. *Diabetes, Obestiy and Metabolism* Nov;2 Supplement 2,S6–S10, 2000.
20. C. S. Dewa and E. Lin. Chronic physical illness, psychiatric disorder and disability in the workplace. *Social Science and Medicine* Jul;51(1),41–50, 2000.
21. P.E. Greenberg, T. Sisitsky, R.C. Kessler, S.N. Finkelstein, E.R. Berndt, J.R. Davidson, et al. The economic burden of anxiety disorders in the 1990s. *Journal of Clinical Psychiatry* Jul;60(7),427–435, 1999.
22. R. J. Wyatt and I. Henter. An economic evaluation of manic-depressive illness—1991. *Social Psychiatry and Psychiatric Epidemiology* Aug;30(5),213–219, 1995.
23. P. Kind and J. Sorensen. The costs of depression. *International Clinic of Psychopharmacology* Jan;7(3-4),191–195, 1993.
24. A. Stoudemire, R. Frank, N. Hedemark, M. Kamlet, and D. Blazer. The economic burden of depression. *General Hospital Psychiatry* Nov;8(6),387–394, 1986.
25. D.R. Gwatkin and M. Guillot. *The Burden of Disease Among the Global Poor.* World Bank: Washington D.C., 2000.

26. M. Bartley. Unemployment and ill health: understanding the relationship. *Journal of Epidemiology and Community Health* 48,333–337, 1994.
27. J.E. Ritsher, V. Warner, J.G. Johnson, and B.P. Dohrenwend. Inter-generational longitudinal study of social class and depression: A test of social causation and social selection models. *British Journal of Psychiatry* Apr;178(40,S84–S90, 2001.
28. S. Soepatmi. Developmental outcomes of children of mothers dependent on heroin or heroin/methadone during pregnancy. *Acta Paediatrica* Nov; 404 (Supplement),36–39, 1994.
29. B. Maughan and G. McCarthy. Childhood adversities and psychosocial disorders. *British Medical Bulletin* Jan;53(1),156–169, 1997.
30. B.T. Zima, K.B. Wells, B. Benjamin, and N. Duan. Mental health problems among homeless mothers: Relationship to service use and child mental heatlh problems. *Archives of General Psychiatry* Apr;53(4),332–338, 1996.
31. G. Scambler and A. Hopkins. Being epileptic; coming to terms with stigma. *Social Health and Fitness* 8,26–43, 1986.
32. E. Friedson. *Profession of Medicine: A study of sociology of applied knowledge.* Russell Sage: New York, 1970.
33. G.L. Albrecht, V.G. Walker, and J. A. Levy. Social distance from the stigmatized: A test of two theories. *Social Science and Medicine* 16(14),1319–1327, 1982.
34. G.L. Birbeck. Barriers to care for patients with neurologic disease in rural Zambia. *Archives of Neurology* Mar 57(3),414–417, 2000.
35. A. Jablensky, J. McGrath, H. Herrman, D. Castle, O. Gureje, M. Evans, et al. Psychotic disorders in urban areas: An overview of the Study on Low Prevalence Disorders. *Australian and New Zealand Journal of Psychiatry* 34,221–236, 2000.
36. R. Padmavathi, S. Rajkumar, N. Kumar, A. Manoharan, and S. Kamath. Prevalence of schizophrenia in an urban community in Madras. *Indian Journal of Psychiatry* 31,233–239, 1987.
37. B.S. Singhal. Neurology in developing countries. *Archives of Neurology* 55,1019–1021, 1998.
38. M. Gourie-Devi, P. Satishchandra, and G. Gururaj. National workshop on public health aspects of epilepsy. *Annals of the Indian Academy of Neurology* 2,43–48, 1999.
39. L. Jilek-Aall, W. Jilek, J. Kaaya, L. Mkombachepa, and K. Hillary. Psychosocial study of epilepsy in Africa. *Social Science and Medicine* 45,783–795, 1997.
40. S.D. Shorvon and P.J. Farmer. Epilepsy in developing countries: a review of epidemiological, sociocultural, and treatment aspects. *Epilepsia* 29(1),S36–S54, 1988.
41. P. Jallon. Epilepsy in developing countries. *Epilepsia* 38(10),1143–1151, 1997.
42. K. K. Hampton, R.C. Peatfield, T. Pullar, H.J. Bodansky, C. Walton, and M. Feely. Burns because of epilepsy. *British Medical Journal* 296(11),16–17, 1988.
43. H.T. Rwiza, I. Mtega, and W.B. P. Matiya. The clinical and social characteristics of epilepsy patients in the Ulanga District, Tanzania. *Journal of Epilepsy* 5,162–169, 1993.
44. M. Berrocal. Burns and epilepsy. *Acta Chirurgiae Plasticae* 39(1),22–27, 1997.
45. L. Jilek-Aall. Morbus sacar in Africa: Some religious aspects of epilepsy in traditional cultures. *Epilepsia* Mar;40(3),382–386, 1999.
46. World Bank. *World Development Report.* World Bank: Washington D.C., 2000.
47. M. Sundar. Suicide in farmers in India (letter). *British Journal of Psychiatry* 175,585–586, 1999.

48. V. Patel, R. Araya, M.S. Lima, A. Ludermir, and C. Todd. Women, Poverty and Common Mental Disorders in four restructuring societies. *Social Science and Medicine* 49,1461–1471, 1999.

49. D. Sinha. Psychological concomitants of poverty and their implications for education. In: *Perspectives on Educating the Poor*. Atal, Y. ed. Abhinav Publications: New Delhi , pp. 57–118, 1997.

50. G. Halliday, S. Banerjee, M. Philpot, and A. Macdonald. Community study of people who live in squalor. *Lancet* Mar 11;355(9207),882–886, 2000.

51. M. Olfson, S. Shea, A. Feder, M. Fuentes, Y. Nomura, M. Gameroff, et al. Prevalence of anxiety, depression, and substance use disorder in an urban general medicine practice. *Archives of Family Medicine* Sep–Oct;9(9),876–883, 2000.

52. G.R. Glover, M. Leese, and P. McCrone. More severe mental illness is more concentrated in deprived areas. *British Journal of Psychiatry* Dec;175,544–548, 1999.

53. H. Freeman. Mental health and the environment. *British Journal of Psychiatry* Feb;132,113–124, 1978.

54. D.K. Pal, A. Carpio, and J.W. Sander. Neurocysticercosis and epilepsy in developing countries. *Journal of Neurology, Neurosurgery, and Psychiatry* Feb;68(2),137–143, 2000.

55. A.J. McMichael. The urban environment and health in a world of increasing globalization: issues for developing countries. *Bulletin of the World Health Organization* 78(9),1117–1126, 2000.

56. S. Tong, Y.E. von Schirnding, and T. Prapamontol. Environmental lead exposure: A public health problem of global dimensions. *Bulletin of the World Health Organization* 78(9),1068–1077, 2000.

57. R. Perez-Escamilla and E. Pollitt. Causes and consequences of intrauterine growth retardation in Latin America. *Bulletin of the Pan American Health Organization* 26(2),128–147, 1992.

58. N.M.J. Van der Put, F. Gabreels, E.M.B. Stevens, J.A.N. Smeitink, F. J. M. Trijbels, and T.K. A. P. Eskes, et al. A second common mutation in the methylenetetra hydrofolate reductase gene: An additional risk factor for neural-tube-defects? *American Journal of Human Genetics* 62, 1044–1051, 1998.

59. B. Lozoff, E. Jimenez, and A.W. Wolf. Long-term developmental outcome of infants with iron deficiency. *New England Journal of Medicine* 325(10),687–694,1991.

60. WHO (World Health Organization). *ICD-10:International statistical classification of diseases and related health problems, 10th revision*. World Health Organization: Geneva, 1992.

61. A. Sommer and K. P. West, Jr. The duration of the effect of Vitamin A supplementation. *American Journal of Public Health*. Mar; 87(3),467–469, 1997.

62. N. Scheper-Hughes. The madness of hunger: Sickness, delirium, and human needs. *Culture, Medicine and Psychiatry* Dec;12(4), 429–458, 1988.

63. N. Scheper-Hughes. *Death Without Weeping: The Violence of Everyday Life in Brazil*. University of California: Berkeley, p. 547, 1992.

64. B. A. de Santana, M. M. Fukujima, and R.M. de Oliveiria. Socioeconomic characteristics of patients with stroke. *Arq Neuropsichiatr* [Portugese]54(3),428–432, 1996.

65. V. Patel, J. Perieira, L. Coutinho, R. Fernandes, J. Fernandes, and A. Mann. Psychological disorder and disability in primary care attenders in Goa, India. *British Journal of Psychiatry* 171,533–536, 1998.

66. V. Patel, E. Simunyu, and F. Gwanzura. The pathways to primary mental health care in Harare, Zimbabwe. *Social Psychiatry and Psychiatric Epidemiology* 32,97–103, 1997.
67. K. Saeed, R. Gater, A. Hussain, and M. Mubbashar. The prevalence, classification and treatment of mental disorders among attenders of native faith healers in rural Pakistan. *Social Psychiatry and Psychiatric Epidemiology* Oct;35(10),480–485, 2000.
68. G.L. Birbeck. Seizures in rural Zambia. *Epilepsia* Mar;41(3),277–281, 2000.
69. A. Singh and A. Kaur. Epilepsy in rural Haryana–Prevalence and treatment seeking behaviour. *Journal of the Indian Medical Association* Feb;95(2),37–39, 1997.
70. A. F. Mirsky. Perils and pitfalls on the path to normal potential: The role of impaired attention. *Journal of Clinical Experimental Neuropsychology* 17(4),481–498, 1995.
71. J.E. Miller. Developmental screening scores among preschool-aged children: The roles of poverty and child health. *Journal of Urban Health* 75(1),135–152, 1998.
72. M. Haq and K. Haq. *Human Development in South Asia: The Education Challenge.* Oxford University Press: Karachi, 1999.
73. V. McLoyd. Socioeconomic disadvantage and child development. *American Psychologist* 53(2),185–204, 1998.
74. I. Heath, A. Haines, Z. Malenica, J. Oulton, Z. Liepando, D. Kaseje, et al. Joining together to combat poverty. *Croatian Medical Journal* Online (http://www.vms.cmj.2000/410104.htm), 2000.
75. G. Alvarez. The neurology of poverty. *Social Science and Medicine* 16(9),945–950, 1982.
76. J. L. Aber, N. G. Bennett, D. C. Conley, and J. Li. The effects of poverty on children's health and development. *Annual Review of Public Health* 18,468–483, 1997.
77. E. Pollitt. Poverty and child development: Relevance of research in developing countries to the United States. *Child Development* 65,283–295, 1994.
78. R. J. Hackett, L. Hackett, and P. Bhakta. The prevalence and associated factors of epilepsy in children in Calicut District, Kerala, India. *Acta Paediatrica* 86(11),1257–1260, 1997.
79. D.J.P. Barker and C. Osmond. Infant mortality, childhood nutrition, and ischaemic heart disease in England and Wales. In: D.J.P. Barker, ed. *Fetal and Infant Origins of Adult Disease.* British Medical Journal: London, 1992.
80. T. A. Pearson. Cardiovascular disease in developing countries: Myths, realities, and opportunities. *Cardiovascular Drugs and Therapy* 13,95–104, 1999.
81. G. Lewis, P. Bebbington, T.S. Brugha, M. Farrell, B. Gill, R. Jenkins, et al. Socioeconomic status, standard of living and neurotic disorder. *Lancet* 352,605–609, 1998.
82. B.P. Dohrenwend, I. Levav, P.E. Strout, S. Schwartz, S. Naveh, B.G. Link et al. Socioeconomic status and psychiatric disorders: The causation-selection issue. *Science* Feb 21;255(5047)946–952, 1992.
83. S. Weich and G. Lewis. Poverty, unemployment and the common mental disorders: A population-based cohort study. *British Medical Journal* 317,115–119, 1998.
84. G. Lewis and A. Sloggett. Suicide, deprivation and unemployment: Record linkage study. *British Medical Journal* 317,1283–1286, 1998.
85. S. V. Thomas and V. B. Bindu. Psychosocial and economic problems of parents of children with epilepsy. *Seizure* 8,66–69, 1999.
86. E. Bahar, A.S. Henderson, and A.J. Mackinnon. An epidemiological study of mental health and socioeconomic conditions in Sumatera, Indoniesia. *Acta Psychiatrica Scandinavica* 85(4),257–263, 1992.

87. D.J. Gunnell, T.J. Peters, R.M. Kammerling, and R.J. Brooks. Relation between parasuicide, suicide, psychiatric admissions, and socioeconomic deprivation. *British Medical Journal* 311,226–230, 1995.

88. S. Jejeebhoy. Wife-beating in rural India: A husband's right? Evidence from survey data. *Economic and Political Weekly* (3), 855–862, 1998.

89. D. B. Mumford, K. Saeed, I. Ahmad, S. Latif, and M. Mubbashar. Stress and psychiatric disorder in rural Punjab: A community study. *British Journal of Psychiatry* 170,473–478, 1997.

90. J. Broadhead and M. Abas. Life events and difficulties and the onset of depression among women in a low-income urban setting in Zimbabwe. *Psychological Medicine* 28,29–38, 1998.

91. J. Cooper and N. Sartorius, eds. *Mental Disorder in China*, Gaskell: London, 1996.

92. M. Gibbon. The use of romal and informal health care by female adolescents in eastern Nepal. *Health Care for Women International* Jul–Aug;19(4),343–360, 1998.

93. R. Warner. *Recovery from Schizophrenia: Psychiatry and Political Economy*. Routledge and Kegan Paul: London:, 1985.

94. C.E. Okojie. Gender inequalities of health in the Third World. *Social Science and Medicine* 39(9),1237–1247, 1994.

95. S. Malik. Women and mental health. *Indian Journal of Psychiatry* 35,3–10, 1993.

96. V. Pearson. Goods on which one loses: Women and Mental Health in China. *Social Science and Medicine* 45,1159–1173, 1995.

97. B. Davar. *The Mental Health of Indian Women: A Feminist Agenda*. Sage: New Delhi, 1999.

98. G. W. Brown and T.O. Harris. *Social Origins of Depression: A Study of Psychiatric Disorder in Women*. Free Press: New York, 1978.

99. S. Guatam. Post partum psychiatric syndromes: Are they biologically determined? *Indian Journal of Psychiatry* 31,31–42, 1989.

100. G.W. Brown, M. Bhrolchain, and T. Harris. Social class and psychiatric disturbance among women in an urban population. *Sociology* 9,225–257, 1975.

101. V. Makosky. Sources of stress: events or conditions? In: *Lives in Stress: Women and Depression*. Belle, D., ed. Sage Publications: Beverly Hills, California, pp.35–53, 1982.

102. I. Blue, M.E. Bucci, S. Jaswal, A. Ludermir, and T. Harpham. The mental health of low-income urban women: case studies form Bombay, India; Olinda, Brazil; and Santaigo, Chile. In: *Urbanization and Mental Health in Developing Countries*, Harpham, T., Blue, T., eds. Avebury: Aldershot, pp.75–101, 1995.

103. R. Kessler. The effects of stressful life events on depression. *Annual Review of Psychology* 48,191–214, 1997.

104. A. Kleinman, J. Kleinman, and L. Sing. The Transforming of Social Experience in Chinese Society. *Special Issue of Culture, Medicine, and Society* 23(1),1–156, 1999.

105. V. Hendrick, L.L. Altshuler, and R. Suri. Hormonal changes in the postpartum and implications for postpartum depression. *Psychosomatics* Mar–Apr;39(2),93–101, 1998.

106. P.J. Lucassen, F. J. Tilders, A. Salehi, and D. F. Swaab. Neuropeptides vasopressin (AVP), oxytocin (OXT) and corticotropin-realesing hormone (CRH) in the human hypothalamus: Activity changes in aging, Alzheimer's disease and depression. *Aging* (Milano) 9(4),48–50, 1997.

107. L. Dennerstein, J. Astbury, and C. Morse. *Psychosocial and Mental Health Aspects of Women's Health.* World Health Organization: Geneva, 1993.
108. M.C. Inhorn. Kabsa (a.k.a. mushahara) and threatened fertility in Eygpt. *Social Science and Medicine* Aug;39(4),487–505, 1994.
109. R. Kumar. Postnatal mental illness: A transcultural perspective. *Social Psychiatry and Psychiatric Epidemiology,* Nov;29(6),250–264, 1994.
110. S. Nhitawa, V. Patel, and S.W. Acuda. Predicting postnatal mental disorder with a screening questionnaire: A prospective cohort study from a developing country. *Journal of Epidemiology and Community of Health* 52,262–266, 1998.
111. Y.A. Aderibigbe, O. Gureje, and O. Omigbodun. Postnatal emotional disorders in Nigerian women. *British Journal of Psychiatry* 163,645–650, 1993.
112. M. E. Reichenheim and T. Harpham. Maternal mental health in a squatter settlement in Rio de Janeiro. *British Journal of Psychiatry* 159,683–690, 1991.
113. L. Murray and P. Cooper. The impact of postpartum depression on child development. *Internal Review of Psychiatry* 8,55–63, 1997.
114. P. Cooper, M. Tomlinson, L. Swartz, M. Woolgar, L. Murray, and C. Molteno. Postpartum depression and the mother-infant relationship in a South African peri-urban settlement. *British Journal of Psychiatry* 175,554–558, 1999.
115. J. Holden. The role of health visitors in postnatal depression. *International Review of Psychiatry* 8,79–86, 1996.
116. R. L. Fishbach and B. Herbert. Domestic violence and mental health: Correlates and conundrums within and across cultures. *Social Science and Medicine* 45,1161–1170, 1997.
117. M.K. Chapo, P. Somse, A.M. Kimball, R.V. Hawkins, and M. Massanga. Predictors of rape in the Central African Republic. *Health Care forWomen International* Jan-Feb;20(1),71–79, 1999.
118. E. Mulugeta, M. Kassaye, and Y. Berhane. Prevalence and outcomes of sexual violence among high school students. *Ethiopian Medical Journal* Jul;36(3),167–174, 1998.
119. D.M. Menick and F. Ngoh. [Sexual abuse in children in Cameroon]. *Médecine tropicale: Revue du corps de santé colonial* 58(3),249–252, 1998.
120. A.L. Coker and D.L. Richter. Violence against women in Sierra Leone: Frequency and correlates of intimate partner violence and forced sexual intercourse. *African Journal of Reproductive Health* Apr;2(1),61–72, 1998.
121. R. Knight, A. Hotchin, C. Bayly, and S. Grover. Female genital mutilation—Experience of The Royal Women's Hospital, Melbourne. *Autralian New Zealand Journal of Obstetrics and Gynecology* Feb;39(1),50–54, 1999.
122. K. Jain, K.A. Maheshwari, and N. Agarwal. Genital injuries in sexually abused young girls. *Indian Pediatrics* Dec;35(12),1218–1220, 1998.
123. M. D. Stein and L. Hanna. Use of mental health services by HIV-infected women. *Journal of Women's Health* 6,569–574, 1997.
124. F. K. Judd and A.M. Mijch. Depressive symptoms in patients with HIV infection. *Australian and New Zealand Journal of Psychiatry* 30,104–109, 1996.
125. A. J. Leblanc, S. A. London, and C. S. Aneshensel. The physical costs of AIDS care-giving. *Social Science and Medicine* 45,915–923, 1997.

126. M. Mbizvo, A. Mashu, T. Chipato, E. Makura, R. Bopoto, Fotrell. Trends in HIV-1 and HIV-2 prevalence and risk factors in pregnant women in Harare, Zimbabwe. *Central African Journal of Medicine* 42,14–21, 1996.

127. D. Sonali. *An Investigation into the Incidence and Causes of Domestic Violence in Sri Lanka.* Women in Need (WIN): Colombo, Sri Lanka, 1990.

128. S. Toft, ed. *Domestic Violence in Papua New Guinea.* Law Reform Commission Occasional Paper NO. 19, Port Moresby, Papua New Guinea, 1986.

129. S. Valdez and E. Shrader-Cox. *Estudio Sobre la Incidencia de Violencia Domestica en una Microregion de Ciudad nezahualcoyotl.* Centro de Investigacion y Lucha Contra la Violencia Domestica: Mexico City, 1991.

130. N. Almeida-Filho, J. J. Mari, E. Coutinho, J. F. Franca, J. Fernandes, S. B. Andreoli, and E. A. Busnello. Brazillian multicentric study of psychiatric morbidity. Methodological features and prevalence estimates. *British Journal of Psychiatry* 171,524–529, 1997.

131. J.C. Campbell and L.A. Lewandowski. Mental and physical health effects of intimate partner violence on women and children. *Psychiatric Clinics of North America* 20,353–374, 1997.

132. N. Malhotra and M. Snood. Sexual assault—A neglected public health problem in the developing world. *International Journal of Gynaecology and Obstetrics* Dec;71(3),257–258, 2000.

133. G.M. Carstairs. *Death of a Witch: A Village in North India,1950–1981.* Hutchinson: London, 1983.

134. L. Cohen. *No Aging in India.* University of California Press: Berkeley, 1998.

135. E. Chinyadza, I. M. Moyo, T. M. Katsumbe, D. Chisvo, M. Mahari, D. E. Cock, O. L. Mbengeranwa. Alcohol problems among patients attending five primary health care clinics in Harare city. *Central African Journal of Medicine* 36,26–32, 1993.

136. T. F. Babor and M. Grant. *Programme on Substance Abuse. Project on identification and management of alcohol-related problems.* World Health Organization: Geneva, 1992.

137. C. Pritchard. Suicide in the People's Republic of China categorized by age and gender: Evidence of the influence of culture on suicide. *Acta Psychiatrica Scandinavica* May;93(5),362–367, 1996.

138. M.M. Khan and H. Reza. The pattern of suicide of Pakistan. *Crisis* 21(1),31–35, 2000.

139. A. Alem, D. Kebede, L. Jacobsson, and G. Kullgren. Suicide attempts among adults in Butajira, Ethiopia. *Acta Psychiatrica Scandinavica* (supplement);397,70–76, 1999.

140. C. La Vecchia, F. Lucchini, and F. Levi. Worldwide trends in suicide mortality, 1955–1989. *Acta Psychiatrica Scandinavica* Jul;90(1),53–64, 1994.

141. World Health Organization (WHO). Stroke trends in the WHO MONICA Project. *Stroke* 28,500–506, 1997.

142. P. Thorvaldsen, K. Asplund, K. Kuulasmaa et al. Stroke incidence, case fatality, and mortality in the WHO MONICA project. World Health Organization Monitoring Trends and Determinants in Cardiovascular Disease. *Stroke* 26,361–367, 1995.

143. Bulletin of the Indian Academy of Neurology Nov/Dec 8(3) Bangalore, India, 1999.

144. R.S. Murthy. Rural psychiatry in developing countries. *Psychiatric Services* Jul;49(7):967–969, 1998.

145. V. Patel. Personal communication, 2000.
146. Data from the African Medical and Research Foundation, http://www.amref.org/, 2000.
147. Data from the HR Program (Observatory) at Pan American Health Organization (PAHO), 2000.
148. Koon Sik Min. Data from the Sam Yook Rehabilitation Center. Personal communication, 2000.
149. Hisao Sato, Japan College of Social Work, 2000.
150. B.S. Singhal. Bombay Hospital Institute of Medical Sciences, personal communication, 2000.
151. A. Gallo Diop. Centre Hospitalier Universitarie De Fam, Dakar, Senegal. Personal communication, 2000.
152. Annual Congress of the Neurology Association of South Africa, 1998.
153. *CIA World Fact Book*, 2000.
154. Pan American Health Organization Scientific Publication, 561.
155. Data from the Uruguay Medical Society, 2001.
156. Meeting on Promotion of Psychiatry and Mental Health in Africa, 2000.
157. World Bank. Entering the 21st Century World Development Report 1999/2000. Oxford University Press: New York, 2000.
158. A. Alem. Human rights and psychiatric care in Africa with particular reference to the Ethiopian situation. *Acta Psychiatrica Scandinavica* (supplement) 399,93–96, 2000.
159. A. Mohit, K. Saeed, D. Shahmohammadi, J. Bolhari, M. Bina, R. Gater, et al. Mental health manpower development in Afghanistan: A report on a training course for primary health care physicians. *Eastern Mediterrean Health Journal* Mar;5(2),373–377, 1999.
160. V. Ganju. The mental health system in India. History, current system, and prospects. *International Journal of Law and Psychiatry* May-Aug;23(3–4):393–402, 2000.
161. Data from the Institute of Psychiatry, Ain Shams University. Cairo, Egypt, 2000.
162. WHO Estimates of Health Personnel in http://who.int.org.

SUMMARY OF FINDINGS:
Integrating Care of Brain Disorders into Health Care Systems

- Although most developing countries have a system of primary health care, the services available vary widely among communities. They may involve private care (specialists, physicians, or traditional healers) or care provided by governmental or nongovernmental organizations (specialists, physicians, nurses, and other health care workers). Specialists are few and physicians limited; both are concentrated in the cities.

- Successful management of brain disorders through community-based primary care clinics requires guidance and training of health care workers. This must be followed by monitoring, continuing education, and periodic and continued support of clinics and their staffs by secondary and tertiary facilities, such as district hospitals and centers for training and research.

- Cost-effectiveness studies using established methods can best guide public investments in management of brain disorders. Optimal approaches to prevention and treatment of these disorders will vary with local needs and costs.

- Primary health care requires the support of robust national and local policies to adequately address the specific needs of different communities.

- International expertise and resources will be needed from development banks, international organizations, nongovernmental organizations, health professionals, research institutions, and others to establish comprehensive health care for brain disorders in developing countries.

3
Integrating Care of Brain Disorders into Health Care Systems

This chapter describes the most promising vehicle for reducing the burden of brain disorders in developing countries: a comprehensive system of primary health care—primary care services supported by secondary and tertiary care facilities, physicians, and specialists. More detailed information on the challenges and opportunities for caring for specific brain disorders is presented in Part II of this report.

THE ROLE OF PRIMARY CARE IN ADDRESSING BRAIN DISORDERS

Over the last century, health care has increasingly been based on a public health approach that promotes health through prevention as well as treatment of disease. In developing countries, the need to provide affordable, accessible care for whole populations has guided the development of health systems based on primary care. The 1978 International Conference on Primary Health Care produced the Alma-Alta Declaration—a strategy promoting health for all that has been broadly accepted by both developing and developed countries. Under this strategy, primary health care is defined as essential health care based on practical, scientifically sound, and socially acceptable methods and technology, made universally accessible to individuals and families in the community through their full participation, and at a cost that the community and country can afford to maintain at every stage of their development, in the spirit of self-reliance and self-determination. Primary health care forms an integral part both of a country's health system, of which it is the central function and main focus, and of the overall social and economic development of the community.[1,2]

Prior to the Alma-Alta declaration, an Expert Committee on Mental Health was convened by the World Health Organization (WHO) in 1974.[3] This committee recognized the scarcity of trained mental health professionals and the need for a tiered approach to treatment that is grounded in communities served by nonspecialized health workers and primary care nurses and physicians linked to specialist resources. Epidemiological research and programmatic development over the last 25 years have been guided by these findings.[4]

Delivery of health care in developing countries varies with needs and resources, as well as with the availability of various types of medical professionals. However basic the staff and facilities, primary care represents the point of entry for the vast majority of people seeking medical care—and for many people, their sole access to medicine.[5] Thus, primary care is the logical setting in which brain disorders can begin to be addressed. Including care for brain disorders in the primary care agenda represents the surest way to promote their prevention, early detection, and timely treatment.[4,6,7]

The incorporation of neurological and psychiatric care into the public health system is widely recognized as a way to improve coverage by providing a low-cost, accessible service that involves families and the community in patient care.[8–11] The integration of neurological and psychiatric services with primary health care is already a significant policy objective in developed and developing areas of the world.[12–18] Examples of this integration are found in low-income countries; one such example is described in Box 3-1. Other programs organized at both the national and local levels have been developed in India, Colombia, China, Iran, Malaysia, Tanzania, and Brazil.[19–24]

Additional features of primary health care systems contribute to their potential for reducing the impact of neurological, psychiatric, and developmental disorders. As noted in Chapter 2, very few medical specialists practice in developing countries (see Figure 2-2). In China, for example, there are approximately 10 psychiatrists for every million people,[22] 5 psychiatrists are available for the 30 million people of Tanzania,[25] and in Ethiopia, about 10 neurologists serve a nation of more than 53 million.[22] Most of these specialists practice in urban settings, further reducing their availability to rural populations. Thus, most people in need of treatment for brain disorders must receive it at community health centers.

As the gateway to health services in most middle- and low- income settings, primary care centers are well placed to recognize brain disorders and facilitate diagnosis and treatment of coexisting diseases. Research indicates that people with severe mental illness suffer higher-than-average rates of mortality from cardiovascular and respiratory diseases, cancer, and—in low-income countries—infectious diseases.[26–31] Additionally, findings show that patients

BOX 3-1 Integration of Mental Health Services and Primary Care in Guinea-Bissau

After Guinea-Bissau became independent from Portugal in 1974, the government established a decentralized, preventive health policy implemented through a nationwide primary health care system. Before developing a plan to add mental health care, researchers conducted epidemiological, sociological, and anthropological studies to determine the prevalence of certain brain disorders, understand community attitudes toward treatment of them by traditional and orthodox practitioners, and assess the abilities of village health workers to diagnose and treat mental disorders and epilepsy.

The researchers then established priorities for the training of Guinean health personnel to address psychiatric emergencies, including acute psychoses and agitation; depression and other neurotic disorders; and seizures, particularly those attributable to epilepsy. Training was focused on staff members (mainly nurses) at health centers, some of whom then trained and supervised volunteer village health workers. Flowcharts and role-playing vignettes were used to instruct personnel in the diagnosis and management of common mental disorders and seizures. After the seminar, the nurses received quarterly supervision focusing on case management and the use and distribution of medications.

The training improved the health workers' abilities to diagnose major mental disorders and epilepsy from 31 to 75 percent and their prescription of appropriate treatment for psychosis and depression from 0 to 75 percent. Nurses were even more successful in learning to recognize and treat epilepsy; after 4 hours of instruction, they were able to correctly diagnose 95 percent of cases of generalized epileptic convulsions and treated 90 percent correctly. In 1985, 2 years after the start of the program, WHO declared Guinea-Bissau to be the first "third world" country to succeed in integrating a social psychiatric program into its basic health care services. Each dollar invested in primary mental health care in Guinea-Bissau served more than 50 citizens for a year. The cost was modest because the program was designed to meet local needs, was built on a solid foundation of primary health care, and was monitored for improvement. Since then, structural adjustment programs have adversely affected the supply and cost of antipsychotics and anti-epileptic drugs. Though no analysis has been conducted, one could presume that the overall costs of the program have increased as a result of changes in the drug supply.

Continuing supervision by nurses and physicians from secondary medical centers was an essential component of program success. Many of the newly trained workers in the villages only began to implement their knowledge and skills after the initial visits with these professionals. This indicates the importance of supervision in the development of similar programs elsewhere.

Source: [22]

BOX 3-2 A Community-Based Rural Mental Health Program in Pakistan

A demonstration project in Rawalpindi began in 1985 with the following objectives:

- To determine the feasibility of integrating mental health care into the primary care system.
- To involve the community in the planning and delivery of mental health services.
- To promote collaboration across sectors (e.g., health, education, local government, nongovernmental organizations [NGOs], religious healers).
- To establish two-way referral systems between primary health care providers and specialists.

In the first phase of the program, researchers collected socioeconomic and demographic information. Then, primary health care staff were trained to provide care under supervision. Finally, a system of monitoring and evaluation of service delivery was put in place. Following adoption of a national mental health program by the government of Pakistan in 1987, the demonstration project was extended to all four districts of Rawalpindi (population 7.5 million).

Compared to districts with no mental health component, the four districts showed the following results:

- Use of primary health care facilities (particularly by males) increased.
- Pregnancy rates consistently declined.
- Use of antenatal clinics increased and was accompanied by a significantly higher rate of assisted deliveries; infant and maternal mortality rates were reduced by nearly one-third and one-half, respectively.
- Immunization rates for children rose steadily.
- Detection rates of mental illnesses were significantly higher.

As a result of these accomplishments, the incorporation of mental health care into primary care has been made a national priority and has been assigned specific funding. Additional benefits of this initiative include the indigenous development of teaching and training modules and information systems for use at all levels of primary health care, as well as the establishment of referral mechanisms.

Sources: [38–41]

with psychiatric disorders seek care from primary providers with greater-than-average frequency because of both increased physical illness and somatization of psychiatric illness.[32–37] Moreover, because they work in the community, primary care teams are well placed to recognize factors such as stigma, family problems, and cultural factors that affect treatment for brain disorders.

DEVELOPING A SYSTEM OF CARE

Primary Care

Provision of services for brain disorders in conjunction with established primary care services builds on existing human and financial resources to promote practical clinical and social outcomes for these disorders.[52] Limited yet significant evidence from developing countries that have established such programs indicates that a feasible and cost-effective means to meet this goal may be to provide diagnosis and, in many cases, treatment for brain disorders at the first point of entry into medical care, in conjunction with secondary and tertiary support.[43–45] Such a system of care should be staffed by appropriately trained personnel whose level of training and responsibility will vary with the needs and resources of different communities and countries and is best determined by rigorous operational research. Limitations in the diagnostic and treatment skills of nonspecialized providers of mental health care have been observed in several studies in both developed [46–50] and developing countries.[51–54] To guide the development of efficient and effective training methods, similar such assessments must be made as programs develop. Following are descriptions of several essential personnel in such systems.

Community health workers. In some communities, community health workers provide primary care services. These workers need a minimum of some high school education; basic training in health care; and additional training in the diagnosis and treatment of brain disorders, the dispensing and monitoring of medication, support for community rehabilitation, prevention of disorders, and means of reducing stigma and discrimination. Their role is to recognize patients who may need neurological or psychiatric care, to consult regularly on such cases with a specialist nurse or physician, and to provide care under the supervision of a physician or specialist at the closest secondary care center.

Nurses. In some communities, nurses provide primary care services under the supervision of a physician or specialist at the closest secondary care center (see Box 3-2). Their qualifications typically include a high school education, general nursing training, and some specific training in neurological and psychiatric care. Specialist nurses have extensive training in neurological and psychiatric care, and in some countries provide oversight of primary care clinics, making monthly or other regular visits.

General physicians. Since it is not possible to assign physicians or specialists to many primary care facilities, physicians and specialists at secondary and tertiary centers have an essential role in the planning, training, and oversight of each primary care center. The same physicians provide care for severe or complex cases and, whenever possible, initial diagnosis and treatment of critical or chronic cases.

Specialists. Specialists in neurology, pediatrics, psychiatry, and related fields, such as psychology, physiotherapy, social work, occupational therapy, and speech therapy, have important roles. They can contribute to the formulation of relevant health care policies, bringing to bear their specialized knowledge about cost-effective methods of control, treatment, and rehabilitation. They may also oversee policies and procedures at health care facilities and staff training programs.

In several developing countries, mental health care has been organized in line with the principles of public health.[22,24,42,55] Key features of the WHO model guiding primary mental health care may be adapted to address the broader range of brain disorders and may include the following objectives[56]:

- Formulation of a national policy on brain health and establishment of a national or regional brain health department;
- Financial provision for the employment and training of personnel;
- An adequate supply of essential medicines;
- A network of facilities linked by appropriate transportation;
- Data collection to support planning of programs, monitoring of outcomes, and epidemiological research;
- Integration of care for brain disorders with general health services and collaboration with relevant nonmedical agencies;
- Use of workers without specialization in brain disorders, including primary health care workers, nurses, medical assistants, and physicians, for basic care; and
- Training of brain health professionals who train and support nonspecialized health workers.

BOX 3-3 Role of Nurses in Primary Health Care in South Africa

In the mid-1990s the Hlabisa district in KwaZulu-Natal, South Africa, used a nurse-led primary health care program to target four major noncommunicable diseases: hypertension and diabetes (key risk factors for stroke), as well as epilepsy and asthma. Nurses at primary care clinics in the mostly rural region coordinated management of these disorders with a goal of increasing adherence to treatment.

The Hlabisa district, with a population of 250,000, was served in 1993 by a 300-bed district hospital, 10 satellite village clinics staffed by nurses and visited once monthly by a doctor, and a nurse-staffed mobile clinic service. The Zulu population lived in scattered rural homesteads and was dependent on subsistence farming, pensions, or migrant work. Patients in the district could attend the primary care clinic of their choice for a fee of US$0.75 per consultation, which covered tests and prescribed drugs.

Nurses at the primary care clinics were trained to use diagnostic and treatment algorithms for hypertension, diabetes, asthma, and epilepsy, based on the available evidence, clinical experience, and, when available, WHO protocols or national guidelines adapted to local conditions. The algorithms provided clear descriptions of essential aspects of diagnosis, monitoring, and treatment adherence for each disease.

Upon seeing a new patient with one of these disorders, the nurse made a provisional diagnosis using the algorithm and recommended a plan for initial management, including referral to the district hospital if necessary. The patients were subsequently seen by a doctor at the primary care clinic to confirm the diagnosis and check for complications. Complex cases werre reviewed by a doctor until they were under control. Once a patient's condition was controlled, he or she received a prescription card that could be used to obtain medications for 6 months, after which time the case was reviewed and the treatment adjusted, if necessary.

Primary care nurses were authorized to prescribe a limited list of drugs for hypertension, asthma, and non-insulin-dependent diabetes. Doctors prescribed additional medications for these conditions, if needed, as well as all drugs for insulin-dependent diabetes and epilepsy.

During the first 2 years of the program, nurses using the protocol achieved a control rate of 68 percent for hypertension cases (this later increased to 92 percent); for non-insulin-dependent diabetes, 82 percent (which increased to 96 percent); and for asthma, 84 percent (which increased to 97 percent). Doctor-led treatment controlled 80 percent of epilepsy cases and 83 percent of cases of insulin-dependent diabetes; thereafter, these cases were managed by nurses. Adherence to treatment, as measured by patients' reports, occurred at a rate of 79 percent after the first visit and increased to 87 percent after a later visit.

This model demonstrates that nurses supervised by physicians can manage some common brain disorders appropriately, even in a resource-poor setting. The simplification and rationalization of diagnosis and treatment allowed patients to be seen and their conditions managed through local clinics. This approach made optimal use of limited health care resources, and provided accessible care for chronic, often asymptomatic disorders, thereby increasing patient adherence to treatments.

Source: [57]

The Role of Secondary and Tertiary Care

Primary care centers are limited in their ability to adequately diagnose and treat certain brain disorders. The complexity and chronicity of some of these disorders necessitates access to medical expertise and technology that are not ordinarily available in a primary care setting, particularly in developing countries.[58–60] When possible such cases can be recognized in a primary care setting and referred for early intervention to a higher secondary level of care to provide the best chance for successful treatment or rehabilitation. Early recognition and intervention can prevent the costly complications that arise when these more serious conditions are not addressed until they become critical.[61,62]

Secondary care is provided in district or regional hospitals. These are usually staffed by several general physicians, medical technicians, and nurses. These facilities are capable of treating severe or complex medical conditions and may contain computed tomography (CT) scanners, heart monitors, incubators, and laboratory facilities for blood analysis. District and regional hospitals can also support care for a broader range of illnesses than can be treated in primary care alone. Neurologists in India have proposed that district hospitals provide essential medicines and mobile care teams to improve the ability of community health care workers to identify, diagnose, and treat epilepsy.[63] This approach could be adapted to include care for schizophrenia, depression, and other disorders, along with the provision of periodic and continued supervision and training.

Secondary care centers could also provide technical and administrative support for primary care clinics in their district or region. Continuing education, which has been shown to improve the performance of community health workers, should include instruction on the symptoms of major brain disorders and ways to help patients maintain proper treatment.[24,64,65] This training could be provided by medical professionals from secondary facilities who, during regular visits to primary care centers, also monitor the care provided by primary care workers and consult on specific cases.

Tertiary care is the most specialized form of diagnosis, treatment, and rehabilitation, and is often provided in teaching hospitals. Tertiary care hospitals also serve as facilities for clinical research, collection of epidemiological data, and the creation and distribution of health educational materials.

Because resources are limited and the operating costs of tertiary centers are high, most developing countries can support only a few such centers. However, studies conducted at these influential institutions—on such topics as identification of risk factors, prevention strategies, and treatment options, can provide the evidence base for determining national health priorities and community health care. The training curricula developed at these centers can also be adapted for health care personnel at secondary and primary care levels.[66]

Health systems vary immensely within and among countries.[67] The capacity of the current health care infrastructure, local health priorities, and financial resources will play a major role in determining the extent and speed with which neurological and psychiatric care can be incorporated into the primary care system. In many communities, primary care providers have rudimentary training and few essential medicines and diagnostic tools. Yet even under these circumstances, primary care may have the ability to fulfill its mission, given sufficient support, training, and supervision by medical professionals at secondary and tertiary facilities.[22,24,55,68,69]

BUILDING CAPACITY THROUGH TRAINING

Training of staff is a key aspect of expanding existing health care services to address brain disorders. Since the responsibilities of community health workers, nurses, and physicians vary widely, the training must be tailored to the needs of specific countries or regions. A general training framework would be based on existing evidence regarding the provision of health care. The existing body of evidence is described and cited below. However, additional operational research is needed to identify cost-effective ways of training health care personnel at all levels to provide appropriate care for brain disorders.

Community health workers. As front-line caregivers in countries such as Botswana,[11] Guinea Bissau,[22] India,[70] Iran,[71] Nepal,[72] and Tanzania,[55] community health workers need to receive both basic training and regular continuing education in basic diagnostic skills and basic treatment and rehabilitation protocols. Basic training in neurological and psychiatric care should cover general skills, such as interviewing a patient, recording appropriate information, referring a patient to a higher level of care, and consulting with a physician who oversees operations, diagnosis, and management of specific disorders, including the use of medication and monitoring for side effects. Such training should also address daily responsibilities, increase awareness, and improve management skills while avoiding unnecessary details and technical jargon. WHO training manuals are a useful source of training guidelines.[73,74]

Although it should be directed more toward improving skills than enhancing knowledge, training should raise health workers' awareness of the importance of psychosocial factors in health and disease. Flowcharts and simple screening devices can be effective in training primary care providers to recognize developmental disabilities,[75] depression,[33] schizophrenia,[10] and epilepsy.[43] Health care workers can be trained to use a simple screen to detect significant deviations from developmental norms or milestones as well as sensory or motor impairments, such as cerebral palsy.[70,76–78] They can also be trained to identify common mental disorders [20] and stroke.[78] However, it is essential that diagnostic and management tools be adapted to local conditions.[43,70] It is also important to recognize that primary care providers are likely to find assessment tools, such as symptom and behavior checklists more useful than instruments (such as intelligence tests) that do not indicate the action needed.[79] It is important to note as well that in many cases, primary care providers should be trained to recognize the need for referral to more specialized treatment rather than trying to make a diagnosis.

Nurses. Primary health care in low-income countries has always relied heavily on nurses, but they could play an even larger role in the system of care envisioned here (see Box 3-3). Physicians in secondary care facilities in developing countries may spend only a few minutes per patient visit. Under these conditions, it is unrealistic to expect them to diagnose any but the most overt cases of brain disorder. Nurses trained to conduct more detailed first interviews may be better able to recognize common mental disorders, such as depression, and to identify risks for stroke, such as hypertension and diabetes.[57,80,81]

In regions where there are few physicians in primary care, specialist nurses may be called on to diagnose and treat brain disorders; however, such efforts are likely to fare best if overseen by neurologists and psychiatrists. In a specialized psychiatric treatment center, periodic visits from psychiatrists were found to improve the ability of psychiatric nurses working in the Botswana bush to care for chronically ill patients, a finding that may apply in the primary care setting as well.[82] Other experience indicates that primary care nurses , using appropriate guidelines provided through a program of continuing education, can also provide effective management for mental disorders.[62,65,83]

Primary care nurses also have many opportunities to promote brain health, and it is appropriate that they receive instruction in simple techniques for managing emotional distress (e.g., physical activity, talking over problems, assertiveness training, and relaxation techniques), and for giving advice on cessation of smoking and adhering to a healthy diet. Similarly, providing mental health education to nurses who serve as birth attendants could help improve the rates of diagnosis and treatment referral for postpartum psychosis and severe depression.

Physicians. Physicians get most of their medical training in teaching hospitals, where tertiary health care is emphasized. Since the cases that present in a hospital are generally more complex and may be further complicated by nosocomial factors, physicians who supervise primary health care personnel must have experience with the diagnosis and treatment at that level.[15,26,61] Training should emphasize preventive measures against such brain disorders as mental retardation and stroke, and provide interview skills that can facilitate the diagnosis of depression and other psychological disorders.[5,84] General physicians should be able to evaluate and treat common neurological and psychiatric disorders as well as respond to emergencies, such as head injury, stroke, epileptic seizure, and psychotic episodes. A program to improve training in neurological disorders for primary care physicians in developing countries was launched in 1997 by WHO and the World Federation of Neurologists.[85–87]

Physicians who supervise or train other primary care providers also need instruction in effective communication skills in order to develop the skills of community health care workers. The supervising physician should regularly work alongside health workers and receive case referrals from them. Given the increasing recognition of the common origins of many brain disorders, psychiatrists should be conversant in neurology and exposed to patients with neurological disorders, while neurologists should have a basic command of psychiatry and experience with patients suffering from major mental disorders.[88]

COLLABORATION WITH OTHER HEALTH AND NONHEALTH SECTORS

The formation of alliances between public health care providers and private physicians, schools and educators, community-based rehabilitation (CBR) programs, other community organizations, and traditional healers is another way of improving health care.[89] Their roles in primary care are discussed below.

Private Physicians

Decentralization of health care services in many developing countries has been required by numerous development programs over the last two decades. The growth in private health care facilities as a result of these initiatives has created an important role for this sector in addressing brain disorders. In India, private practitioners are estimated to provide half of all primary care, and up to 80 percent in some states.[90] Many of the rural and urban poor consult with private practitioners because of their relatively low consultation fees and accessibility, as well as negative perceptions of the quality of public health care. The recent imposition of user fees for public health care services in India is likely to increase the proportion of care provided by private practitioners.

In the least-developed regions of India and sub-Saharan Africa, which tend to be underserved by government-provided health care, the principal providers of health care are community-based NGOs, which offer such care as part of a broader development agenda. Some NGO providers focus on specific psychiatric and neurological problems, attempting to fill needs unmet by either public or private providers.[91] In many developing countries, outreach to and participation by private physicians will be important to the success of public education, prevention, and treatment initiatives aimed at brain disorders. Comprehensive operational research to establish appropriate training requirements, cost-effective interventions, and future research needs will be most useful when the services provided by private physicians are considered jointly with public health system measures.[92,93]

Schools and Educators

When developmental and other brain disorders occur in children, educators may be the first to recognize them. Such vigilance can be encouraged through consultations between teachers and primary care providers. Research is needed on how teachers can best facilitate the early diagnosis and treatment of brain disorders in children. Schools can also include neurological and mental health education, as they do physical health education, in their curricula.[5] In India and Pakistan, school children who have been taught basic skills play an important role in identifying adult relatives with epilepsy, schizophrenia, and other disorders and bringing them to medical attention.[92]

Community-Based Rehabilitation Programs

CBR programs are a low-cost way to coordinate medical guidance and community resources in the rehabilitation of disabled people, allowing them to live as normally as possible.[94,95] Some of the most successful CBR programs work to mainstream disabled children into public education at the earliest opportunity and to assist them in the transition from school to employment (see Chapter 6 for a detailed discussion of CBR for developmental disabilities). In addition to providing long-term care and support, CBR addresses the isolation and stigma experienced by disabled people. The program can be linked to and supported by institutional and hospital-based programs, thereby creating a comprehensive rehabilitation service (see Box 3-4). Additionally, CBR programs should consider the needs of both children and adults who require mental and physical rehabilitation.

BOX 3-4 Psychiatric Rehabilitation Villages in Tanzania

Tanzania, a country that spends only about US $1.33 per capita annually on health care, has created several self-sustaining facilities for the care of people with chronic psychiatric disorders. Modeled after the pioneering Aro Village in Abeokuta, Nigeria,[96] the Tanzanian villages were established in the late 1960s to provide a socially stimulating environment for patients who require extended rehabilitation. Rehabilitation villages offer psychiatric services similar to those available in hospitals, but in an environment intended to duplicate the social and economic milieu of a rural community. By providing agricultural plots where patients can be engaged according to their abilities and stages of motivation, the villages encourage patients' personal growth and independence.

Hombolo psychiatric village, the first to be established in central Tanzania in 1969, was built by patients with assistance from the staff of Mirembe Psychiatric Hospital, a large mental health institution. During the 1970s and 1980s, 11 psychiatric rehabilitation villages were developed in Tanzania to meet growing demand, and more villages have followed. In 1992, the villages cared for 450 patients.[23]

Vikuruti village, located 18 kilometers south of Dar es Salaam on 75 hectares of land, is a typical rehabilitation village. Most of the land is used for horticulture, coconut and citrus plantations, and animal husbandry. The village houses 32 patients in eight cottages and has a kitchen, dining hall, three staff houses, offices, and a hostel to house students and patients' relatives, who are encouraged to visit and take part in the activities.

The afflictions of patients include schizophrenia, alcohol dependence syndrome, epilepsy complicated by psychotic illness, and bipolar disorders. The staff has three agricultural and livestock field officers, two nurses, nursing assistants, three artisans who perform occupational therapy, a driver, and three security staff, all of whom are supervised by a psychiatrist at Muhimbili University College of Health Sciences in Dar es Salaam. Traditional healers may play a role in therapy if a patient requests it. With the assistance of the psychiatrist and a medical social worker who visit weekly, the team works with patients and relatives on rehabilitation plans and counseling support. Patients participate in the village's token-economy system and take part in the management of community life, including the election of a village government.

Patients generally reside at the rehabilitation villages for 3 months to 2 years, during which time they make more rapid progress than similar patients in hospital environments. Cost-effectiveness studies would be useful to review alternative uses of resources and consider recruiting of additional professionals.

Sources: [23,96,96]

Community Organizations

Although relatively few and often poorly funded, local groups can facilitate mutual support and sharing of experience among patients, families, and caregivers. NGOs and parent groups together can establish facilities, such as vocational training centers, day care centers, and supported living facilities, most of which are staffed by community volunteers. Groups such as the Kenya Association for the Welfare of Epileptics and Zimcare, an organization for the support of persons with mental handicaps in Zimbabwe, can work to change social attitudes and draw the attention of policy makers to patients with disabilities.

Traditional Healers

In some countries, many people—perhaps a majority—seek care for brain disorders from traditional healers.[98–100] These practitioners are therefore likely to influence health care delivery in the developing world for some time to come.[5,101,102] Although a scientific basis and empirical evidence of their effectiveness may be lacking, there is little doubt that some aspects of traditional healing benefit patients.[103] Most community health workers and other care providers in developing countries come in regular contact with traditional healers and are aware of their practices.[89,104,105] They may even rely on traditional healers for their own mental health care [8] and experience conflict between traditional and biomedical explanations of disorders.[103,106]

In determining their relationship with traditional healers, providers of biomedical care must address several issues. First, they must determine how to protect patients from intrinsically harmful traditional practices. Patient education about the negative effects of some traditional treatments can be an important role for physicians, nurses, and health care workers. Second, they must establish dialogue to determine whether patients are simultaneously taking orthodox and traditional medicines.[107] Some herbal medicines have pharmacological effects similar to those of orthodox medicines and may thereby inadvertently cause overdose or dangerous side effects. Conversely, traditional practices that are benign or potentially helpful [108–111] can be incorporated into protocols for care.[112] Malaysia has established a specific research framework to evaluate traditional medicines.[113,114]

Some developing communities have determined that the most effective route to good health care lies in creating alliances between biomedical care providers and traditional healers.[115] In the mid-1980s, such informal collaborations emerged in Brazil.[16] In Nepal, where allopathic psychiatric care coexists with traditional healing, healers attend community education courses on mental health that are organized by nongovernmental organizations (NGOs).[72] Through such courses in Nigeria, healers have been trained to recognize and manage cases of psychiatric disorder and refer them to community health workers.[105] In Zimbabwe, psychiatrists work with the two leading associations of traditional healers to assist in HIV/AIDS prevention and treatment. Operational research on such collaborative efforts may identify opportunities in other countries seeking to facilitate constructive cooperation with traditional healers.

Where resources for primary health care are extremely limited, traditional healers, who vastly outnumber community health workers, can be recruited and trained to provide primary care.[96,116–118] Additional training for those who currently provide care can be the fastest way to increase the capacity to treat brain disorders.[22,92]

THE COST OF INTEGRATING SERVICES

Current estimates of the significant disease burden imposed by brain disorders (see Chapter 2), along with evidence of cost-effective interventions that have been implemented in a limited number of health care programs in developing countries, argue for action to reduce this burden. The existing limited evidence, coupled with further operational research, can guide public investment to permit the expansion of primary health care to include care for brain disorders.[92,119,120] Timely investments in personnel, training, drugs, and infrastructure are key to preventing or reducing the impact of these disorders on individuals, their families, and society. Treatment of these disorders is also the surest means of reducing the stigma associated with them and replacing archaic beliefs with contemporary understanding.

Determination of the appropriate level of effective, affordable care for brain disorders should be based on cost-effectiveness analyses for a range of treatments in different systems of health care. Considerable variability among communities in their perception of neurological and psychiatric illness, their expectations of what medical care should provide, and the cost of drugs and other services complicates choices for good-quality, affordable services. Optimal approaches to treatment and prevention need to reflect local costs and benefits.

Evaluations of cost-effectiveness may be based on costs to the patient alone or may include costs to the family and the community. The cost to an individual of being unemployed is direct and measurable; therefore, when treatment permits a return to employment, this benefit is measurable as well. But to society, the loss of productivity due to the disability of a single worker may be small if unemployment is high. Where treatments can be shown to benefit society and the economy as well as individuals and their families, the case for treatment will be more compelling.

Health care economists generally agree on the methodology for establishing the cost-effectiveness of alternative approaches to health care delivery.[120–122] Briefly, such analyses compare interventions for health promotion, prevention, diagnosis, and treatment and rehabilitation on the basis of outcome and cost. They also evaluate different systems of primary care, including the routine use routine use of primary care workers with oversight from secondary routine use of primary care workers with oversight from secondary care facilities. These assessments should be addressed from the perspective of the community; thus, they should employ a common descriptive terminology and express the costs of health care in terms of purchasing power.

Analyses depend on data, however, little of which is currently available. Appropriate databases for systemic analyses of cost-effectiveness in primary care can be built through a review of existing data, followed by establishment of a multinational collection of information based on a common framework. New information should be collected in local studies that include comparisons of financing, costs, and service utilization, as well as rigorous assessments of cost-effectiveness.[123]

Once neurological and psychiatric care have been incorporated into a system of health care, maintaining a cost-effective program will require monitoring, evaluation, and comparison with new alternatives. Research to establish the cost-effectiveness of treating brain disorders will be a key element in persuading governments, donor missions, and NGOs that incorporating these services into health care programs is affordable and necessary for the health and well-being of individuals, families, and the community.

BOX 3-5 Cost-Outcome Study in India and Pakistan

A recent study in India and Pakistan developed and tested methods for economic analysis of community health programs. The Pakistan program was described in Box 3-2. Researchers screened four rural populations (two in India and two in Pakistan) for psychiatric morbidity to estimate the prevalence of common mental disorders and the patterns of health care-seeking behavior. Between 12 and 39 percent of participants at each site were found to have a diagnosable mental disorder and were invited to seek treatment. They were then assessed prospectively as to their symptoms, disability, quality of life, and resource use.

In three of the four locales studied, treatment of mental disorders improved patients' symptoms, reduced their disability, and increased their quality of life, all of which resulted in reduced costs to the overall economy. The evaluation was based on data on the relative costs and benefits of alternative responses to mental disorders in the community and thereby identified opportunities for improvement in the health care system.

This general study design could be adapted for use in other countries. To that end, the authors prepared a brief set of guidelines for the economic evaluation of mental health care. These guidelines and sample surveys appear in Appendix D.

Source: [90]

BUILDING RESEARCH CAPACITY THROUGH
COLLABORATION

The expansion of primary health care services to include cost-effective neurological and psychiatric care demands an increased capacity not only for delivery of care, but also for research. A robust research agenda to inform and support primary care should include operational studies to test techniques and strategies for their effectiveness in the local setting, along with epidemiological surveillance. Such a program could also promote the development of an international cadre of neurological and psychiatric professionals focused on these issues in developing countries. A successful model for such a research program, the WHO Special Programme for Research and Training in Tropical Diseases, could be adapted for this purpose (see Box 3-6).

BOX 3-6 The WHO Special Programme for Tropical Disease Research

The WHO Special Programme for Research and Training in Tropical Diseases (TDR) was established in 1975 through a joint effort of the United Nations Development Programme, the World Bank, and WHO. TDR has produced many successful partnerships in a broad variety of international organizations, and its collaborators include more than 5,000 scientists in 160 countries.

TDR acts as a global facilitator of research and training in tropical disease management by selecting, guiding, funding, and developing research on 10 major tropical diseases: malaria, schistosomiasis, African trypanosomiasis, leishmaniasis, dengue, lymphatic filariasis, Chagas disease, onchocerciasis, leprosy, and tuberculosis. The program's goal is to support the development of safe, acceptable, and affordable methods of prevention, diagnosis, treatment, and control of target diseases, as well as training that strengthens the capability of developing disease-endemic countries to undertake the research required to develop new methods and strategies for disease control.

Partners with TDR in fulfilling these goals include governments and ministries of health in disease-endemic countries such as Cameroon, India, Malaysia, and Nigeria; research institutions, including the Liverpool School of Tropical Medicine and the London School of Hygiene and Tropical Medicine; NGOs, such as the Wellcome Trust; and industry. Financial contributors include both developed and developing nations and an international roster of foundations and associations.

Research and training activities are organized into four main areas, each overseen by a committee. The section on Basic and Strategic Research funds the use of cutting-edge technology and social, economic, and behavioral research to develop tools for long-term control of target diseases.

Product Research and Development focuses on the identification of novel drugs, vaccines, and diagnostics for target diseases, as well as their development from clinical trials through to regulatory approval and registration. Intervention Development and Evaluation supports the evaluation of existing programs related to target diseases and the development, implementation, and evaluation of new control strategies. In the area of Research Capability Strengthening, TDR seeks to fund institutional development and technology transfer in countries where its target diseases are endemic. It also aims to build links between institutions in endemic and nonendemic countries, train individual researchers and research groups from disease-endemic countries, and strengthen computing capabilities and Internet access in these countries.

Scientists from all countries, especially those where TDR diseases are endemic, are eligible to receive research and training grants from the program. Funding is available for a wide variety of purposes, including collaborative research, project development, research capability strengthening, and research training.

Source: [124]

In addition to large-scale international collaborations such as TDR, efforts to increase health research capacity in developing countries include national and local programs that focus existing scientific expertise on particular health problems. For example, the Research Institute of Tropical Medicine has established institutional links between the University of the Philippines and several governmental and nongovernmental organizations. A similar program of transdisciplinary research collaboration among experts in Uganda was found to be a low-cost means of increasing research capacity on AIDS.[125] Participants in collaborative efforts to build the capacity for health care delivery and operational research can also contribute to the improvement of national and local policies and programs. Support from the Carnegie Corporation funded health and behavior research training in East Africa out of the University of Nairobi and University of Dar es Salaam from 1990 to 1999. Similar research training was supported by the Freeman Foundation in Southeast Asia in conjunction with Harvard Medical School.[126]

Several participants in collaborative efforts to build health care research and delivery capacity in developing countries have emphasized the importance of involving local researchers and policy makers in program design and implementation.[66,127–130] A key means of accomplishing this goal is through the training of local researchers to assume responsibility for directing and sustaining national research programs. Moreover, as members of USAID's Applied Diarrheal Disease Project have discovered, such training programs afford increased access to local knowledge that can immediately improve researchers' ability to apply their findings productively.[128] The ultimate goal of training, however, should be the establishment of research institutions in developing countries that can grow, mature, and participate as equals in international networks of scientific exchange.[33,131]

Two principal means of collecting epidemiological data for health care planning purposes are surveys and record keeping at the primary care level.[113] Given the diverse means by which people in developing countries obtain primary care, surveys that attempt to determine the extent to which patients with brain disorders make use of various health care providers,[132,133] as well as surveys of the prevalence of specific neurological and psychiatric disorders among the general population, should prove especially useful. Research on pathways to health care can reveal areas for improvement in the efficiency of treatment and referral in health care systems.[105,132,133] A program designed to improve the basic epidemiological research skills of clinicians in developing countries for such research efforts is the International Clinical Epidemiology Network. The program and suggested mechanisms for its role in research for brain disorders are described in Box 3-7.

POLICY IMPLICATIONS

Policies designed to support the expansion of health care services to address neurological, psychiatric, and developmental disorders in developing countries will need to be advanced at every level of governement, from local communities to international bodies. This section examines the national and local policy implications of addressing brain disorders in developing countries, while the next section describes potential international contributions to this effort.

National Policy

In formulating health care policy, governments rarely start with a clean slate. It is therefore important not only to appraise national needs for the care of brain disorders, but also to identify resources and strengths that can be directed toward new goals. Experience even in resource-poor countries such as Botswana,[11] Guinea Bissau,[59] and Tanzania [55] indicates that when a robust national policy of primary care is in place, it can be expanded successfully to address additional types of care. As discussed previously, established mental health programs represent the logical starting point for addressing a broader spectrum of brain disorders. Additionally, where collaborative efforts exist between the health and nonhealth sectors (e.g., education, environment, social welfare), these relationships should be reinforced and expanded.[5,61,70]

Many developing countries have made significant investments in specific disease-control initiatives and in primary care infrastructure for infectious diseases and maternal and child health.[98,99] They have also expanded these pro-grams to meet broader health care needs. In Iran, for example, a program of childhood immunization that began as a vertical, stand-alone project achieved greater success when integrated into the existing system of primary health care.[100] Such programs of integrated care could, with appropriate expertise and oversight, be augmented to include the prevention, identification, treatment, rehabilitation, and surveillance of brain disorders.

BOX 3-7 The International Clinical Epidemiology Network

Since 1980, the International Clinical Epidemiology Network (INCLEN) has worked to establish training programs in developing countries through which clinicians can learn basic epidemiological research skills. The organization specifically seeks to improve physicians' abilities in the following areas:

- Making clinical decisions when treating patients;
- Analyzing the cost-effectiveness of interventions;
- Designing clinical trials of medicines and treatments;
- Evaluating diagnostic tests; and
- Appraising the medical literature.

The ultimate goal of this effort is the creation of a worldwide network of physicians, statisticians, and social scientists to build and sustain institutional capacity for clinical epidemiology in research and medical education.

To date, INCLEN has helped found and support more than 31 clinical epidemiology units (CEUs) in 16 countries and has trained more than 300 clinical epidemiologists and health specialists. They in turn train students and assist their colleagues with research projects; many also serve as advisors to ministers of health in their countries. With the founding of the INCLEN Trust in 2000, the organization has adopted a governing structure based in the developing world and spearheaded by regional leaders of its units in Africa, India, China, Southeast Asia, Latin America, and the Mediterranean.

INCLEN represents a promising potential collaborator in efforts to integrate care for neurological, psychiatric, and developmental disorders into existing heath care services in developing countries. One starting point might be the few CEUs that currently offer training on epidemiological strategies specific to mental health. Programs at these sites could be expanded to include other topics relevant to brain disorders, then reproduced throughout the established INCLEN system.

Sources: [134]

An effective system of primary care requires periodic and continued supervision and oversight from medical specialists, a system of referral, and guidelines for good practice. At the national level, policies to implement the integration of care for brain disorders into primary health care must address a variety of issues, including those detailed below.

Strategies for prevention. Prevention is generally the most cost-effective means of reducing disease burden. Two basic approaches to preventing brain disorders require the support of national policy: public education and reduction of known risk factors.[58] Although education occurs at the community level, national policy should support the training of community health workers in educating their clients about the nature and causes of brain disorders. Such programs can promote prevention by alerting the public to avoidable risk factors, and also reduce the stigma associated with such disorders as epilepsy and schizophrenia.

National public health policy should seek as well to control known and preventable risk factors for brain disorders, many of which are common in developing countries (see Part II for discussion of risk factors associated with specific disorders). Likewise, national governments can lead efforts to identify and strengthen factors that protect against these disorders. For example, future research could include studies to determine whether literacy campaigns, such as the National Literacy Campaign in northern India, effectively discourage risk-taking behavior or increase the use of appropriate health facilities for neurological and psychiatric conditions.[141]

Strategies for intervention. While each community should define its health care priorities, national policy can support this process by establishing uniform standards and protocols for the care of specific disorders based on best-practice guidelines, and by undertaking data collection and information distribution. Capacity and resources may be too limited to permit the complete fulfillment of internationally established practice guidelines; however, the implementation of all feasible component practices is likely to increase the cost-effectiveness of treatment.

Governments should also coordinate care among all tiers of the health care system, recognizing the importance of oversight of primary care centers and their connection to secondary and tertiary care by physicians or specialists at district or national facilities.[11,21,59,76,136] Policy should guide the progress of patients who need advanced care along established pathways that will ensure the earliest appropriate intervention.

Priority setting. To make optimal use of limited health care resources, countries may find it beneficial to enact policies that will guide each community in formulating and updating its health care strategy. To the extent possible, these policies should be based on evidence of cost-effectiveness. Since early detection and treatment of many brain disorders, for example, tends to reduce their severity and prevent recurrence, training guidelines for community health workers should stress the importance of these practices.[61] Likewise, policies that target people at high risk for brain disorders are likely to make the most efficient use of limited resources. For example, people who have recently experienced important or catastrophic life events (e.g., childbirth, unemployment, war, natural disaster) would benefit from screening for and prompt treatment of depression.[137,138] Similarly, early detection and control of hypertension and diabetes is key to preventing stroke, as well as other complications.[43] The treatment and, especially, prevention of brain disorders in children should receive particular emphasis, since these are an important means of reducing long-term disability and overall disease burden.[139]

Training. Governments should establish standards for the training of health care personnel at all levels to build a strong foundation for a primary care system. National training policies should also reflect the importance of continuing professional education for primary caregivers, as demonstrated in several studies in developing countries.[8,20,65,140] Although such training may be organized by local health services, it could be encouraged through national policies that make available such resources as quality instruction, access to journals, distance learning, lectures, and workshops. Primary care and other staff will need to be released for training courses and given funds for travel and subsistence for the time they are away. They may also be rewarded with small incentive payments to encourage high participation.[92]

Education. National policies supporting school-based efforts to recognize common brain disorders among children would improve their early diagnosis and treatment.

Monitoring of health care delivery and outcomes. The surveillance of brain disorders and their care, including data collected in primary care settings, provides a basis for evaluating the effectiveness of prevention, diagnosis, and treatment practices. National policy should therefore support the collection, analysis, and dissemination of information on health care outcomes.[140]

Local Policy

Rather than simply reacting to health care policy set by the national government, communities are best served when they determine their own priorities. Community involvement in the development of health services tends to promote self-reliance and has been shown to increase demand for health care services.[24] Because district medical officers and their staffs play a vital role in determining local priorities and implementing plans, brain disorders should have a regular place on the agendas of these officials. Some needs may be met through collaborations between health care and other social services and NGOs—for example, through the creation of day care and rehabilitation facilities, crisis centers, and halfway homes. Areas best addressed by community-level policy include the following.

Education. Community education about the nature of brain disorders can reduce stigmatization and facilitate care. Programs should be adapted to community needs, as determined through empirical methods. Explanations of brain disorders should make use of culturally appropriate idioms and constructs to clearly describe the causes of the disease, means of prevention and treatment, and expected outcomes.

Community education programs should be aimed at abolishing harmful local practices and beliefs, such as the ascription of epilepsy, schizophrenia, and other disorders to supernatural beings or demons, ancestral spirits, sorcery, or witchcraft, as well as the use of dangerous medicinal preparations or ritual treatments.[8,10,11,61,120] In some communities, educators may also need to promote public health care so that more people with neurological and psychiatric disorders will make use of this resource. Policy that guides training for educators may include programs to develop their ability to recognize certain brain disorders in children, such as epilepsy, vision or hearing impairments, and depression.

Access to care. In many communities, especially rural ones, primary care teams require transportation if they are to conduct outreach (to reach many of their clients), as do patients who may need to travel relatively long distances to access both primary and secondary care. Appropriate transportation for health care workers and patients may need to be provided or subsidized by both the community and the health service.

Family care. In the vast majority of cases of psychiatric and neurological disorders in both the developing and developed worlds, the patient's family provides most of the necessary care and in many cases, makes all care decisions on behalf of the patient. Thus, strengthening the ability of families to support people with brain disorders—and when possible, enabling families to play an active role in the control and management of illness—represents a key strategy in reducing the global impact of these diseases. This could be accomplished in part by designing family-based interventions, such as the program for schizophrenia described in Box 3-8.

INTERNATIONAL SUPPORT FOR SYSTEMS OF
PRIMARY CARE

The international implications of addressing brain disorders in developing countries are similar to those for a variety of health concerns, many of which are best addressed through the creation of comprehensive community-based health care.[3] Building such capacity in developing countries, as well as attaining the more specific goal of reducing the disease burden due to neurological and psychiatric disorders, will require international contributions of expertise and resources.[91] Two areas in which international support could be especially effective are described below.

The Role of Professional Societies and International Organizations

The international community of health care professionals can make significant contributions by assisting in the formulation of relevant health care policies that can benefit from their specialized knowledge concerning effective and cost-efficient methods of control, treatment, and rehabilitation of brain disorders. Policy makers are often pessimistic about the likelihood that disorders such as schizophrenia and epilepsy can be treated successfully.[101] They may also assign low priority to rehabilitative efforts for these disorders if they believe

---

BOX 3-8 Family-Based Intervention for Schizophrenia Patients in China

In 1993, more than 90 percent of the approximately 4.5 million people with schizophrenia in China were estimated to live with their families, and nearly all their outpatient visits included family members. Encouraged by this situation, a team of researchers from Shashi City Veterans Psychiatric Hospital and Harvard Medical School worked intensively with 30 families of schizophrenic patients to test and adapt Western techniques of family-based interventions for use in China.

The researchers quickly discovered that Western approaches to family therapy rely on assumptions that do not hold in China, such as the acceptance of counseling and the goal of encouraging greater independence for individuals with mental disorders. Nevertheless, the team was able, through trial and error, to develop a comprehensive, ongoing program appropriate for the family relationships and social environment of China. The intervention included monthly 45-minute counseling sessions on how to manage social and occupational problems, medication, family education, family group meetings, and crises.

The intervention program was then compared with standard hospital-based treatment for schizophrenia through a series of blind follow-up evaluations after 6, 12, and 18 months. Compared with patients who received standard treatment for schizophrenia, those who participated in the family-based intervention were rehospitalized less often and for shorter periods of time, and they were employed for longer periods. The family-based intervention was also found to be less costly than standard treatment, saving an estimated US $149 per family, equivalent to nearly 1.5 percent of China's expenditure for health care in 1991. Similar programs in Shanghai, Beijing, and Nanjing have been evaluated as effective.

Source: [141]

patients are not likely to be economically productive. Medical professionals can provide a realistic perspective on these issues.[136]

The medical community can also advocate that brain disorders receive health policy attention commensurate with the contribution of those disorders to the overall burden of disease. This is particularly important where patients are stigmatized. In recent years the World Psychiatric Association, the World Federation of Mental Health, and WHO's Nations for Mental Health of Underserved Populations Action Program (see Box 3-9) have battled against the stigma associated with most psychotic disorders. These efforts could be extended through participation by other professional organizations [87].

Collaborative efforts to control these disorders are most likely to succeed if they involve experts from other than psychiatry and neurology, fields such as public health, obstetrics, pediatrics, and social welfare. One such program, the Out of the Shadows campaign for epilepsy awareness, is led by the International League Against Epilepsy, the International Bureau of Epilepsy, and WHO. Similar efforts for other disorders have been organized by NGOs such as MINDS, the International League of Societies for Persons with Mental Handicap, and the March of Dimes.

BOX 3-9 Nations for Mental Health

Nations for Mental Health is an Action Programme of WHO, developed in collaboration with the Department of Social Medicine of Harvard Medical School. Its main aims are to raise awareness among the people, communities, and governments of the world regarding the effects of mental, neurological, and behavioral problems (e.g., substance abuse) on psychosocial well-being and physical health; promote and support the implementation of mental health policies around the world; and create country-level demonstration projects to serve as models for larger-scale implementation.

Nations for Mental Health is an initiative primarily for underserved populations and therefore includes disadvantaged persons in addition to those suffering from mental disorders. The two groups have much in common, including the need for common solutions that address specific situations. As such, disadvantaged persons and many of those with mental disorders form a broad virtual nation of underserved people dispersed throughout the world.

Nations for Mental Health's intervention model includes the following key elements:

• Stimulating political awareness, political will, and commitment;
• Utilizing existing knowledge to create a sound theoretical framework;
• Developing the necessary human capital;

- Supporting local demonstration projects; and
- Providing financial and human resources.

Direct technical support to countries is provided by WHO. WHO also works collaboratively with partner organizations in the United Nations to maximize the efficient use of technical and financial resources. In addition, WHO provides seed money to initiate demonstration projects and assists country authorities in raising additional support from funding bodies to achieve agreed-upon objectives.

Topical areas for intervention within Nations for Mental Health are listed below. Each involves research, dissemination, education and training, and communication:

- National plans for mental health;
- Promotion of mental health and prevention of mental disorders;
- Improved services and treatments;
- Human rights and legislation;
- Empowerment of consumers and families; and
- Special programs for indigenous populations and refugees.

Nations for Mental Health was conceived as a vehicle for multidisciplinary and interorganizational work. There is close collaboration among WHO Headquarters, regional offices, and country representatives, as well as many other important entities, including the United Nations system; multilateral organizations such as the World Bank; and academic institutions and NGOs, such as Harvard Medical School, the London Institute of Psychiatry, the World Federation for Mental Health, the World Psychiatric Association, the World Association for Psychosocial Rehabilitation, the Red Cross, the Geneva Initiative, and the Carter Center.

Source: [142]

WHO has championed many activities designed to improve the services available for people with brain disorders. WHO's primary care protocols could be adapted and applied in more communities. Similarly, UNICEF and the United Nations Development Program (UNDP) have supported the Expanded Program on Immunization and the supplying of essential vaccines to developing countries, as well as research and development programs aimed at combating tropical diseases. Both organizations could also take an active role in dealing with vaccine-preventable diseases that cause developmental disabilities.

By supporting the Global Burden of Disease Study, the World Bank fostered new insights into the worldwide social and economic impacts of neurological and psychiatric disorders. The World Bank and other development banks could advance this frontier by supporting efforts to better estimate the disease burden in different cultures, and by contributing to the building of infrastructure needed to reduce the burden of brain disorders in developing countries.

Provision of Essential Drugs

The efforts of donors and NGOs are needed to improve the availability of essential medications for neurological and psychiatric disorders in developing countries.[61] The WHO (1998) List of Essential Drugs contains 302 products "that satisfy the health care needs of the majority of the population and should therefore be available at all times in adequate amounts and in appropriate dosage forms." Yet one-third of the world's population, most of whom live in developing countries, does not have access to these drugs.[23,96]

About 90 percent of the essential drugs are off-patent and available at reasonable prices. The availability of these relatively affordable drugs could be increased through a combination of targeted aid programs and systematic improvements in developing countries' purchasing and distribution systems.[143] Every country needs to have in place an effective screening/approval mechanism for new drugs, a cost-effective purchasing mechanism, an efficient distribution system, and local health care providers capable of getting drugs to the people who need them. To this end, model programs and international purchasing cooperatives should be encouraged.[143,144]

Because of patent protections, several highly effective medications for disorders such as depression, schizophrenia, and epilepsy are priced beyond the reach of most people in developing countries. In Nigeria, for example, a public worker's minimum monthly wage will purchase only a 10-day supply of the antipsychotic drug risperidone.[145] Scarcity of foreign exchange and general budgetary restrictions prevent developing countries from purchasing adequate quantities of these drugs. Innovative procurement and partnership strategies designed to ease these problems for certain drugs for which there is no alternative treatment have been developed in cooperation with a number of manufacturers and are currently being tested (see Table 3.1). Others have proposed that developing countries, or an international agency purchasing on their behalf, guarantee the purchase of a certain quantity of a drug at a high price in exchange for giving low-income countries the option of purchasing additional quantities at a substantial discount.

Partnerships with the private sector, particularly pharmaceutical and medical device companies, could further support and sustain programs in developing countries. As socioeconomic development gradually progresses in developing countries, it is likely that the pharmaceutical and medical devices industry will increasingly influence the nature and adequacy of care among these populations. Efforts to initiate constructive working relationships may help promote a sense of responsibility within private industry and secure strong commitments into the future.

TABLE 3-1 Philanthropic drug donation program

Drug Company	Drug and target disease(s)	Public health goal	Program manager	Major partners[A]
Merck	Mectizan: Onchocerciasis, Lymphatic filariasis[B]	Elimination of onchocerciasis (and lymphatic filariasis in Africa)	Mectizan Donation Program, in the Task Force for Child Survival and Development (Carter Center)	Merck, Carter Center, WHO, Africa Programme for Onchocerciasis Control
Pfizer	Zithromax: Trachoma	Elimination of blinding trachoma	International Trachoma Initiative	Pfizer, Edna McConnell Clark Foundation, WHO
SmithKline Beecham	Albendazole: Lymphatic filariasis	Elimination of lymphatic filariasis	WHO	SmithKline Beecham, WHO
GlaxoWellcome	Malarone: Malaria	Control of drug-resistant malaria	Task Force for Child Survival and Development (Carter Center)	GlaxoWellcome, Carter Center, Task Force for Child Survival and Development, WHO-Roll Back Malaria

Source: [146]

[A] In each case, many more partners are involved than are shown on these illustrative lists.
[B] An additional commitment by Merck, Source: ref. 5.

NATIONAL CENTERS FOR TRAINING AND RESEARCH

Many organizations make important individual contributions to strengthening health care in developing countries. However, a coordinated effort is needed to support comprehensive health care systems that address brain disorders.

Centers for such coordinated efforts have been established in a limited number of developing countries.[9] Evidence for the successful development of research and intervention programs resulting from these initiatives indicates that similar centers could be adapted by other countries consistent with their national priorities and resources. The development of similar national centers for training and research is proposed for the provision of a range of services for brain disorders currently under way at existing centers:

- Organization of protocols and procedures for the care of brain disorders in primary, secondary, and tertiary care;
- Initial and continuing training of instructors, who in turn train community health care workers in basic care for brain disorders;
- Operational research to evaluate the effectiveness of treatments and delivery systems;
- Surveillance and monitoring of brain disorders and their risk factors;
- Data collection and analysis to support health planning and policy development at the community, primary care, specialist, and national levels; and
- Demonstration projects for evaluating the quality of care provided for brain disorders and its cost-effectiveness in various settings.

By serving as resources for knowledge regarding effective prevention and intervention strategies, training programs, and research findings, and by disseminating this information locally, nationally, and internationally, national centers would facilitate the exchange of information among medical professionals and policy makers. This process could be further advanced by collaboration between centers in developing countries and their counterparts in developed countries. The focus of the centers would be on the adaptation of effective programs and procedures to national and local settings.

A particularly promising paradigm for research conducted at such centers, known as health systems research (HSR), emphasizes the solving of problems that weaken locally available health care resources—technical, human, and fi-

---

[9] These centers include the National Institute of Mental Health and Neurosciences Department of Psychiatry, Bangalore, India; WHO Collaborating Centre for Mental Health Teheran Institute of Psychiatry, Islamic Republic of Iran; Institute of Mental Health, Beijing Medical College, People's Republic of China; Institute of Psychiatry, Ain Shams University, Cairo, Egypt; WHO Collaborating Centre for Research and Training in Mental Health, Rawalpindi, Pakistan; Program of the Ministry of Health of Mozambique, Africa; WHO Collaborating Centre for Research and Training in Mental Health, Porto Alegre, Brazil; and Center for Mental Health, Ministry of Health and Social Welfare, Mongolia.

nancial. The methodologies of HSR are influenced by existing medical knowledge as well as sociocultural factors and represent an attempt to facilitate communication between health care providers and patients.[93] Thus, one tenet of HSR is the need to understand patient-explanatory models, since simple agreement on a diagnostic label for a patient's condition may be no guarantee of agreement on the condition's etiology or treatment; on the contrary, it may give a false impression of consensus.[93] HSR also emphasizes implementing research programs in representative settings as well as focusing on mitigating the social risk factors for disease, such as poverty. By stressing the use of HSR in the study of neurological and psychiatric disorders in particular, centers for training and research could not only foster greater awareness and provision of services for brain disorders in developing countries, but also lead to the evolution of strategies with international relevance.

A crucial step toward developing a worldwide network of national centers for training and research is to secure initial funding. Given their broad role, these centers should attract funding from a wide variety of sources, including international donor agencies, foundations, NGOs, development banks, industry, and health care advocacy groups. Two initiatives established by WHO in 1997—the Action Program on Mental Health for Underserved Populations [93] and the Global Initiative on Neurology and Public Health [3]—could be key resources. It will be important to ensure, however, that funding for the centers is not diverted from funding for local health services. Strengthening local health care capacity and quality is the fundamental goal. With the commitment of the best specialists, these centers could advance the effort to reduce the total burden of disease in the developing world by championing cost-effective treatment and prevention of long-neglected brain disorders.

CONCLUSION

Integrating care for neurological, psychiatric, and developmental disorders into primary care-based health systems stands as the central challenge in reducing the impact of these disorders in developing countries. Given the existing constraints on resources, building comprehensive health care systems capable of addressing increasingly prevalent brain disorders must proceed gradually in most settings. However, intermediate steps toward this goal appear likely to provide rewards that can encourage further progress. Several programs in developing countries have achieved a successful, if limited, integration of neurological or psychiatric care into primary care services. The successes and limitations of these programs suggest what needs to be done in the future.

International collaborations and partnerships can play an important role by increasing the capacity of developing countries for delivery of neurological and psychiatric care as well as for locally relevant research on brain disorders. Local evaluations of priorities and resources can best guide communities and countries in their choices of appropriate interventions, local staffing, and oversight. Effective primary care programs will require strong support and periodic and continued supervision from providers of secondary and tertiary care, particularly where resources are limited. The balance between primary and higher care levels should be determined by rigorous programmatic evaluation on the basis of cost-effectiveness.

It is crucial that such programs—and indeed all future efforts to reduce the impact of brain disorders—include the capacity for rigorous evaluation. Providing optimal care for these often complex and difficult disorders will necessarily involve an iterative process of testing a program, evaluating it, and redesigning it for improvement. There is no endpoint in this process: demand, delivery, and innovation must be constantly monitored and incorporated to provide the best possible health care to the greatest number of people.

REFERENCES

1. WHO (World Health Organization). Alma-Ata Declaration. *International Conference on Primary Health Care*, 1978.
2. T.B. Üstün and R. Gater. Integrating mental health into primary care. *Current Opinion in Psychiatry* 7:173–180, 1994.
3. M. Isaac, A. Janca, and J.A. Costa e Silva. A review of the World Health Organization's work on primary care psychiatry. *Primary Cae Psychiatry* 1:179–185, 1995.
4. World Health Organization. Organization of mental health services in the health services in the developing countries. Technical Report Series 564. Geneva: WHO, 1975.
5. R. Jenkins. Mental health and primary care-implications for policy. *International Review of Psychiatry* 10:158–160, 1998.
6. R. Giel and T.W. Harding. Psychiatric priorities in developing countries. *British Journal of Psychiatry* 128:513–522, 1976.
7. A. Mehryar and F. Khajavi. Some implications of a community mental health model for developing countries. *The International Journal of Social Psychiatry* Winter-Spring;21(1):45–52, 1974–1975.
8. O. A. Abiodun. Knowledge and attitude concerning mental health of primary health care workers in Nigeria. *International Journal of Social Psychiatry* 37:113–120, 1991.
9. M. Freeman. *Mental health care in crisis in South Africa*. Center for the Study of Health Policy, Johannesburg. Johannesburg: Witwatersrand, 1989.
10. V. G. Ngubane and L. R. Uys. The social support network for black psychiatric inpatients. *Curationis* 17(2):6–9, 1994.
11. D. I. Ben-Tovim. A psychiatric service to the remote area of Botswana. *British Journal of Psychiatry* 142:199–203, 1983.
12. M. Shepherd. Mental health as an integrant of primary medical care. *Journal of the Royal College of General Practitioners* 30:657–664, 1980.
13. B.J. Burns, D.A. Regier, and A.M. Jacobson. Factors relating to the use of mental health services in a neighborhood health center. *Public Health Report* 93(3):232–239, May-Jun 1978.

14. R. Jenkins. Developments in the primary care of mental illness—A forward look. *International Review of Psychiatry* 4:237–242, 1992.
15. J. La Grenade. Integrated primary mental health care. *West Indies Medical Journal* 24 (Supplement 4):31–33, 1998.
16. M. Richeport. Strategies and outcomes of introducing a mental health plan in Brazil. *Social Science and Medicine* 3:261–271, 1984.
17. G. Norquist and S.E. Hyman. Advances in Understanding and Treating Mental Illness: Implications for policy. *Health Affairs* Sep/Oct 18(5):32–47, 1999.
18. M.F. Hogan. Public-Sector Mental Health Care: New Challenges. *Health Affairs* Sept/Oct 18(5):106–111, 1999.
19. T.G. Sriram, C.R. Chandrashekar, M.K. Issac, R. S. Murthy, and V. Shanmugham. Training primary care medical officers in mental health care: An evaluation using a multiple-choice questionnaire. *Acta Psychiatrica Scandinavica* 81:414–417, 1990.
20. A. Mohit. Mental health in the Eastern Mediterranean Region of the World Health Organization with a view to future trends. *Eastern Mediterranean Health Journal* 5(2):231–240, 1999.
21. C.E. Climent, M.V. de Arango, and C.A. Leon. Capacitatión en psiquiatríc de grupos de salud en Colombia [Psychiatric Training of Health Organizations in Columbia] *Educacion médica y salud* 17(1):40–53, 1983.
22. J. de Jong. A comprehensive public mental programme in Guinea-Bissau: A useful model for African, Asian, and Latin American countries. *Psychological Medicine* 26:97–108, 1996.
23. G.P. Kilonzo. The Challenges of Rehabilitation Psychiatry–The Tanzanian Experience. *Medicus* 11(6):14–18, 1992.
24. G. P. Kilonzo and N. Simmons. Development of mental health services in Tanzania: A reappraisal for the future. *Social Science and Medicine* Aug 47(4):419–428, 1998.
25. Sylvia Kaaya, Professor, Department of Psychiatry. Muhimbili University College of Health Science, Personal communication, 2000.
26. IOM. Control of Cardiovascular Disease in Developing Countries. C.P. Howson, K. S. Reddy, T.J. Ryan, and J.R. Bale, eds. National Academy Press, Washington, D.C., 1998.
27. J.G. van Manen, P.J. Bindels, C.J. Ijzermans, J.S. van der Zee, B.J. Bottema, and E. Schade. Prevalence of comorbidity in patients with a chronic airway obstruction and controls over the age of 40. *Journal of Clinical Epidemiology* Mar; 54(3):287–293, 2001.
28. R.B. Lydiard. Social anxiety disorder: Comorbidity and its implications. *Journal of Clinical Psychiatry* 62 Supplement 1:17–23; discussion 24, 2001.
29. M. Berk and H. Plein. Platelet supersensitivity to thrombin stimulation in depression: A possible mechanism for the association with cardiovascular mortality. *Clinical Neuropharmacology* Jul–Aug;23(4):182–185, 2000.
30. V.K. Lim. "Non-infectious" syndromes associated with infectious agents. *Medical Journal of Malaysia* Sep;55(3):389–397, 2000.
31. K.B. Wells, A. Stewart, R.D. Hays, M.A. Burnam, S.W. Rogers, M. Daniels, et al. The functioning and well-being of depressed patients: Results from the Medical Outcomes Study. *Journal of the American Medical Association* 262:914–919, 1989.
32. W. J. Hueston. Personality disorder traits: Prevalence and effects in primary care patients. *International Journal of Psychiatry in Medicine* 29:63–74, 1999.

33. D. Gunnell and T. Frankel. Prevention of suicide: Aspirations and evidence. *British Medical Journal* 308:1227–1233.
34. M. Von Korff, J. Ormel, W. Katon, and E. Lin. Disability and depression among high utilizers of health care: A longitudinal analysis. *Archives of General Psychiatry* 49:91–100, 1997.
35. M. Dhadphale, R.H. Ellison, and L. Griffin. The frequency of psychiatric disorders among patients attending semi-urban and rural general out-patient clinics in Kenya. *British Journal of Psychiatry* 142:379–383, 1983.
36. O. Gureje and B. Obikoya. Somatization in primary care: pattern and correlates in a Nigerian clinic. *Acta Psychiatrica Scandinavica* 86:223–227, 1992.
37. M. Dhadphale and R.H. Ellison. The frequency of mental disorders in the outpatients of two Nyanza hospitals. *Central African Journal of Medicine* 29:29–32, 1983.
38. M.H. Mubbashar, S.I. Malik, J.R. Zar, and N. N.Wig. Community-based mental health care programme report of an experiment in Pakistan Medicine. Region Health Services Journal 1:14–20, 1986.
39. A. Rahman, M. Mubbashar, R. Gater and R. Goldberg. Randomized trial of impact of school mental health programme in rural Rawalpindi, Pakistan. *Lancet* Sept 26;352, 1022–1025, 1998.
40. K. Saeed, R. Gater, M.H. Mubbashar, and N. Maqsood. Mental health, the missing link of primary care. *Hospital das Forcas Armadas* (Brazil), revised 2000.
41. A. Rahman, M. Mubbashar, R. Gater, and D.P. Goldberg. Through the eyes and ears of the community: The impact of a school mental health programme. *Lancet*, 1998.
42. R. S. Murthy. Rural psychiatry in developing countries. *Psychiatric Services* 49(7):967–969, 1998.
43. N. Poungvarin. Stroke in the developing world. *Lancet* 352:19–22, 1998.
44. G. Cohen, N. Sartorius, and T.W. Harding. The WHO collaborative study on strategies for extending mental health care, I: The genesis of the study. *American Journal of Psychiatry* 140:1470–1473, 1983.
45. R. Giel, E. d'Arrigo Busnello, C.E. Climent, A.S.E.D. Elhakim, H.H.A. Ibrahim, L., Ladrigo-Ignacio, et al. The classification of psychiatric disorder: A reliability study in the WHO Collaborative Study on Strategies for Extending Mental Health Care. *Acta Psychiatrica Scandinavica* 63:61–74, 1981.
46. J. Coyne, T. Schwenk, and S. Fechner-Bates. Nondetection of depression by primary care physicians reconsidered. *General Hospital Psychiatry* 17:3–12, 1995.
47. L. Eisenberg. Treating depression and anxiety in primary care: Closing the gap between knowledge and practice. *New England Journal of Medicine* 326:1080–1084, 1992.
48. J. Ormel, W. Van den Brink, M.W. Koeter, R. Giel, K Van Der Meer, G. Van De Willige, et al. Recognition, management and outcome of psychological disorders in primary care: A naturalistic follow-up study. *Psychological Medicine* 20:909–923, 1990.
49. J. Ormel, M. Koeter, W. Van den Brink, and G. Van De Willige, et al.Recognition, management, and course of anxiety and depression in general practice. *Archives of General Psychiatry* 48:700–406, 1991.
50. K. Wells and M. Burnam. Caring for depression in America: Lessons learned from early findings of the medical outcomes study. *Psychiatric Medicine* 9:503–513, 1991.
51. O.A. Abiodun. A study of mental morbidity among primary care patients in Nigeria. *Comprehensive Psychiatry* 34:10–13, 1993.

52. H. Al-Jaddou and A. Malkawi. Prevalence, recognition and management of mental disorders in primary health care in Northern Jordan. *Acta Psychiatrica Scandinavica* 96:31–35, 1997.

53. R. Kempinski. Mental health and primary health care in Tanzania. *Acta Psychaitrica Scandinavica* 83(supplement)364:112–121, 1991.

54. C. Wright, M.K. Nepal, and W.D.A. Bruce-Jones. Mental health patients in primary care services in Nepal. *Asia-Pacific Journal of Public Health* 3:224–230, 1989.

55. F. Schulsinger and A. Jablensky. The national mental health programme in the United Republic of Tanzania: A report from WHO and DANIDA. *Acta Psychiatrica Scandinavica* 83(364):1–132, 1991.

56. WHO (World Heath Organization). Mental health care in developing countries. Report of A WHO Study Group. Technical Report Series 698. Geneva: World Health Organization, 1984.

57. R. Coleman, G. Gill, and D. Wilkinson. Noncommunicable disease management in resource-poor settings: A primary care model from South Africa. *Bulletin of the World Health Organization* 76(6):633–640, 1998.

58. B.S. Singhal. Neurology in developing countries. *Archives of Neurology* 55:1019–1021, 1998.

59. A. Perra and A.M. De L Costello. Efficacy of outreach nutrition rehabilitation centers in reducing mortality and improving nutritional outcome of severely malnourished children in Guinea-Bissau. *European Journal of Clinical Nutrition* 49:353–359, 1995.

60. E. Lin, W. Katon, M. von Korff, J. Russo, and G. Simon. Relapse of depression in primary care: Rate and clinical predictors. *Archives of Family Medicine* 7:443–449, 1998.

61. D.P. Goldberg and P. Huxley. *Common mental disorders—A biosocial model.* London: Routledge and Kegan Paul, 1980, 1992.

62. D.C. Bergen. Preventable neurological diseases worldwide. *Neuroepidemiology* 17:67–73, 1998.

63. M. Gourie-Devi, P. Satishchandra, and G. Gururaj. National workshop on public health aspects of epilepsy. *Annals of the Indian Academy of Neurology* 2:43–48, 1999.

64. B. Saraceno, R.A. Briceno, F. Asioli, A. Liberati, and G. Tognoni. Cooperation in mental health: An Italian project in Nicaragua. *Social Science and Medicine* 31(9):1067–1071, 1990.

65. N. E. Sokhela. The Integration of Comprehensive Health Care into the Primary Health System: Diagnosis and Treatment. *Journal of Advanced Nursing,* 1999.

66. M. Lansang and R. Olveda. Institutional linkages: Strategic bridges for research capacity strengthening. *Acta Tropica* 57 (1994): 139–145, 1994.

67. B. Saraceno, E. Terzian, F.M. Barquero, and G. Tognoni. Mental health care in the primary health care setting: A collaborative study in six countries of Central America. *Health Policy and Planning* 10(2):133–143, June, 1995.

68. R. Alarcon and S. Aguilar-Gaxiola. Mental health policy developments in Latin America. *Bulletin of the World Health Organization* 78:483–490, 2000.

69. O. Gureje and A. Alem. Mental health policy development in Africa. *Bulletin of the World Health Organization* 78:475–482, 2000.

70. G.P. Mathur, S. Mathur, Y. D. Singh, K. P. Kushwara, and S. N. Lee. Detection and prevention of childhood disability with the help of Anganwadi workers. *Indian Pediatrics* 32:773–777, 1995.

71. R. Corney. The effectiveness of counseling in general practice. *International Review of Psychiatry* 4:331–338, 1992.
72. S. Acland. Nepal: Mental health program. In: A. Cohen, A. Kleinman, and B. Sarceno, eds. World Mental Health Casebook. New York: Plenum Press, In press.
73. K. Meursing and V.B. Wankiiri. Use of flow-charts by nurses dealing with mental patients: An evaluation in Lesotho. *Bulletin of the World Health Organization* 66:507–514, 1988.
74. R. Serpell, L. Margia, and K. Harvey. Mental retardation in African countries: Conceptualization services and research. *International Review of Research in Mental Retardation* 19:1–40, 1993.
75. Z. Stein, M. Durkin, L. Davidson et al. Guidelines for identifying children with mental retardation in community settings. In: Assessment of people with mental retardation. Geneva: World Health Organization, 1992.
76. B. S. Schoenberg. Clincial neuroepidemiology in developing countries. Neurology with few neurologists. *Neuroepidemiology* 1:137–142, 1982.
77. B. O. Osuntokun, A. O. G. Adeuja, B. S. Schoenberg, O. Bademosi, V. A. Nottidge, A. O. Olumide et al. Neurological disorders in Nigerian Africans: A community-based study. *Acta Neurologica Scandinavica* 75:13–21, 1987.
78. M. E. Cruz, B. S. Schoenberg, J. Ruales et al. Pilot study to detect neurologic disease in Ecuador among a population with high prevalence of endemic goiter. *Neuroepidemiology* 4:108, 1985.
79. N. Poungvarin, A. Viriyavejakul, and C. Komontri. Siriraj stroke score and validation study to distinguish supratentorial intracerebral hemorrhage from infarction. *British Medical Journal* 302:1565–1567, 1983.
80. L. Ladrigo-Ignacio, C.E. Climent, M.V. de Arango, and J. Baltazar. Research screening instruments as tools in training health workers for mental health care. *Tropical and Geographical Medicine* 35:1–7, 1983.
81. R.S. Murthy and N.N. Wig. The WHO collaborative study on strategies for extending mental health care, IV: A training approach to enhancing the availability of mental health manpower in a developing country. *American Journal of Psychiatry* 140:1486–1490, 1983.
82. D.I. Ben-Tovim. *Development psychiatry: Mental health and primary health care in Botswana.* London: Tavistock Publications, 1987.
83. V.B. Wankiiri. Training of community mental health nurses in Botswana. *World Health Forum* 15(3):260–261, 1994.
84. T. A. Badger, J. M. Cardea, I. J. Biocca, and M. H. Mishel. Assessment and management of depression: An imperative for community-based practice. *Archives of Psychiatric Nursing* 4:235–241, 1990.
85. A. Janca, L. Prilipko, and J.A. Costa e Silva. The World Health Organization's work on public health aspects of neurology. *Journal of Neurology, Neurosurgery, and Psychiatry* 62(Supplement 1) 6–7, 1997a.
86. A. Janca, L. Prilipko, and J. A. Costa e Silva. The World Health Organization's global initiative on neurology and public health. *Journal of the Neurological Sciences* 145: 1–2, 1997b.
87. J. A. Aarli. Ncurology and public health: Strategy and perspectives. *Journal of the Neurological Sciences* 145:3–4, 1997.

88. B.H. Price, R. D. Adams, and J. T. Coyle. Neurology and psychiatry: Closing the great divide. *Neurology* 54:8–14, 2000.

89. V. Patel, E. Simunyu, and F. Gwanzura. The pathways to primary mental health care in high density suburbs of Harare, Zimbabwe. *Social Psychiatry and Psychiatric Epidemiology* 32:97–103, 1997.

90. D. Chisholm, K. Sekar, K.K. Kumar, K. Saeed, S. James, M. Mubbashar, et al. Integration of mental health care into primary care. Demonstration cost-outcomes in India and Pakistan. *British Journal of Psychiatry* Jun;176:581–588, 2000.

91. V. Patel and R. Thara, eds., *Meeting the Mental Health Needs of Developing Countries: NGO Innovations in India*. India: Sage, In press.

92. D. Chisholm, M. R. J. Knapp, H. C. Knudsen, F. Amaddeo, L. Gaite, and B. van Wijngaarden. The Client Socio-Demographic and Service Receipt Inventory: Development of an instrument for international research. EPSILON study 5. *British Journal of Psychiatry*, 177(39), 2000.

93. V. Patel. Health Systems Research: A pragmatic model for meeting mental needs in low-income countries. In: G. Andrews and S. Henderson, eds., *Unmet Need in Psychiatry*. Cambridge, U.K.: Cambridge University Press, 2000.

94. ILO, UNESCO, and WHO. *Community Based Rehabilitation for and with people with Disabilities*. Joint Position Paper p 4E., 1994.

95. E. Helander, P. Mendis, and G. Nelson. *Training Disabled People in the Community*. WHO: Geneva, 1983.

96. T.A. Lambo. The village of ARO. *Lancet* 2:513–514, 1964.

97. R. Lambo. *Treating the long-term mentally ill: Beyond deinstitutionalization*. London: Jossey-Bass, 1982.

98. A. Nicoll. Current issues in tropical pediatric infectious diseases. *Transactions of the Royal Society of Tropical Medicine and Hygiene* 94:9–11, 2000.

99. A. E. Shearley. The societal value of vaccinations in developing countries. *Vaccine* 17:S109–112, 1999.

100. C.M. Winston and V. Patel. Use of traditional and orthodox medicine in urban Zimbabwe. *International Journal of Epidemiology* 24:1006–1012, 1995.

101. K. Nasseri, B. Sadrizadeh, H. Malik-Afzali, K. Mohammad, M. Chasma, M. T. Cheraghchi-Bashi et. al. Primary health care and immunization in Iran. *Public Health* 105:229–238, 1991.

102. C.M. Winston, V. Patel, T. Musonza, and Z. Nyathi. A community survey of traditional care providers in Harare. *Central African Journal of Medicine* Sep;41(9):278–283, 1995.

103. A.M. Kleinman and J. L. Gale. Patients treated by physicians and folk healers: A comparative outcome study in Taiwan. *Culture, Medicine and Psychiatry* 6(4):405–420, 1982.

104. M. Tausig and S. Subedi. The modern mental health system in Nepal: Organizational persistence in the absence of legitimizing myths. *Social Science and Medicine* 45(3):441–447, 1997.

105. O. Gureje, R. A. Acha, and O. A. Odejide. Pathways to psychiatric care in Ibadan, Nigeria. *Tropical and Geographical Medicine* 47: 125–129, 1995.

106. J.R. Dale and D.I. Ben-Tovim. Modern or traditional? A study of treatment preference for neuropsychiatric disorders in Botswana. *British Journal of Psychiatry* Aug;187–192, 1984.

107. S.X. Li and M.R. Phillips. Witch doctors and mental illness in mainland China: A preliminary study. *American Journal of Psychiatry* Feb;147(2):221–224, 1990.

108. R. Gater, B. de Almeida e Sousa, G. Barrientos, J. Caraveo, C. R. Chandrashekar, et. al. The pathways to psychiatric care: A cross-cultural study. *Psychological Medicine* 21:761–764, 1991.

109. E. Ovuga, J. Boardman, and E. Oluka. Traditional healers and mental illness in Uganda. *Psychiatric Bulletin* 23:276–279, 1999.

110. W.G. Jilek. *Salish Indian Mental Health and Culture Change: Psychohygienic and Therapeutic Aspects of the Guardian Spirit Ceremonial.* Toronto: Holt, Reinhart & Winston, 1974.

111. V. Crapanzano. *Tuhami, Portrait of a Moroccan.* Chicago: University of Chicago Press, 1980.

112. K. Finkler. *Spiritualist Healers in Mexico.* New York: Praeger, 1985.

113. Health Ministry of Malaysia. *Straits Times.* Kuala Lumpur, Malaysia, Nov. 14, 2000.

114. G. Bodeker. Lessons on integration from the developing world's experience. *British Medical Journal* 322:164–167, 2001.

115. W. Jilek and L. Jilek-Aall. Traditional medicine and mental health care. *Arctic Medical Research* Supplement;303–308, 1991.

116. A. Kleinman. *Patients and Healers in the Context of Culture.* Berkeley: University of California Press, 1980.

117. World Health Organization. *The education of mid-level rehabilitation worker, recommendations from country experiences.* Geneva:World Health Organization, 1992.

118. V. Patel. Recognizing common mental disorders in primary care in Africa: Should we drop "mental" altogether? *Lancet* 347:742–744, 1996.

119. C.J. Murray and A.D. Lopez. *The Global Burden of Disease.* Boston: Harvard School of Public Health, 1996.

120. D. Chisholm. Challenges for the international application of mental health economics. *Epidemiologia e Psychiatria Sociale* 8:1, 1999.

121. M. F. Drummond, B. O'Brien, G. L. Stoddart, and G. W. Torrance. *Methods for the Economic Evaluation of Health Care Programmes.* Oxford: Oxford Medical Publication 2nd edition, 1997.

122. M. R. Gold, J. E. Siegel, L. B. Russell, and M. C. Weinstein. *Cost-effectiveness in Health and Medicine.* Oxford: Oxford University Press, 1996.

123. W. Gulbinat, R. Manderscheid, A. Beigel, and J. A. Costa e Silva. A multinational strategy on mental health policy and care. A WHO collaborative initiative and consultative program. In: M. Moscarelli, A. Rupp, and N. Sartorius, eds. *Handbook of Mental Health Economics and Health Policy.* Volume 1, Schizophrenia. Chichester: John Wiley & Sons, 1996.

124. The Special Programme for Research Training in Tropical Diseases, (http://www.who.int/tdr/). Geneva: World Health Organization, 2000.

125. J.F. Kengaya-Kayondo. Transdisciplinary research: Research capacity building in developing countries at low cost. *Acta Tropica* 57:147–152, 1994.

126. Arthur Kleinman, Maude and Lillian Presley Professor of Medical Anthropology and Psychiatry, Harvard Medical School, personal communication, 2000.

127. S.A. Okuonzi and J. Macrae. Whose policy is it anyway? International and national influences on health policy development in Uganda. *Health Policy and Planning* Jun;10(2):122–132, 1995.

128. M.I. Good. Factors affecting patient dropout rates. *American Journal of Psychiatry* Feb;149(2):275–276, 1992.
129. R. Maclure. Primary health care and donor dependency: A case study of nongovernment assistance in Burkina Faso. *International Journal of Health Services* 25(3):539–558, 1995.
130. T.J. Partanen, C. Hogstedt, R. Ahasan, A. Aragon, M.E. Arroyave, J. Jeyaratnam, et al. Collaboration between developing and developed countries and between developing countries in occupational health research and surveillance. *Scandinavian Journal of Work, Environment and Health* Jun;25(3):296–300, 1999.
131. R.H. Morrow and M. A. Lansang. The role of clinical epidemiology in establishing essential national health research capabilities in developing countries. *Infectious Disease Clinics of North Am*erica Jun;5(2):235–246, 1991.
132. S. A. Al-Shammari, T. A. Khoja, and S. A. Rajeh. Role of primary care physicians in the care of epileptic patients. *Public Health* 110:47–48, 1996.
133. J.James. Community involvement towards community objectives. *Soz Praventivemed* 37(5):218–222, 1992.
134. S.B. Macfarlane, T.G. Evans, F.M. Muli-Musiime, O.L. Prawl, and A.D. So. Global health research and INCLEN. International Clinical Epidemiology Network. *Lancet* Feb 6;353(9151):503, 1999.
135. S.R. Mazta and S.K. Ahelluwalia. Literacy campaign and health education go hand in hand. *World Health Forum* 16(2):184–185, 1995.
136. C.A. Leon. Outlook of community mental health in Latin America. *Boletin de la Oficina Sanitaria Panamericana* Aug;81(2):122–138, 1976.
137. R. Kessler. The effects of stressful life events on depression. *Annual Review of Psychology* 48:191–214, 1997.
138. S. Weich. Prevention of the common mental disorders: A public health perspective. *Psychological Medicine* 27:757–764, 1997.
139. P. J. Mrazek and R. J. Haggerty, eds. *Reducing Risks for Mental Disorders*. Washington, D.C.: National Academy Press, 1994.
140. T. Lorenzo. The identification of continuing education needs for community rehabilitation workers in a rural health district in the Republic of South Africa. *International Journal of Rehabilitation* Research 17:241–250, 1994.
141. W. Xiong, M.R. Phillips, R. Wang, Q. Dai, J. Kleinman, and A. Kleinman. Family-based intervention for schizophrenic patients in China: A randomized controlled trial. *British Journal of Psychiatry* 165:239–247, 1994.
142. Nations for Mental Health. (http://www.who.int/msa/nam1.htm). Geneva: World Health Organization, 2000.
143. M.R. Reich. The global drug gap. *Science* Mar 17;287(5460):1979–1981, 2000.
144. WHO. *The Use of Essential Drugs, (Tenth Model List of Essential Drugs)*. WHO Technical Report Series No. 882, Eighth Report of the WHO Expert Committee. Geneva: WHO, 1998.
145. T.G. Suleiman, J.U. Ohaeri, R.A. Lawal, A.Y. Haruna, and O.B. Orija. Financial cost of treating out-patients with schizophrenia in Nigeria. *British Journal of Psychiatry* Oct;171:364–368, 1997.
146. M. R. Reich. Public-private partnerships for public health. *Nature Medicine* Jun 6(6): 617–620, 2000.

Strategies For Addressing Brain Disorders

To reduce the disease burden now:

- Increase public and professional awareness and understanding of brain disorders in developing countries, and intervene to reduce stigma and ease the burden of discrimination often associated with these disorders.

- Extend and strengthen existing systems of primary care to deliver health services for brain disorders. Secondary and tertiary centers should train and oversee primary care staff, provide referral capacity, and provide ongoing supervision and support for primary care systems in developing countries.

- Make cost-effective interventions for brain disorders available to patients who will benefit. Financial and institutional constraints require selectivity and sequencing in setting goals and priorities. The continued implementation of these interventions should also be informed by ongoing research to reveal the applicability and sustainability of such programs.

To create options for the future:

- Conduct operational research to assess the cost-effectiveness of specific treatments and health services in local settings, along with epidemiological research to monitor the incidence, prevalence, and disease burden of brain disorders in developing countries.

- Create national centers for training and research on brain disorders in developing countries. Link these centers with institutions in high-income countries through multicenter research projects, staff exchanges and training, and Internet communication.

- Create a program to facilitate competitive funding for research and for the development of new or enhanced institutions devoted to brain disorders in developing countries. This effort should be global, and spearheaded by the Global Forum for Health Research, the World Health Organization, and well-funded research centers, such as the U.S. National Institutes of Health and the Centers for Disease Control and Prevention. To ensure the sustainability of the program, major donors—such as the World Bank, foundations, and governmental and nongovernmental aid organizations—must commit initial investments to this effort, and longer-term annual budgets must be established.

4

Findings and Future Strategies

The high economic and social costs of ignoring neurological, psychiatric, and developmental disorders include lost work time, reduced productivity, and the increased cost and difficulty of treating conditions that have become more debilitating. While these outcomes have their profound effects on patients and their families, they also impede economic development to an extent that warrants the attention of national and international policy makers. Their leadership is crucial to the identification of affordable solutions for addressing brain disorders and to the enlistment of health care professionals in implementing such strategies.

Brain disorders—neurological, psychiatric, and developmental—account for a significant proportion of the global burden of disease (see Chapter 2). Growing recognition of the prevalence of brain disorders, as well as the availability of cost-effective treatments, may now lead to the adoption of measures designed to achieve significant reductions in the disease burden due to these disorders. This is true even where resources for health care are limited. The strategies proposed in this chapter highlight the actions needed to achieve this goal and describe the additional analyses required for implementation and research.

Though brain disorders have been largely neglected by health planners and practitioners throughout the developing world, a limited number of innovative programs have been implemented in countries and communities with varying levels of resources. In most cases, these programs have not been extensively evaluated for cost-effectiveness or long-term sustainability. However, a review of the existing evidence permits examination of these programs as preliminary models for the development of other programs and future planning (components of these programs are described in Chapter 3 and throughout Chapters 5 through 10).

A review of programs in several countries reveals that there are effective interventions for brain disorders. However, the existence of a successful intervention in one setting does not ensure its programmatic success in other, even similar, settings. It is clear that the design and implementation of such programs should be tailored to each country's needs and resources. Successful programs will meet the neurological and psychiatric health needs of at-risk groups within both resource constraints and the local cultural context, and will reflect consideration of a country's or community's capacity to implement and sustain the interventions.

Building on the evidence of a limited range of programs, this report proposes strategies for operational research in conjunction with the provision of care. Both therapies and health care delivery systems should be assessed and guided by an iterative process developed to improve clinical care in the local setting while maintaining its affordability. The six general strategies described in this chapter represent key steps toward reducing the burden of brain disorders in the developing world. They were developed by the committee based on a review of current literature, workshop deliberations, and background papers that provided the evidence for the discussion in Chapters 2 and 3. The first three actions can be undertaken now; the last three provide for the creation of better options in the future. Recommendations that address specific brain disorders are presented in Part II of the report and should be viewed in the context of the strategies presented here.

REDUCING THE DISEASE BURDEN NOW

Increasing Awareness

Despite the existence of low-cost preventive and treatment interventions for many neurological and psychiatric disorders, the human, economic, and social burdens associated with these conditions remain high and are increasing in developing countries. In many cases the public and even the health community are unaware that effective treatments are available for certain disorders.

Individuals with brain disorders and their families are subjected to stigmatization and discrimination generated by ignorance, misconceptions, and misplaced beliefs about certain of these disorders (see Chapter 2). In addition to care for those afflicted, community education is needed to counter these misperceptions and false beliefs. The knowledge that effective treatments are available is, in itself, an important tool for reducing the stigma. Awareness programs aimed at reducing stigmatization by disseminating information about available treatments have the added effect of stimulating health care-seeking behavior at earlier, more manageable stages of disease.

Educational programs should be tailored to the needs of local communities. Local thinking can be changed by educational messages delivered in written materials, oral presentations in schools and workplaces, movies with clear messages, street theater depictions, and religious forums. In several developing countries, advocacy groups, educators, religious leaders, and traditional healers have been effective in delivering this information (see Chapter 3).

Governments should facilitate and advance efforts aimed at increasing public awareness and understanding of brain disorders and, in the absence of community and advocacy groups, provide such messages. These efforts can be reinforced by laws that protect people with brain disorders from abusive practices, provide access to health care, and prevent discrimination in education, employment, housing, and other opportunities.

> **Strategy 1. Increase public and professional awareness and understanding of brain disorders in developing countries, and intervene to reduce stigma and ease the burden of discrimination often associated with these disorders.**

Utilizing Existing Health Systems

Modest investments in and reorientation of existing systems of health care could make it possible to provide and monitor needed treatments for brain disorders and thus substantially reduce the associated disease burden. Integration of care for brain disorders into the primary health care system should occur as part of a national policy to provide comprehensive health care (see Chapter 3). Even in the absence of national policies, however, provision of neurological and psychiatric care should be encouraged, since dedicated professionals can effect important changes despite a limited set of interventions.

Most countries have established specific disease-control initiatives and primary care infrastructures for infectious diseases and maternal and child health. Care for brain disorders should be incorporated into these existing programs. Additional resources will be required to train primary care staff in the prevention, diagnosis, treatment, and rehabilitation of brain disorders, and to provide diagnostic tools and essential treatments. Cooperative funding for this additional care should involve national and local governments, international nongovernmental organizations (NGO), and development agencies. Local support and participation should be sought from private physicians, nurses, social workers, traditional healers, and teachers. The basic components of comprehensive primary care for brain disorders include prevention, interventions, and community-based rehabilitation.

Prevention should focus on reducing risk factors for these disorders in patients who are or could be at risk. Examples include perinatal and other injury to the brain, which can lead to developmental disabilities and epilepsy; vaccination and other measures to prevent infectious causes of developmental disability and epilepsy; and healthy diets and active lifestyles to protect against stroke.

Interventions should include diagnosis and treatment of brain disorders. Where routine care is provided by trained community health workers, physicians or specialist nurses at secondary centers should support primary care with regular shared consultations, supervision, and continuing training of community health workers. A reliable supply of appropriate medications should be maintained at the primary care center. Primary care providers must understand drug indications, dosages, outcomes, and side effects, and be able to monitor drug levels in the blood. They must also be trained to handle problems of compliance associated with long-term or lifetime use of medication.

Community-based rehabilitation supports families in the appropriate care of patients to minimize further disability and encourage optimal development so that patients can resume lives that are as normal as possible. The role of primary health services is generally to provide guidance, knowledge, and encouragement to programs that are developed and maintained by the community.

Since the diagnosis and treatment of some brain disorders demand specialized skills and facilities, primary care centers must have a direct link to a district hospital or other secondary facility for guidance and referral. While secondary and tertiary facilities are key to the provision of appropriate care, such facilities may prove too expensive for efforts aimed at expanding cost-effective routine case management. Routine care can be provided in primary care centers, overseen by skilled staff from higher-level centers. Oversight might involve monthly visits from a neuropsychiatric nurse or specialist, or less frequent visits supplemented by regular telephone review of cases. Urgent and severe cases would be referred to the district hospital for diagnosis and treatment, and then returned to the community primary care setting for maintenance therapies.

The level of government investment in specialized care should be determined according to local priorities and resource availability, aided by the findings of operational research on cost-effectiveness. In general, the activities of a well-supported primary care facility (prevention, early recognition of potential cases, and routine case management) deserve high priority.

> **Strategy 2. Extend and strengthen existing systems of primary care to deliver health services for brain disorders. Secondary and tertiary centers should train and oversee primary care staff, provide referral capacity, and provide ongoing supervision and support for primary care systems in developing countries.**

Expanding Use of Cost-Effective Interventions

Perhaps the single most encouraging finding of this report is that highly cost-effective interventions exist that can be used to address the enormous disease burden due to brain disorders. As noted, however, the public and even health professionals are often unaware of effective treatments for these disorders, and few such interventions have been adapted for use in developing countries or communities. Evidence presented in Chapters 5–10 on specific disorders reveals a range of effective, low-cost interventions (see Table 4-1).

To the extent possible, treatment programs for brain disorders should follow best-practice guidelines. Where this is not possible because of capacity and resource limitations, however, implementation of component practices is likely to be cost-effective relative to inaction. Initial demonstration projects that encompass these interventions should include evaluation of their cost and effectiveness in various geographic and resource settings to determine long-term implementation guidelines.

Inadequate supplies of low-cost, widely available medications continue to handicap many developing countries. One-third of the world's population does not have access to medications that appear on the World Health Organization's (WHO) List of Essential Drugs (which includes treatments for brain disorders). About 90 percent of the essential drugs are off-patent and available at reasonable prices. The availability of these relatively affordable drugs could be increased through a combination of targeted aid programs and systematic improvements in the purchasing and distribution systems of developing countries. Every country needs to have in place an effective screening/approval mechanism for new drugs, a cost-effective purchasing mechanism, and an efficient distribution system, with local health care providers being able to get the drugs to the people who need them the most. To this end, model programs and international purchasing cooperatives should be encouraged.

Education and rehabilitation strategies are likely to be most cost-effective when linked to existing public and/or private programs with similar objectives. This is especially true for strategies that seek to enable people with brain disorders to attend regular schools or training programs and obtain employment.

Strategy 3. Make cost-effective interventions for brain disorders available to patients who will benefit. Financial and institutional constraints require selectivity and sequencing in setting goals and priorities. The continued implementation of these interventions should also be informed by ongoing research to reveal the applicability and sustainability of such programs.

TABLE 4-1 Cost-Effective Interventions for Management of Brain Disorders*

Condition(s)	Primary and secondary prevention goals	Treatment and management modalities
Developmental Disabilities	• Provision of folic acid and iodine supplements to women of child bearing age • Expansion of vaccination programs and other proven methods of infectious disease control	• Early detection and treatment of infections that threaten the nervous system • Implementation of prenatal, newborn, and developmental screenings
Epilepsy	• Public education to destigmatize the disorder and to create awareness of available treatments • Prevention and treatment of cystircercosis • Reduce incidence of head injury, brain infection, and parasitosis	• Phenobarbital and phenytoin • Low-cost carbamazepine and valproate
Schizophrenia	• Public education to destigmatize the disorder • Suicide prevention • Relapse prevention	• Low-cost antipsychotic drugs, such as chlorpromazine and haloperidol • Community rehabilitation programs for patients to improve social and occupational skills • Psychosocial interventions to reintegrate patients into family and community life
Major Depression	• Public education to destigmatize the disorder and to create awareness of available treatments • Early identification and counseling of high-risk individuals • Suicide prevention • Relapse prevention	• Tricyclic antidepressants and, where available, low-cost SSRIs • Adjunctive problem-solving and interpersonal psychotherapy
Bipolar Disorder	• Early identification and counseling against substance abuse among high-risk individuals • Relapse prevention	• Long-term treatment with lithium, carbamazepine, valproate, or other agents • Adjunctive psychosocial treatments
Stroke (Cerebrovascular Disorders)	• Use of public health and education strategies for lowering stroke-related risk factors (e.g., hypertension, smoking, diet, and exercise)	• Control of hypertension with low-dose thiazide, beta-blockers, and low-cost statins and ACE inhibitors • Sulphonylureas with metformin if needed for diabetes

* Supporting evidence for these recommended interventions is derived from research in both developed and developing countries. Specific discussion of the evidence base for each of these interventions appears in Part II of the report.

CREATING OPTIONS FOR THE FUTURE

Applied Research

Because of limited knowledge and experience in the delivery of care and interventions for brain disorders in developing countries, the integration of neurological and psychiatric care into health systems must be accompanied by rigorous evaluation. Both health care delivery systems and therapies should be tested and compared for cost-effectiveness in a variety of settings and refined on an ongoing basis. Planning, implementing, and evaluating interventions for the prevention, treatment, and rehabilitation of brain disorders will require a range of local and national research programs:

- Controlled trials to evaluate specific therapies, training programs, and models of care delivery;
- Surveillance of the incidence and burden of specific brain disorders;
- Monitoring of risk factors and the effects of interventions designed to reduce them; and
- Identification of and strategies to overcome nonfinancial barriers to implementation (e.g., inadequate training or misbeliefs about disease origins).

In the interest of cost-effectiveness, surveillance may be restricted to obtaining data that can be used to improve the effectiveness of local and national care for brain disorders. Such data collection would address local environmental and genetic risk factors, the cost and effectiveness of treatment and rehabilitation interventions, the overall burden of brain disorders, and the gap between health needs and the services provided.

Providing cost-effective neurological and psychiatric care that is judged to be at the level of "best practice" is a long-term goal. This goal may be best accomplished through an iterative process of evaluation and improvement directed by secondary or tertiary centers and at the national level. Involving nonhealth sectors—particularly education, industry, and environment—in the development of intervention and research programs can help advance progress toward this goal.

Strategy 4. Conduct operational research to assess the cost-effectiveness of specific treatments and health services in local settings, along with epidemiological research to monitor the incidence, prevalence, and disease burden of brain disorders in developing countries.

Capacity Strengthening

Addressing needs for the care of brain disorders should be viewed as an essential component of a comprehensive agenda for public health interventions, research, and policy. To develop the leadership, training, and operational research required to accomplish the first four strategies, the creation of national centers for training and research on brain disorders should be initiated. Staff members of these centers would be trained in all aspects of the care of brain disorders. They would serve as the trainers of staff at primary and secondary care centers, and as one level of support for primary care staff. Where existing centers already address infectious disease, maternal and child health, or other health problems, specific issues for brain disorders should be integrated into their initiatives.

The specific projects undertaken at national centers would be expected to vary, depending on the needs, priorities, and resources of their host countries, but would probably include the following basic functions:

- Developing national priorities and strategies for integrating the care of brain disorders into existing health systems;
- Establishing locally relevant treatment and training guidelines for primary and higher-level care;
- Training medical professionals who supervise community-level care and who train community-level care providers;
- Supporting primary care centers by providing referral care, clinical guidelines, and regular clinical consultation for brain disorders;
- Conducting operational research on brain disorders—including demonstration projects with strong evaluative components—to inform the ongoing improvement of health planning and the delivery of care;
- Conducting surveillance to support health planning and policy development by national and local governments;
- Preparing and disseminating educational materials about brain disorders to health ministries, medical schools, community public health programs, physicians, primary care workers, traditional healers, schools, and workplaces;
- Building networks to enable researchers and health care professionals to exchange information via the Internet;
- Conducting operational research to evaluate the cost-effectiveness of available therapies and delivery systems;
- Sponsoring methodological development, epidemiological surveillance, and other locally relevant research concerning the risk factors for brain disorders as well as research on cost-effective models of care management;
- Contributing to the creation of medical and nursing curricula that are sensitive to local health priorities and cultural practices regarding health care and health-seeking behavior; and
- Collaborating with nongovernmental and community organizations that provide or promote health services for brain disorders.

Strategic collaborations should be developed between centers in industrialized and developing countries. Centers should also be linked to international efforts, such as the Nations for Mental Health Initiative (sponsored by WHO, the World Bank, and Harvard Medical School) and INCLEN (the International

Clinical Epidemiology Network). Models for national centers with strong international cooperation include the Research Institute for Tropical Medicine in the Philippines, the Triangle Program at the University of Peradeniya in Sri Lanka, and the Ministry of Health in Uganda (see Chapter 3). Collaborative research with institutions in industrialized countries would provide an opportunity for complementary research activities that would utilize the advantages of each center while eliminating the misuse of limited resources for redundant efforts.

The focus of a national center should be on training staff who provide support for primary care workers and conducting operational research on the delivery of cost-effective care for brain disorders in primary care centers. The national centers would also support secondary care centers in their capacity of overseeing primary care centers. Care would be necessary to avoid using limited resources for tertiary care or for expensive or sophisticated therapies that are unlikely to be cost-effective by serving the needs of most patients.

Building on recent international commitments to increase access to the Internet and other digital technology, a centralized site should be established to serve as a repository of information on brain disorders. This gateway site should enlist the participation of professionals, public health organizations, and advocates throughout the world. It could include recent research findings, standardized versions of diagnostic and assessment tools, treatment and program guidelines for common disorders and different settings, evaluations of interventions for cost-effectiveness, and access to distance learning training packages. Additionally, the site could facilitate communication among health care providers, researchers, and policy makers at national centers and in the communities they serve.

To encourage the training of medical specialists and researchers in the care of brain disorders and to strengthen local capacity in developing countries, the U.S. National Institutes of Health, Fogarty Center for International Training and Research Program, and similar programs at other research institutions should be established to provide training and initial research support. Under such programs, researchers, clinicians, and other health professionals from developing and developed countries could receive training in epidemiology, biostatistics, clinical trials, genetics, ethics, health policy, health communication, and culturally informed management. Long-term research and training collaborations with mentors in the United States and other countries could be established. To ensure that research and training agendas focus on important local issues, the experience of these investigators should be directly linked to—and, when possible, conducted in—the national centers for training and research. Long-term funding commitments will be necessary for these programs to build sustainable and high-quality levels of scientific expertise. Such centers can provide the knowledge needed to develop local policies, health care programs, and ongoing clinical and community studies.

Based on the findings presented in this report, opportunities for such collaborative research on brain disorders in developing countries might include the following:

- Evaluation of low-cost rehabilitation programs for mental retardation, disability after stroke, and long-term mental illness;
- Support for clinical trials of new drugs that offer promise for patients in developing countries;
- Research and clinical studies aimed at better understanding genetic risk factors for certain disorders, as well as the role of gene-environment interactions;
- Development of long-term follow-up cohort studies of the natural history of psychoses, prevention of stroke, prevention of developmental disabilities, and therapies for epilepsy; and
- Health systems research on pilot programs providing health care services, their sustainability over time, and their cost-effectiveness in different settings.

Strategy 5. Create national centers for training and research on brain disorders in developing countries. Link these centers with institutions in high-income countries through multicenter research projects, staff exchanges and training, and Internet communication.

The Role of International Aid

Integrating care for brain disorders and related operational research into existing health systems in developing countries will require broad international support and multiple funding sources. The sponsors of this report—the Global Forum for Health Research, the U.S. National Institutes of Health, and the U.S. Centers for Disease Control and Prevention—should spearhead this effort, along with research centers in other developed countries. Partnerships between institutions in developed and developing countries will be needed to establish health care services and support their development.

Substantial and long-term funding will be essential to develop a worldwide network of national centers for training and research and to enable significant participation by researchers in developing countries. A priority for international aid efforts directed at brain disorders should be the creation of a mechanism for competitive funding of research, training, and institutional development. To create the basis for a sustainable program, initial investments must be committed by major donors to this international effort, and longer-term annual budgets must be established.

This support should be tailored to specific country needs and capabilities. In-country analysis, coupled with timely, ongoing feedback and the flexibility to change programs as indicated, will be important in determining overall program targets, modifying implementation elements, and keeping programs efficient and effective. Support should also be maintained for a sufficient and plausible period of time to show success in achieving program goals within the framework of the host country's development plan. The availability of short-term, goal-oriented, program-specific external funding should not be the primary factor driving the development of intervention programs.

A broad spectrum of organizations should be enlisted for technical and financial support for this worldwide effort to provide comprehensive health care for brain disorders:

- National health and finance ministries;
- National agencies for international development (such as the U.S. Agency for International Development, Canadian International Development Agency, and Swedish Economic Development Agency);
- Foundations (such as the Wellcome Trust, Gates Foundation, Open Society Foundation, and Rockefeller Foundation);
- Nongovernmental organizations;
- Research and medical universities;
- Multilateral development banks;
- Industry;
- Professional societies;
- Advocacy groups; and
- Consumer and patient groups.

Strategy 6. Create a program to facilitate competitive funding for research and for the development of new or enhanced institutions devoted to brain disorders in developing countries. This effort should be global, and spearheaded by the Global Forum for Health Research, the World Health Organization, and well-funded research centers, such as the U.S. National Institutes of Health and the Centers for Disease Control and Prevention. To ensure the sustainability of the program, major donors—such as the World Bank, foundations, and governmental and nongovernmental aid organizations—must commit initial investments to this effort, and longer-term annual budgets must be established.

CONCLUSION

With effective, affordable treatments available, current health care services can be extended to encompass neurological, psychiatric, and developmental disorders. For the most part, these treatments have been used infrequently, leaving millions of people to endure unnecessary hardship and impaired productivity. This report describes strategies for redressing this mismatch between opportunity and action. Specific diseases require specific responses, which this report identifies, for settings with limited resources. The above strategies provide a starting point for the delivery of affordable, accessible, and effective care. Each needs to be evaluated and refined through an iterative process to meet good-practice guidelines and the varying needs of each community. International efforts will be needed to catalyze the actions required to reduce the impact of brain disorders now and those required to develop improved options for the future. Through such efforts, affordable reductions in the level of suffering from brain disorders can be achieved in the developing world.

Part II

INTRODUCTION

In addition to reviewing the overall burden of disease attributable to brain disorders and formulating a strategic framework to reduce that burden in developing countries, presented in Part I of this report, the committee was also charged to address specifically the following group of representative disorders: developmental disabilities, epilepsy, bipolar disorder, schizophrenia, unipolar depression, and stroke. The committee reviewed evidence of the impact of each of these disorders in developing countries and identified strategies to reduce that impact through prevention and low-cost treatment, research and development, and capacity building. The results of this process are presented in the next six chapters, which comprise Part II of this report.

Several factors were considered in selecting these particular disorders for study. First, each ranks among the most prevalent of neurological, psychiatric, or developmental disorders worldwide and is known to cause significant disability. Second, these disorders represent a spectrum of disease affecting people at every stage of life, from fetal development through old age; their order of presentation in the following chapters, which begins with developmental disabilities and concludes with stroke, reflects this chronological progression. Finally, these particular classes of disorder appeared to be strong candidates for cost-effective interventions, and therefore critical targets for reducing the overall burden of disease associated with brain disorders. It is hoped that future studies on other brain disorders of public health significance, such as Alzheimer's disease, injuries to the central nervous system, substance abuse, and posttraumatic stress disorder, will build on this initial effort.

The framework for studying each of the selected disorders or groups of disorders included an overview of the available epidemiological parameters, a review of the existing knowledge base to support intervention, and projections of the feasibility, cost, and expected impact of proposed interventions. Wherever possible, the committee based its review and recommendations on evidence from a broad range of settings in the developing world; unfortunately, due to the limited available research on most brain disorders in developing countries, they were frequently forced to make qualified extrapolations based on data from the developed world. In most cases, direct correlations appear to exist between developed and developing countries. For example, many proven risk factors for stroke have been established in developed countries (such as hypertension, high-fat and sodium diets, and diabetes), and these risk factors are of growing concern in developing countries. Though extensive data do not exist on prevention methods for controlling or eliminating these risk factors in developing countries, it can be said that such efforts would bear similar reduction in stroke mortality as has been observed in developed countries. In the few instances where correlations might be skewed by differences between developed and developing countries, these limitations are clearly noted.

As one might expect, several observations regarding the impact and outlook for reducing the burden of specific disorders presented in the chapters of Part II mirror comments in Part I that pertain to many or all brain disorders. These points are reiterated in order to build the most complete picture possible of each individual disorder. However, since the discussions of specific brain disorders presented in Part II are ultimately intended to be viewed in the context of the general discussion and strategies that appear in Part I, readers are advised to familiarize themselves with the introductory chapters of this report before proceeding to the chapters in Part II.

Summary of Findings:
Developmental Disabilities in Developing Countries

- Developmental disabilities impose enormous personal, social, and economic costs due to their early age of onset and frequent result of lifetime dependency.

- The magnitude of the impact of developmental disabilities is largely unknown and unrecognized in low-income countries today, where more than 80 percent of the world's children are born.

- The prevalence of many of the specific causes of developmental disabilities (including genetic, nutritional, infectious, and traumatic causes) appears to be elevated in low-income countries.

- Numerous prevalent diseases and common environmental factors have been found to contribute to or increase the risks for developmental disabilities. Many of these causes—including nutritional deficiencies, infection, environmental toxins, and perinatal complications—are preventable, either by controlling the underlying condition, or by treating illness or injury to prevent progression to long-term disability.

- Rehabilitation for developmental disorders is likely to be cost-effective given the benefits of reduced dependency and improved productivity and quality of life. Models of low-cost rehabilitation include community-based rehabilitation, school-based models, institution- and hospital-based models, and various primary health care models and national strategies, all of which can be integrated into low-cost comprehensive treatment programs.

5

Developmental Disabilities

DEFINITION

Developmental disabilities include limitations in function resulting from disorders of the developing nervous system. These limitations manifest during infancy or childhood as delays in reaching developmental milestones or as lack of function in one or multiple domains, including cognition, motor performance, vision, hearing and speech, and behavior. Table 5-1 provides a listing of the major categories of developmental disability with corresponding *International Classification of Diseases* (ICD)-10 codes.[1]

To varying degrees, the causes of many other neurological and psychiatric disorders not typically designated as developmental disabilities may also be traced to early neurodevelopment. For several of the disorders discussed in subsequent chapters—specifically epilepsy, depression, and schizophrenia—evidence indicates such a causal relationship.[2–11]

The clinical features of developmental disabilities are variable in severity as well as in the specific areas of function that are limited. Brief descriptions of the clinical features of each of the broad categories of developmental disability are provided below. It may be noted that children with developmental disabilities are often affected in multiple domains of function because of the nature and extent of brain impairment or increased susceptibility to other causes of disability (e.g., malnutrition, trauma, infection) among children with a single disability.

TABLE 5-1 Major Categories of Developmental Disability with Corresponding ICD-10 Diagnostic Codes (when available)

	ICD-10 Code
Cognitive	
Mental Retardation	
Mild (IQ approximately 50–69)	F70
Moderate (IQ approximately 35–49)	F71
Severe (IQ approximately 20–34)	F72
Profound (IQ below 20)	F73
Specific Learning Disabilities	F81
Reading (Dyslexia)	F81.0
Mathematics (Dyscalculia)	F81.2
Other	
Motor	
Cerebral Palsy	G80
Post-Polio Paralysis	B91
Muscular Dystrophies	G71.0
Spina Bifida	Q05
Spinal Muscular Atrophies	G12
Other	M01–M03, Q65–Q79
Vision	
Refraction Disorders	H52
Cataract, infantile and juvenile	H26.0
Chorioretinal Inflammation, infectious or parasitic	H32.0
Nightblindness, due to vitamin A deficiency	E50.5
Other	Q10–Q15
Hearing	
Conductive and Sensorineural	H90
Other	Q16
Hearing and Speech	
Specific Speech Articulation Disorder	F80.0
Expressive Language Disorder	F80.1
Receptive Language Disorder	F80.2
Behavior	
Attention-Deficit Hyperactivity Disorder	F90.0
Pervasive Developmental Disorder, including autism	F84
Other	F80–F98

Source: [1]

Cognitive Disabilities

Cognitive disabilities in children include mental retardation as well as specific learning disabilities in children of normal intelligence. Mental retardation is defined as subnormal intelligence (intelligence quotient [IQ] more than two standard deviations below that of the population mean), accompanied by deficits in adaptive behavior. Grades of mental retardation are typically defined in terms of IQ. Children with mild mental retardation, the most common form, are limited in academic performance and consequently have somewhat limited vocational opportunities. Adults with mild mental retardation typically lead independent lives. Children with more severe grades of mental retardation (moderate, severe, and profound) are more likely to have multiple disabilities (e.g., vision, hearing, motor, and/or seizure in addition to cognitive disability) and to be dependent on others for basic needs throughout their lives.

In contrast, specific learning disabilities result not from global intellectual deficit, but from impairments in one or more of the specific "processes of speech, language, reading, spelling, writing or arithmetic resulting from possible cerebral dysfunction."[12] Children with specific learning disabilities are usually identified as such only after entering school, where a significant discrepancy is noted between their achievements in specific domains and their overall abilities. With special educational accommodations, these children may learn to overcome their limitations and demonstrate normal or even superior levels of achievement.

Motor Disabilities

Motor disabilities include limitations in walking and in use of the upper extremities (arms and/or hands). Some motor disabilities also affect speech and swallowing. Severity can range from mild to profound. Motor disabilities diagnosed in infancy or childhood include cerebral palsy, which results from damage to motor tracts of the developing brain; paralysis following conditions such as poliomyelitis and spinal cord injuries; congenital and acquired limb abnormalities; and progressive disorders, such as the muscular dystrophies and spinal muscular atrophies. Cerebral palsy results from a permanent, nonprogressive damage or insult to the developing brain. Affected children therefore may manifest a variety of motor dysfunctions, depending on the specific location of the damage. Involvement of the motor cortex produces spasticity, while involvement of the cerebellum results in hypotonia with or without ataxia. Involvement of the basal ganglia leads to dyskinesia and dystonia. Individuals with cerebral palsy often have other disabilities as a result of concomitant insults to various areas of the brain. Such disabilities include mental retardation, learning disabilities, epilepsy, language disorders, and behavioral problems. Similarly, some of the progressive motor disorders, such as muscular dystrophy, can be accompanied by cognitive disabilities. In contrast, in many forms of paralysis, such as that due to poliomyelitis or spinal cord injury, and congenital or acquired limb abnormalities, the disability is more likely to be restricted to motor skills or mobility.

Vision, Hearing and Speech Disabilities

The prevalence of low vision, blindness, and hearing loss increases with age, making these disabilities conditions that affect primarily adults. A number of important causes of vision as well as hearing disability have their onset early in life, however, and may be considered neurodevelopmental (as discussed further below). Refractive errors, the most common form of vision impairment, are especially problematic for children in low-income countries because eyeglasses and basic vision care services are unavailable to many. However, refractive errors are readily amenable to low-cost methods of diagnosis and intervention, which can become a component of primary care screening services.[13–18]

Learning to speak depends on the ability to hear and repeat sounds. The optimal period for speech acquisition is the first 2 years of life; a child who does not speak by the age of 5–6 will have difficulty developing intelligible speech thereafter. It is therefore important to screen young children for hearing impairment and to evaluate the hearing of a child who is suspected of having mental retardation or delay in speech development.

Behavioral Disorders

In most of the developing world, resources for mental health care are far more limited than those for physical care. Therefore, the majority of children with psychological or behavioral disorders go undiagnosed or untreated. Although formal data are lacking, it is probable that behavioral problems are more common in low-income than in wealthier countries because of the excess prevalence of poverty, war, famine, and natural disasters in the developing world.[19,20] Moreover, recent social transformations and rapid urbanization in many low-income countries have produced adverse effects, such as residential displacement and disruption of traditional family systems, that have in turn resulted in large numbers of homeless and displaced children. Behavioral disorders not necessarily linked to psychosocial precursors include autism and attention-deficit and hyperactivity disorders. These disorders can have profound effects on academic achievement and on families. Current research is seeking to identify structural and functional correlates in the brain for a range of behavioral disorders.

SCOPE OF THE PROBLEM

Developmental disabilities impose enormous personal, social, and economic costs because of their early onset and the lifetime of dependence that often ensues. Children with disabilities often have limited educational opportunities, and as they grow older, limited employment options, productivity, and quality of life. Yet the costs of developmental disabilities are difficult to quantify in settings where relevant data and services are lacking. As a result, in low-income countries today, where more than 80 percent of the world's children are born, the magnitude of the impacts of developmental disabilities on individuals, families, societies, and economic development remains largely unrecognized and has yet to be addressed from a policy perspective.

While disability-adjusted life years (DALYs; for definition see Chapter 2) have been computed for some of the specific causes of developmental disability, such as meningitis and iodine deficiency,[1] these figures do not convey the full proportion of cases within a given category of disorder that result in early and lifelong disability or death. Nor are DALY estimates currently available for the broad categories of developmental disability listed in Table 5-1 or for developmental disability as a whole. What is needed before useful DALY or other measures of impact can be calculated for developmental disabilities is accurate and up-to-date information from low-income countries on the prevalence and impacts of long-term functional limitations originating early in life as a result of both known and unknown causes. These data would allow an assessment of the costs and impacts of developmental disabilities against the costs of their prevention, which would in turn facilitate rational decision making and resource allocation with respect to child health and development. Without this information, there is a tendency to conclude that in low-income countries, more pressing issues preclude the allocation of resources for the prevention of developmental disabilities.

While the focus of this report is on the public health dimensions of developmental disabilities in children, including etiology, quantitative indicators, and strategies for prevention, we cannot neglect the fact that the major impacts of developmental disabilities in all countries are borne by families and individuals as a result of experiences that are difficult to quantify. These experiences include stigma, lost hopes and opportunities, discrimination, increased stress and daily challenges brought on by lifelong impairment, handicap, and social isolation. It is hoped that as countries and governments begin to take responsibility for the public health dimensions of developmental disabilities, improved awareness and management of the human dimensions of these disorders will follow.

As societies and economies become increasingly information-oriented and dependent on highly skilled and literate workers, it is critical that children everywhere have an opportunity to attain their optimal levels of cognitive and neurological development. The persistence of excess prevalence rates of developmental disabilities observed in low-income countries today is both a consequence of poverty and poor resource allocation and an impediment to future social and economic development.

---

[1] The most recent DALY figures in low- and middle-income countries for risk factors discussed in this chapter include HIV/AIDS, 5.5 percent; polio, 0.0 percent; measles, 2.4 percent; tetanus, 1.0 percent; meningitis, 0.4 percent; malaria, 3.1 percent; Japanese encephalitis, 0 percent; trachoma, 0.1 percent; protein-energy malnutrition, 1.2 percent; iodine deficiency, 0.1 percent; vitamin A deficiency; 0.2 percent; anemias, 1.9 percent; road traffic accidents, 2.7 percent; homicide and violence, 1.6 percent; war, 1.7 percent.

PREVALENCE AND INCIDENCE

Valid generalizations about the frequency and causes of developmental disabilities are difficult to make for any population because of the lack of true incidence data. Data on incidence (i.e., the frequency of newly occurring cases) are preferable to those on prevalence (i.e., the number of existing cases in a population) for investigating etiology because they allow causes to be distinguished from factors associated with survival. For developmental disabilities, incidence data are not available because only a minority of cases survive long enough to be identified, while for those who do survive, the onset of recognizable disability is often insidious as development unfolds.[21] In relatively wealthy countries, epidemiological studies of developmental disabilities are generally cross-sectional and use service records or registries to ascertain prevalent cases. Thus, in contrast to incidence, a great deal is known about the prevalence of developmental disabilities in populations where affected children receive services.

In populations lacking universal schooling and formal services for children with disabilities, the relatively few prevalence studies conducted to date have employed door-to-door surveys designed to identify all children with developmental disabilities in defined populations. The validity and interstudy comparability of prevalence estimates from these surveys depend on the quality and comparability of the assessment methods and diagnostic criteria used, which can be difficult to appraise from published reports. In addition, even when valid methods have been employed, there may be questions about the cross-cultural appropriateness of standardized tests of intelligence and behavior used to diagnose disabilities in children of diverse cultural and socioeconomic backgrounds.[22]

An additional problem in comparing prevalence studies from developing countries is that elevated infant and child mortality rates may curtail the prevalence of developmental disabilities in the population. If improvements in child survival are made without concomitant reductions in the occurrence of new cases of developmental disabilities, the result will be an increase in the population prevalence of disability due to the increased longevity of children with disabilities.[23–25]

A review of the prevalence studies of developmental disabilities published between 1970 and 1999 shows that most of the available data are restricted to the relatively high-income populations of developed countries in Europe, North America, and eastern Asia. Yet during this period, more than 80 percent of the world's children resided in low- and middle-income countries. This imbalanced knowledge is both a cause and a consequence of the fact that the public health impact of childhood disabilities has received little attention in low-income countries. Available evidence, however, suggests that many of the causes of disability in children are more prevalent in developing than in developed countries.

Prevalence of Cognitive Disabilities

Prevalence data on an aggregate of cognitive disabilities in developing countries are not available. Figure 5-1 summarizes the range of prevalence estimates for severe mental retardation among children in populations throughout the world. The studies are listed in descending order by per capita income of the countries in which they were conducted. These estimates show a clear tendency toward elevated prevalence in low-income countries. In developed countries, the prevalence of severe cognitive disability is consistently found to be in the range of 3 to 5 per 1,000 children. By contrast, the prevalence of severe cognitive disability in developing countries ranges from a low of 2.9 per 1,000 children in Beijing to a high of 22 per 1,000 in slum areas surrounding Lahore, Pakistan. The majority of estimates from low-income countries are above 5 per 1,000, while no estimates from developed countries are this high.

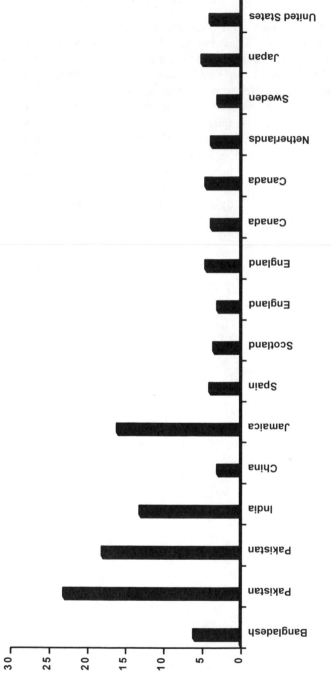

FIGURE 5-1 Prevalence of severe mental retardation in childhood, per 1,000 child population, based on published epidemiological studies after 1970 from selected countries
Source: [26—42]

Prevalence of Motor Disabilities

The prevalence of motor disability among children in developing countries is not well defined. Figure 5-2 provides prevalence data on cerebral palsy from available sources.

Prevalence of Vision Disabilities

The World Health Organization (WHO) estimates the worldwide prevalence of childhood blindness to be 1.5 million, with the numbers of affected children being 1 million in Asia and 0.3 million in Africa. In addition, an estimated 5 million children have low vision.[43,44] The prevalence of blindness in northern Nigeria has been estimated to be 1.5 percent, more than seven times the prevalence in the United Kingdom.[45] Specific prevalence data on vision disorders among children in low-income countries are scarce. Figure 5-3 illustrates the findings of these limited studies. For all ages combined, the prevalence of vision disorders is clearly higher in less developed than in developed countries (see Figure 5-4). Several studies have estimated that as much as 47 percent of blindness and low vision is preventable or curable.[15–18,44,45]

Prevalence of Hearing and Speech Disabilities

Estimates of hearing loss and profound deafness vary from 1 per 1,000 in developed countries to 1.4 to 4 per 1,000 in developing countries. WHO estimates the worldwide prevalence of hearing impairment to be 120 million, with 78 million of those affected living in developing countries.[46] Limited studies from developing countries reflect the frequent variability found in prevalence data on disabilities described earlier due to non-standardized methods of testing and reporting.[47] A study from Kenya revealed rates from 1 to 3 percent while studies in Sri Lanka and Thailand found rates as high as 12 and 13.6 percent, respectively.[48–50] Studies in India have estimated that 80 million individuals suffer from some level of disabling hearing impairment.[51] A 1990 official survey of the handicapped in China reported 23.1 million hearing-impaired individuals among which six million suffered from profound hearing loss.[52] Prevalence rates of profound hearing loss of 2.7 per 1,000 in the Gambia and 4 per 1,000 in Sierra Leone are three to four times the prevalence rates of developed countries.[53–55] Chronic otitis media (CMO) has been determined as the most frequent cause of hearing impairment in many developing countries.[55–59] High prevalence of the infectious diseases that cause CMO, such as meningitis and measles, in developing countries suggests a greater risk for hearing impairment in these populations. Estimates suggest that as much as 50 to 66 percent of all hearing impairment is preventable.[54,60–62]

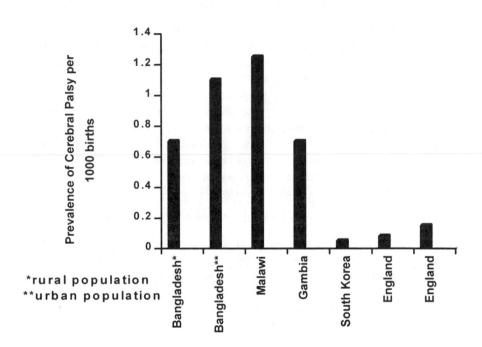

FIGURE 5-2 Prevalence of Cerebral Palsy, a subtype
of motor deficits, in various countries
Source: [63–68]

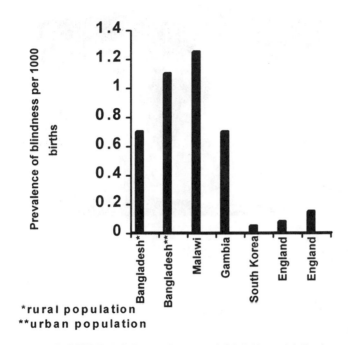

*rural population
**urban population

FIGURE 5-3 Prevalence of Childhood blindness
per 1000 births
Source: [69–73]

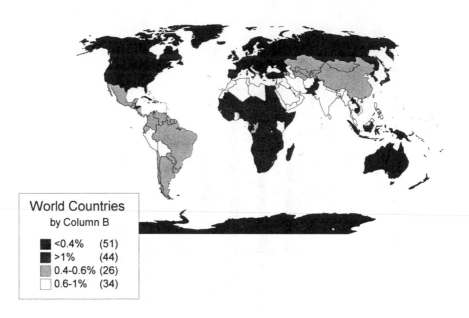

World Countries
by Column B

■ <0.4%   (51)
■ >1%   (44)
▨ 0.4-0.6% (26)
□ 0.6-1%   (34)

FIGURE 5-4 World Prevalence of Blindness
Source: [74]

Prevalence of Behavioral Disabilities

Autism and autistic disorders are relatively rare among the developmental disabilities, affecting fewer than 5 per 1,000 children. Before the advent of explicit diagnostic criteria for autism, this condition was thought to be restricted to severe forms and was found in studies in a number of developed countries to affect about 4 per 10,000 children in the general population.[75,76] More recent prevalence studies based on explicit diagnostic criteria and including Asperger's syndrome report a range of severity with overall prevalence as high as 4 per 1,000 children.[77] Similar studies of the prevalence of autistic disorders in developing countries could not be identified.

Attention-deficit hyperactivity disorder is a common childhood behavioral disorder with increasing recognition and reported prevalence in developed countries. Epidemiological studies in the United States have reported prevalence to be approximately 4 percent, with figures as high as 11 percent in some studies.[78] Studies of the prevalence of attention-deficit hyperactivity disorder in developing countries could not be identified.

RISK FACTORS

The causes of developmental disabilities include damage to or anomalies in the developing nervous system. The human nervous system is especially vulnerable during the period of its most rapid growth, which begins during gestation and extends into early childhood.

A large proportion of developmental disabilities have their origin in inherited or sporadically occurring genetic or chromosomal aberrations or in the combined effects of genetic traits and environmental exposures. Other causes include infections, nutritional deficiencies, and other exogenous insults or exposures during critical periods of neurodevelopment. The consequences of these exposures often depend on the precise timing of the insult to the developing nervous system. For example, maternal rubella infection has devastating effects on the nervous system of the fetus, but only if exposure occurs between the first and thirteenth weeks of pregnancy.

The following subsections describe the major classes of risk factors for developmental disabilities: genetic factors, nutritional deficiencies, infection, exposure to environmental toxins, perinatal and neonatal factors, and poverty and trauma. Rather than providing an exhaustive review, this section highlights risk factors for which evidence exists from developing countries of both (1) high frequency and/or public health and economic impacts, and (2) viable, if unrealized, potential for prevention.

Genetic

Genetic components within the heterogeneous and multifactorial etiology of most developmental disabilities may appear to be overshadowed in low-income countries by the high frequency of infectious, parasitic, and nutritional disorders and traumatic causes. Nevertheless, genetic factors and congenital anomalies are of considerable importance in these countries. In West Africa, 2–3 percent of all children have a serious hemoglobinopathy (sickle cell anemia, thalassaemia).[79–81] Children with hemoglobinopathies are at risk for nervous system complications, the frequency of which may be as high as 12.8 percent.[82] Complications of sickle cell disease in children include mental changes; cerebrovascular accidents (strokes); cranial nerve palsies; dural sinus thrombosis; and increased susceptibility to meningitis, especially salmonella meningitis and pneumococcal meningitis. A recent study in the United States revealed that 33 percent of the children observed with sickle-cell disese were functioning in the range of mild mental retardation.[83]

In populations lacking effective contraception, family planning, and prenatal screening, the proportion of births to women over age 35 and the prevalence of Down syndrome are high. In low-income countries, the proportion of births contributed by mothers over 35 is 11–15 percent, compared with 9 percent in industrialized countries.[84]

Another factor contributing to the high levels of developmental disabilities observed in some populations, notably in South Asia, the Middle East, and North Africa, is the prevalence of consanguineous marriage, resulting in increased homozygosity for deleterious mutations. In some parts of Africa, the Middle East, and South Asia, the prevalence of consanguinity ranges from 25 to 61 percent among all parents.[85–89] Consanguinity has been linked to elevated rates of perinatal mortality and disabling childhood conditions in a number of populations.[90–95]

Some inborn errors of metabolism, such as galactosemia, mucopolysaccharidoses, maple syrup urine disease, and homocystinuria, are occasionally reported from centers in low-income countries with adequate laboratory facilities.[96] Others may be distinctly rare in certain low-income countries. For example, phenylketonuria (PKU) is rare in black African children. By contrast, some dominantly inherited neurocutaneous disorders, specifically neurofibromatosis and tuberous sclerosis, appear to be especially common among black African children.[97–99]

The major genetic causes of childhood motor disability, such as Duchenne muscular dystrophy, are found in virtually all countries. Others, such as the congenital myopathies (central core disease, Nemaline myopathy, myotubular myopathy) have been reported mainly from Southeast Asia, and also among Arabs in the Middle East and North Africa. Spinal muscular atrophies are particularly common in Southern Africa, while congenital muscular dystrophies are very common in North Africa and the Middle East.[100–103]

PKU, a rare defect of amino acid metabolism occurring in 1/15,000 Caucasian live births and somewhat less frequently in Africans,[98,104–106] results from a mutation at the phenylalanine hydroxylase gene and is inherited in an autosomal recessive manner. Deficient metabolism of phenylalanine causes accumulation, which if untreated leads to hyperphenylalaninaemia, progressive damage to the developing brain during the neonatal and postnatal periods, and severe mental retardation in most cases. In populations where newborn screening and dietary treatment for PKU are feasible (as discussed in the following section on interventions), the diet must be continued for females throughout the childbearing years to prevent brain damage in offspring from prenatal exposure to elevated maternal phenylalanine.

Nutritional Deficiencies

Micronutrient Deficiencies

Iodine deficiency occurs on all continents and is associated with a range of adverse reproductive and developmental outcomes, including miscarriage; perinatal mortality; and cognitive, motor, and hearing disabilities.[107] Sustained exposure to severe maternal iodine deficiency through the second trimester of pregnancy can result in cretinism or iodine-deficiency syndrome, a severe form of congenital disability involving cognitive and motor deficits, and often hearing loss and speech impairment. Milder cases of maternal iodine deficiency result in a range of intellectual, motor, and hearing deficits among children in iodine-deficient regions.[108] In addition, continued iodine deficiency in the postnatal period may increase infant mortality [109] and impair mental performance in subsequent years.[110,111]

Vitamin A deficiency contributes to childhood disability in two ways. One is through its effects on ocular tissue. When severe and prolonged, the deficiency leads to xerophthalmia, which ranges in severity from night blindness to permanent corneal scarring and blindness. Vitamin A deficiency also increases the severity of serious childhood infections, such as measles, making the deficiency a major contributor to child mortality in low-income countries and potentially the cause of long-term disability among survivors.[112] WHO (1995) has estimated that 250 million infants and children under age 5 in low-income countries have low vitamin A stores, and an additional 3 million are clinically deficient in vitamin A with evidence of xerophthalmia and are at risk for blindness. In 1992, WHO estimated that at least half of the prevalent cases of childhood blindness worldwide were the result of vitamin A deficiency.[44]

Iron deficiency anemia is a widespread public health problem in low-income countries, where it affects a high percentage of women, infants, and children. Although iron deficiency may not be a sufficient cause of developmental disability, it contributes to the risk of such disability by lowering immunity, impairing fat and vitamin A absorption, impairing thyroid hormone transformation, increasing lead absorption, and increasing the risk for low birth weight.[113,114] Evidence of direct, central nervous system effects of iron deficiency anemia during infancy was recently found in Chile.[115] An association has been observed between iron deficiency anemia in childhood and persistent deficits in cognition, attention, and learning capacity, though confounding effects of socioeconomic disadvantage are difficult to disentangle.[116,117] In addition to dietary iron deficiency, major risk factors for iron deficiency anemia in low-income countries include hookworm and other helminthic infestations, malaria, diarrheal disease, and poverty.[118]

Folate deficiency early in pregnancy contributes to the occurrence of neural tube defects, such as spina bifida, which result in motor disability and in some cases intellectual impairment among surviving infants. Epidemiological studies reveal large geographic differences in the prevalence of neural tube defects, and an association between preconceptional and periconceptional folate consumption during pregnancy and the occurrence of neural tube defects in offspring. This association is due, at least in part, to a gene–environment interaction. Mutations of the methylenetetra hydrofolate reductase gene in the absence of a folate-rich diet is associated with elevated maternal plasma homocysteine and the occurrence of neural tube defects in offspring.[119,120] Supplementation of 400 micrograms of folic acid per day is sufficient to increase the activity of the variant methylenetetra hydrofolate reductase; correct maternal hyperhomocysteine-mia; and, when initiated prior to conception or very early in pregnancy, prevent the occurrence of a substantial portion of neural tube defects.[121]

Protein-Energy Malnutrition

The clinical consequences of severe malnutrition for the developing nervous system may include compromised intersensory integration, poor language development, and retarded behavioral and learning skills.[106,122–124] Malnutrition can also lead to various neuropathies, including tropical ataxic neuropathy and pellagrous neuropathy. Yet the contribution of protein-energy malnutrition to developmental disabilities is less clear than that of micronutrient deficiencies. Animal studies have long shown that nutritional deprivation during the phase of maximum brain growth can adversely and, under some circumstances, irreversibly affect the brain.[125] The effects of such deprivation on behavior in animals, and on mental performance in human beings, are not fully understood, however.[126,127] Poor nutrition is typically confounded with poverty and poor education, two of the strongest predictors of poor mental performance.

Evidence regarding the independent effects of general nutrition on children's mental development suggests that nutritional changes from gestation through 6 months of age, as well as between 42 and 75 months of age, appear to produce no measurable effects on mental performance later in childhood.[126,128–132] Dietary supplementation of undernourished infants and children in Bogota between 6 and 36 months of age was followed by improved mental performance from 12 to 36 months, but follow-up beyond 36 months was not done. If supplementation between 6 and 36 months could be shown to produce persistent gains in mental performance, this would suggest the existence of a critical period when nutrition can affect mental development. If, on the other hand, the effect of early supplementation does not persist, it may be that children need food to perform well on developmental tests,[133] but malnutrition severe enough to retard physical growth does not produce long-term cognitive delay or disability.

On the whole, studies of mental development indicate that the association between socioeconomic deprivation and developmental disabilities is better explained by lack of access to education and intellectual stimulation and by micronutrient deficiencies than by protein-energy malnutrition.[126] Even if irreversible effects of protein-energy malnutrition per se on the developing nervous system of humans cannot be demonstrated, however, it is clear that chronic malnutrition is detrimental to children's survival, growth, and cognitive and physical performance. Prevention of protein-energy malnutrition is therefore a top international priority.[134] Moreover, malnutrition among children with developmental disabilities impacts adversely on survival, as well as on the ability to benefit from educational interventions.[135]

Infection

Numerous prenatal, perinatal, and postnatal infections can damage the developing nervous system or senses and cause long-term disabilities in children, and are important causes of developmental disability in low-income countries. In Nigeria, for example, the majority of cases of blindness and deafness in children are secondary to infections such as measles, rubella, onchocerciasis, meningitis, and chlamydia.[45,136]

Congenital rubella can manifest with deafness, cataract and visual impairment, mental retardation, and failure to thrive. This cause of developmental disability has been virtually eliminated in successfully vaccinated populations, but epidemics of rubella continue to occur in some developing countries.[137–139] **Congenital syphilis** remains rampant in some developing countries, with neurological manifestations that include deafness, interstitial keratitis, and mental retardation.[140–143] **Congenital toxoplasmosis** manifests as necrotizing encephalopathy, microcephaly, cranial nerve palsies, spastic quadriparesis, intracranial calcification, and chorioretinitis; seizures can also be a presenting feature.[144–146] **Congenital cytomegalovirus** infection can result in microcephaly, mental retardation, seizures, and deafness.[147] **Herpes simplex** may be acquired congenitally or during parturition, resulting in microcephaly, intracranial calcification, microphthalmia, and retinal dysplasia.[148]

HIV is now an important cause of developmental disability, particularly in populations where it affects a high proportion of childbearing women and where access to effective antiretroviral therapies and cesarean delivery are not available. In some high-risk populations, the prevalence of infection in women of reproductive age is 20–30 percent or higher.[105,149–151] With the emergence of antiretroviral therapy (zidovudine) to prevent perinatal transmission of HIV,[152] the risk of vertical transmission of the virus from infected mothers to offspring has been reduced from about 25 percent to less than 10 percent in European and North American populations. When treatment is combined with delivery by cesarean section, transmission can be reduced to as low as 2 percent.[153,154] In low-income populations—which include the majority of HIV-infected women worldwide and in which prenatal screening, counseling, and treatment options are limited—the probability of vertical transmission from untreated infected mothers remains as high as 30 to 40 percent. Recently, short-course antiretroviral prophylaxis regimens have been shown to provide a relatively low-cost and effective strategy for preventing vertical transmission of HIV in low-income populations.[155,156] Once a child has been infected, the ensuing effects of pediatric AIDS include central nervous system impairment, acquired microcephaly, and cognitive and movement disabilities in virtually all cases.[157] Thus, HIV infection is now a leading, fatal cause of developmental disability in many populations.

Brain damage from many intrauterine infections (toxoplasmosis, cyto-megalovirus, varicella, HIV) may follow either prenatal or perinatal transmission.[158,159] When exposure occurs during the first or second trimester of pregnancy, several impairments are recognizable at birth, including microcephaly, hydrocephaly, growth retardation, cataracts, seizures, rashes, jaundice, and hepatosplenomegaly.[160,161] Exposure late in pregnancy or during delivery may result in inapparent infection at birth and onset of developmental delay during infancy or childhood.[162] In the case of toxoplasmosis, early detection and treatment (prenatal or neonatal) with antiparasitics is believed to reduce the occurrence of hydrocephalus and cognitive sequelae, though even among treated infants the frequency of severe mental retardation in one follow-up study of infected infants was 21 percent.[163]

Postnatally acquired infections are important causes of developmental disabilities among children in low-income countries, where access to prophylaxis and treatment is often limited and delayed. These infections include malaria, bacterial meningitis, viral encephalitis, measles, poliomyelitis, tetanus, and trachoma.[93,164,165]

Malaria is a public health problem in about 90 countries and is estimated to cause several hundred million cases and approximately 1 million deaths among children each year.[165–167] A major complication of malaria is cerebral malaria, the major clinical manifestations of which are convulsions and an alteration in the level of consciousness that starts as drowsiness and rapidly proceeds to deep coma. Repeated episodes of malaria are responsible for poor school attendance and childhood anemia. During pregnancy, malaria may result in placental parasitemia and intrauterine growth restriction, as well as maternal anemia and death.[168,169]

Meningitis from major bacterial agents probably occurs more commonly in developing than in developed countries, though specific data are lacking. Children under age 5 and especially under age 1, as well as the elderly, are at highest risk.[170–172] In developing countries, pneumonia is the most common presentation of *Haemophilus influenzae* Type b meningitis; it has been estimated that this cause of meningitis in developing countries has a case fatality rate of 30 percent and results in permanent nervous system impairment in 20 percent of survivors.[166,173,174] Meningococcal meningitis occurs sporadically in developed countries, but major epidemics of the disease occur every several years in sub-Saharan Africa and South America.[166] Case fatality exceeds 50 percent in the absence of early and adequate treatment, and it is estimated that 15 to 20 percent of survivors are left with deafness, seizures, and mental retardation.[166] Otitis media is most often secondary to meningitis and the most common cause of hearing loss in many developing countries.[55–59]

Japanese viral encephalitis is the leading cause of **viral encephalitis** in Asia, where it is responsible for at least 50,000 cases of clinical disease each year, primarily among children.[166,175,176] Case fatality is as high as 20 percent, and the frequency of neuropsychiatric sequelae among survivors is high, ranging from 30 to 50 percent in several developing country studies.[176–179] Following an infectious mosquito bite, the virus replicates in the lymph nodes, spreads to the central nervous system, and propagates in the brain, leading to seizures, cognitive and motor disabilities, and progressive coma.[166]

Measles is an acute viral disease that is still a leading cause of death worldwide, largely because of its occurrence among children under age 5 in developing countries.[180–182] Rarely (about 1/1000 cases), measles infection causes encephalitis, which can result in long-term nervous system sequelae among survivors. While Vitamin A deficiency has been shown to increase the severity of measles infection, it is thought the infection can, in turn, exacerbate Vitamin A deficiency and lead to blindness.[183–186]

Following a concerted international initiative, paralytic **poliomyelitis** was eradicated from the Western Hemisphere, the Western Pacific region, and Eastern Europe.[187] This enteroviral disease, however, remains a major problem among children in tropical Africa and to a lesser extent in South and Southeast Asia. Once established in the intestines, poliovirus can enter the blood stream and invade the central nervous system. As it multiplies, the virus destroys motor neurons and leads to irreversible paralysis.

Tetanus, especially neonatal tetanus, is still prevalent in many developing countries. Various studies have shown that it is not only associated with high mortality, but also followed by adverse developmental sequelae in those who survive.[182,188–190] Neonatal tetanus is due mainly to improper management of the umbilical cord, which is often cut by traditional birth attendants with items such as bamboo knives, broken bottles, and unsterilized razors, and dressed with herbal concoctions and cow's dung that are heavily contaminated with *Clostridium tetani*. Tetanus, like poliomyelitis, is preventable by appropriate immunization of infants, while neonatal tetanus can be prevented by immunizing pregnant mothers.[182,188–190]

Trachoma is a bacterial disease of the conjunctiva caused by *Chlamydia trachomatis*.[191] Repeated infections, which often begin in childhood, result in blindness in adulthood. Trachoma is endemic in many impoverished areas of the world where access to clean water is compromised. An estimated 5.9 million people worldwide have become blind or are at immediate risk for blindness as a result of trachoma infection.[191–193]

Environmental Toxins

Children may be exposed to toxins that predispose them to developmental disabilities through a variety of routes. Some, such as lead, are present in either the prenatal (maternal) or postnatal environment. Others may be introduced systemically, as through the maternal use of alcohol or teratogenic medications. Lead, which can be absorbed from paint flakes on the floor or painted toys and from the fumes of burning batteries, has long been known to cause the serious and often fatal condition of lead encephalopathy in children. In low-income countries, children continue to be exposed to lead from gasoline and other sources.[194,195] Persistence of the effects of early lead exposure into adolescence and young adulthood has also been demonstrated.[196,197] Overall, a dose–response relationship between lead exposure in early childhood and mental performance, as well as hyperactivity and other behavioral problems, is well documented.[198]

Heavy alcohol abuse during pregnancy is associated with fetal alcohol syndrome in offspring. This syndrome includes cognitive disability (usually mild to moderate in severity), low birth weight, microcephaly, and subtle facial abnormalities that may diminish over time. Ototoxic drugs capable of causing congenital hearing loss if ingested during pregnancy include streptomycin and salicylates. Thalidomide, a well-documented and once-banned teratogen, has recently been reintroduced in developing countries for patients with leprosy and HIV infection.[199] Without appropriate precautions, this drug could lead to an epidemic of birth defects in low-income countries. In addition, prenatal exposure to ubiquitous environmental contaminants such as polychlorinated biphenyls (PCBs) and tobacco smoke may also have detrimental effects on the developing nervous system.[200,201]

Perinatal and Neonatal

Perinatal events such as preterm birth, low birth weight, intrauterine growth restriction, and birth asphyxia are associated with elevated risk of impaired physical, sensory, and mental development during infancy and childhood.[202] Many factors contribute to the elevated frequency of these events in low-income countries. These factors include the scarcity of resources for obstetrical care and management of complications of labor and delivery; dietary deficiencies, some of which are encouraged by the fear of increased delivery complications associated with larger babies in settings where professional obstetrical services are lacking; anemia; and increased risk of maternal infections, such as malaria and genital tract infections, in some settings.

Perinatal complications are important risk factors for developmental disabilities. For example, retinopathy of prematurity is a leading cause of childhood blindness worldwide.[203] In addition, prematurity is an important risk factor for cerebral palsy and cognitive disabilities in childhood. Yet the etiology of many perinatal complications, as well as the nature and direction of their causal association with developmental disabilities, is often not clear, limiting efforts at prevention. Research is urgently needed on the etiology and prevention of adverse perinatal outcomes such as low birth weight, preterm birth, and intrauterine growth restriction; on the causal relationships between these factors and developmental disabilities; and on the impact of their prevention on the prevalence of neurodevelopmental disabilities in low-income countries.

Neonatal factors that can be devastating to the developing nervous system, resulting in long-term disability, include severe, untreated hyperbilirubinemia and neonatal infections.[204] A cross-sectional, retrospective study in Bangladesh found both of these exposures to be significant risk factors for serious mental retardation in childhood.[205]

Poverty and Trauma

Poverty greatly increases children's risk for developmental disabilities (see Chapter 2). Low socioeconomic status of the family and suboptimal maternal education have both been shown to be associated with deficits in cognitive development among children in developing countries.[88,205] Low socioeconomic status appears to be the strongest and most consistent predictor of mild mental retardation throughout the world.[206,207] Moreover, impoverished physical environments, war, land mines, natural and human-induced disasters, lack of road safety and injury prevention initiatives, and child abuse and neglect together expose children in many low-income countries to excess hazards that potentially contribute to the prevalence of developmental disabilities,[19,208–212] though evidence from follow-up studies linking these exposures to the occurrence of developmental disabilities is lacking.

INTERVENTIONS

Comprehensive prevention of developmental disabilities involves primary prevention, secondary prevention or treatment, and tertiary prevention or rehabilitation.

Primary and Secondary Prevention

Primary prevention includes efforts to control the underlying cause or condition resulting in developmental disability. Examples are vaccination to prevent congenital rubella and salt iodination to prevent iodine deficiency. Secondary prevention is aimed at preventing an existing illness or injury from progressing to long-term disability. Examples of such interventions are newborn screening for PKU, followed by dietary modifications, and emergency medical care for trauma.

Genetic Factors

Expansion of family planning and contraception to prevent unplanned births to women over age 35 is a cost-effective strategy for prevention of mental retardation, specifically of Down syndrome (trisomy 21).

Another clear risk factor for genetic causes of developmental disability— the practice of consanguineous marriage[213]—may be difficult to modify, being integral to the culture, social structure, and land tenure systems of many integral to the culture, social structure, and land tenure systems of many populations. However, educational campaigns and genetic counseling are potential strategies for reducing this important contributor to the prevalence of developmental disabilities in many countries.

In countries with routine newborn screening programs and effective follow-up of affected children, disabilities due to conditions such as hypothyroidism and PKU are rarely seen. Newborn screening and intervention programs for treatable conditions may be cost-effective in low-income countries, as they are in wealthier countries, when weighed against the costs of disability that are incurred when these conditions go undetected and untreated.[105,106,214,215]

Nutritional Deficiencies

There are four broad categories of interventions designed to correct or prevent micronutrient deficiencies: education regarding dietary sources of essential nutrients and strategies for ensuring adequate dietary intake; fortification of the food supply; supplementation to ensure adequate intake by targeted individuals, such as by means of vitamin A capsules or iron tablets; and control of infectious and parasitic diseases that deplete bodily stores or interfere with absorption of micronutrients.[216]

Iodine Deficiency. Correction of maternal iodine deficiency immediately before conception is necessary if the adverse effects of the deficiency on neurodevelopment and cognition are to be prevented in children. The only practical way to achieve this from a public health perspective is through universal dietary fortification. Salt iodination is now being implemented in many developing countries,[217] though difficulties with distribution and quality control remain, and the success of this intervention requires major commitments from governments and international agencies (see Figure 5-5 for the percentage of households worldwide using iodized salt). In 1993, the World Bank estimated a DALY cost of US$8 for elimination of iodine deficiency by means of salt fortification, but this estimate did not take account of the full impact of iodine deficiency disorder on the intellectual capacity of affected populations.[218] Thus, the actual cost per DALY is likely to be even less than US$8. Iodination of drinking water has been shown to be a safe and cost-effective alternative in some settings.[219] Iodine deficiency is still a prevalent cause of developmental disability in many communities, and its elimination will require sustained efforts.[218]

135

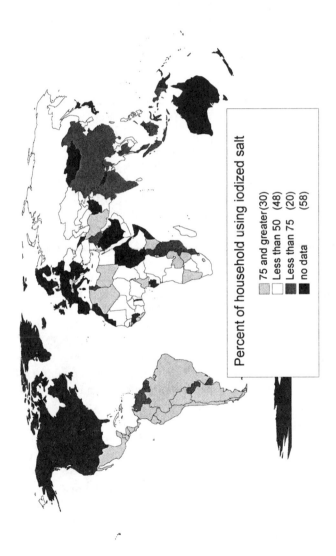

FIGURE 5-5 Percent of household using iodized salt
Source: [220]

Vitamin A. Elimination of blindness due to Vitamin A deficiency is feasible through increased dietary intake of foods naturally rich in the vitamin, fortified foods, and supplements.[216] For economic and cultural reasons, it may not be possible to eliminate vitamin A deficiency through education aimed at promoting dietary intake of foods naturally rich in vitamin A. Fortification of a staple food is a long-term, low-cost intervention. Supplements are also inexpensive, at less than US$0.03 per capsule, and may be cost-effective to implement through immunization and maternal and child health care programs. Control of diarrheal diseases in children is also a necessary component of the prevention and correction of vitamin A deficiency.[221]

Iron. Nutrition education will have limited effectiveness against iron deficiency in populations where this deficiency is prevalent because foods rich in bioavailable iron are not accessible to economically disadvantaged women and children, who are at greatest risk. Fortification of staple foods, such as processed cereals, is feasible and cost-effective in some populations.[222] Fortification is generally not sufficient for preventing or correcting iron deficiency anemia in pregnant women, however, and supplementation is often required. The cost of fortifying cereals or flour is very low in populations where this is feasible, at US$0.05 per person per year.[222] The cost of supplementing women during pregnancy is about US$1.20 for 9 months, and the cost of fortifying infant diets has been estimated to be US$0.20 per person per year. In areas where hookworm or malaria is prevalent, treatment and prevention of these diseases is a necessary component of programs to prevent iron deficiency. Overall, the World Bank has estimated the benefit-to-cost ratio for a comprehensive iron deficiency prevention program to be as high as 500, implying that for the equivalent of every dollar spent on program costs, $500 is saved in costs associated with mortality, morbidity, and reduced functional capacity due to iron deficiency.[222]

Folic acid. Folic acid supplementation or fortification of the food supply is effective against neural tube defects, but only if the folate requirements of childbearing women are met periconceptionally or very early in pregnancy. Folates are present in leafy vegetables, legumes, and citrus, but it is doubtful whether dietary advice alone can result in consumption of sufficient amounts by those at risk. The strategy adopted in the some countries (e.g., the United States, Chile) is to supplement the entire population at an estimated level of 100 micrograms per day by fortifying bread flour with folic acid. Folic acid supplementation of the whole population at the level shown to prevent neural tube defects (i.e., 400 micrograms per day) raises two safety concerns that require monitoring, however. One is that doing so could mask pernicious anemia due to vitamin B_{12} deficiency, allowing neural damage characteristic of pernicious anemia to progress undetected. The other is the potential for drug interaction between high folate levels and certain medications. It has been estimated that folic acid supplementation could prevent 50 to 70 percent of neural tube defects.

Infections

Congenital Rubella. Vaccination of the population against rubella can prevent virtually all cases of congenital rubella. The availability of a combined measles and rubella vaccine increases the feasibility of eradicating rubella infection, though this goal is not currently recognized as a priority in low-income countries.[137] The cost-effectiveness of programs to ensure that all women of childbearing age are vaccinated against rubella has been demonstrated in the United States (benefit-to-cost ratio of 11.1:1), but not specifically in low-income countries.[137]

Malaria. Measures to prevent malaria infection include use of protective clothing, insect repellents, insecticide-treated bednets, and environmental management to control mosquito vectors. Once infection has occurred, chemoprophylaxis may be effective against the development of severe disease. The cost-effectiveness of malaria prophylaxis and treatment programs is well established in populations where malaria is endemic, even without accounting for the potential for long-term neurological deficits in children who survive cerebral malaria.[223,224]

Bacterial Meningitis. Primary prevention of *Haemophilus influenzae* Type b meningitis can be achieved by means of vaccination of all infants or by chemoprophylaxis following close contact with an affected child. Vaccination is the only practical method of preventing infection on a population level. In developed countries where immunization against this disease during infancy is routine, the incidence of *Haemophilus influenzae* Type b meningitis has dropped dramatically [164]. It has been argued that vaccination against *Haemophilus influenzae* Type b infection is cost-effective in developing countries as well,[225] but information on the frequency of the disease and its sequelae in developing countries is needed to guide the implementation of control strategies.[170,171,174]

With regard to meningococcal meningitis, epidemics can be controlled effectively by means of mass immunization campaigns resulting in at least 80 percent coverage, while infection in endemic situations can be prevented by chemoprophylaxis administered to close contacts of patients.[166] Information on the cost-effectiveness of these interventions in developing countries is needed.

Japanese encephalitis. An effective mouse brain-derived vaccine is available against the viral agent that causes Japanese encephalitis, and has been incorporated effectively into the national childhood vaccination program of Thailand.[226] The high cost of this vaccine and the potential for serious neurological sequelae, however, are barriers to its widespread use in endemic and epidemic situations.[226]

Trachoma. Improvements in hygiene, including access to clean water and education to promote frequent face washing, are highly cost-effective in the prevention of blindness due to trachoma.[191,192]

Measles. Vaccination using live, attenuated measles virus produces long-lasting immunity. Eradication of measles is theoretically feasible, given the effectiveness of available vaccines and the likelihood that humans are the only reservoir capable of sustaining transmission of the measles virus. Widespread vaccination has successfully prevented the spread of measles in a number of developing countries, and is considered one of the most cost-effective public health interventions ever undertaken.[183,227,228] However, measles continues to be a major contributor to childhood death and disease worldwide. Global eradication of this cause of developmental disability will require sustained efforts.

Poliomyelitis. Immunization programs have effectively eradicated poliomyelitis from much of the world, but the disease remains endemic in much of sub-Saharan Africa and parts of South and Southeast Asia.[187] Reported immunization coverage with the oral polio vaccine is still low in most African countries.[229] Although worldwide eradication of polio as a cause of childhood paralysis can be achieved by vaccination during infancy, meeting this goal will require major commitments that may be difficult to sustain in the face of the decline of the disease in much of the world.[187,229]

HIV. Efforts must focus on cost-effective and accessible methods of preventing maternal infection, as well as maternal–infant transmission. Low-cost provision of antiretroviral drugs to women infected with HIV in low-income populations should be viewed as an international priority. Vaccine development, the role of breastfeeding in transmission and prevention, and the effectiveness of modified treatment regimens and vaginal antimicrobials are currently areas of active research.[155,230–234]

Environmental Toxins

Preventing childhood lead poisoning should be both universally feasible and cost-effective when balanced against the improved cognition and occupational potential that result.[235] Prevention of lead exposure can be accomplished by controlling lead-based industrial processes, removing lead from gasoline and paint, and maintaining low lead levels in soil. Screening of blood lead levels in young children can be used to monitor risks and identify those requiring intervention. When elevated lead levels are detected, removal of the child from the source of exposure, developmental monitoring, and possibly chelation treatment to increase the excretion level are indicated. In developed countries, universal childhood screening of blood lead levels followed by intervention has proven cost-effective in high-risk populations, while targeted screening based on risk factor profiles is preferable in low-risk populations.[236,237] Research is needed on the feasibility and cost-effectiveness of interventions to prevent lead poisoning in low-income countries. In addition to such measures, prevention of industrial disasters resulting in neurotoxic exposures requires monitoring and enforcement of safety measures.[238]

In view of evidence that alcohol consumption during pregnancy is associated with a variety of adverse fetal outcomes, abstinence or restricted drinking during pregnancy should be a public health objective in all populations. Moreover, education and access regulations are necessary to prevent exposure to teratogenic medications during pregnancy; both of these measures appear to be underutilized in developing countries.[239]

Prenatal Care and Perinatal Services

Several specific interventions discussed in other sections of this chapter that are effective in the primary prevention of developmental disabilities may be implemented through prenatal and perinatal services. These include prenatal and newborn screening and intervention, prevention and treatment of prenatal infections, and avoidance of teratogenic exposures during pregnancy. Other interventions, such as rubella immunization and correction of maternal iodine deficiency, must be undertaken prior to pregnancy or before the initiation of prenatal care, and thus may need to target all women of childbearing age.

Models for providing prenatal care, obstetrical services, and neonatal care in low-income countries have been discussed and developed primarily with two goals in mind: prevention of maternal mortality and prevention of infant mortality.[240,241] Little attention has been given in low-income countries to the role of these interventions in the prevention of developmental disabilities. To some extent, perinatal and neonatal interventions to promote survival are also effective in the prevention of developmental disabilities. For example, effective management of maternal infections, of other complications of labor and delivery such as birth asphyxia, and of neonatal complications may prevent fetal and neonatal brain injuries. However, interventions aimed exclusively at improving survival by increasing the survival of infants with neurodevelopmental disorders can be expected to increase the prevalence of developmental disabilities in the population.[241,242] Research is urgently needed in low-income countries to identify specific causes of adverse perinatal and neonatal outcomes that are amenable to intervention, and to evaluate the effectiveness and cost-effectiveness of alternative interventions in terms of the prevention of not only mortality but also developmental disabilities.

Trauma

Prevention of childhood neurological injuries includes a wide range of measures that have been shown to be effective in developed countries. Notable examples are seat belts, helmets designed for bicycling and certain sports, sidewalks, road safety equipment, education regarding traffic and pedestrian safety, window guards to prevent falls, and playground renovation. Such measures appear to be uncommon in low-income countries, though studies remain to be done in these countries on the incidence of various causes of neurotrauma, on long-term impacts, and on the use and cost-effectiveness of relevant interventions. Effective strategies are needed for the prevention of intentional causes of injury that can result in developmental disabilities, such as child abuse and war-related trauma.

Secondary Prevention

Opportunities abound for secondary prevention of developmental disabilities in low-income countries through early recognition of potentially disabling conditions and interventions aimed at preventing or minimizing disability. These include early identification and correction of vitamin A deficiency and other forms of malnutrition; PKU screening followed by dietary modifications; accurate and early detection and effective management of bacterial infections that can lead to meningitis or hearing loss [51,54]; effective treatment of malaria; provision of vision and hearing screening, eye and ear care, and refractive and hearing aid services at the primary health care level [15,243–249]; improved access to emergency medical services to prevent trauma-associated disability; and educational interventions to overcome specific learning and sensory disabilities.[51,54,250–254]

Children in high-income countries have benefited for decades from interventions such as prenatal and newborn screening, iodine fortification of the food supply, and maternal vaccination to prevent congenital rubella.[223] Recently, antiretroviral therapies have become available in high-income countries to prevent pediatric HIV transmission, but cost barriers prevent access for children at greatest risk in the developing world. Extension of such interventions to low-income countries will be vital to the long-term goal of reducing international inequalities in child health.

> **Recommendation 5-1. Proven methods of preventing developmental disabilities and enhancing children's functioning should be implemented and expanded in low-income countries. These methods should be tailored to local resources and needs, and should include the following:**
>
> - **Nutritional interventions to prevent iodine, vitamin A, iron, and folic acid deficiencies, and to ensure adequate overall nutrition, especially among women of childbearing age, infants, and children.**
> - **Vaccination to prevent conditions such as congenital rubella, bacterial meningitis, pertussis, diphtheria, tuberculosis, tetanus, and poliomyelitis, and commitment of resources to prevent other infectious diseases, such as pediatric AIDS, malaria, and neurocysticercosis (see Annex 5-1 in Chapter 5).**

- Identification of specific causes of adverse perinatal and neonatal outcomes that are amenable to intervention, and evaluation of the effectiveness and cost-effectiveness of alternative interventions in terms of the prevention of developmental disabilities.
- Prenatal, newborn, and childhood screening for potentially disabling conditions that are amenable to intervention, such as sickle cell disease, hypothyroidism, PKU, and vision and hearing impairments.
- Early identification and special educational interventions to improve outcomes for children with cognitive disabilities, including specific learning and sensory disabilities.
- Child injury prevention.

The results of screening will increase recognition of both the impacts of developmental disabilities and the importance of identifying cost-effective interventions. Indicators currently exist for infant, child, and maternal mortality, as well as for numerous other outcomes, bringing visibility to these problems and suggesting priorities for prevention. Comparable indicators are needed for the prevalence of developmental disabilities among surviving children to allow estimates of impact, such as DALYs, which at present cannot be derived for developmental disabilities. Surveillance of developmental disabilities will allow countries to identify locally relevant priorities for prevention, consistent with the risk factor and prevalence patterns of specific populations. Once surveillance data are available, it will be possible to monitor and evaluate trends over time in the prevalence of developmental disabilities, evaluate policies and programs, and identify emerging problems requiring intervention in the future.

Recommendation 5-2. Screening and surveillance of developmental disabilities should be implemented in low-income countries for the purposes of early identification and treatment, as well as generation of the data needed to quantify the prevalence, causes, impacts, and costs of these disabilities.

Rehabilitation

Article 23 of the United Nations Convention on the Rights of the Child states that a child with a disability "should enjoy a full and decent life, in conditions that ensure dignity, promote self-reliance and facilitate the child's active participation in the community."[242] Member states are charged to ensure that a child with a disability "receives education, training, health care services, rehabilitation services, preparation for employment and recreation opportunities in a manner conducive to the child's achieving the fullest possible integration and individual development, including his or her cultural and spiritual development."

While admirable, these goals are ideals yet to be fully realized in any nation. In low-income countries and communities, allocation of the limited resources available for all forms of intervention addressing developmental disorders demands careful consideration and an evidence base that has yet to be developed. Even if rehabilitation proves to be less cost-efficient than primary prevention of disability, however, it is likely to be cost-effective when one considers the benefits of reduced dependency, improved productivity and quality of life, particularly since there are low-cost rehabilitation strategies that can be integrated into comprehensive treatment programs for developmental disabilities in settings where resources are extremely scarce. Though this report focuses on the range of implications of developmental disabilities for children, it is important to note that rehabilitation programs must be extended as well to adult populations that are impaired by these life-long conditions. In many cases, appropriate educational rehabilitation in adults with such conditions as mild mental retardation can vastly increase their ability to function independently and contribute to family and community responsibilities.

Models for Rehabilitation

Multiple models are feasible and may be necessary for providing rehabilitation services to children with developmental disabilities and their families in settings where professional resources are extremely limited. These models include community-based rehabilitation, school-based models, institution- and hospital-based models, and various primary health care models and national strategies.

Community-Based Rehabilitation (CBR). CBR has been defined as a strategy within community development for the rehabilitation, equalization of opportunities, and social integration of all people with disabilities.[255,256] The strategy relies on mobilization of local resources and focuses on families of persons with disabilities as an important resource, seeking to enable people with disabilities and their communities to evolve their own solutions and programs. CBR also aims to eliminate the isolation and stigmatization experienced by people with disabilities, and has as its guiding principal normalization of the lives of people with disabilities and their integration into society. Thus, wherever possible, children should attend normal schools, and the model of institutionalization should be abandoned. Implicit in the CBR approach is the idea that social expectations and environmental constraints contribute to the degree of functional limitation and other consequences experienced by persons with disabilities.[257] This concept is also central to revisions of the Classification of Impairments, Diseases and Handicaps (ICIDHI) currently under consideration.[258] The terms "disability" and "handicap," which have negative connotations, are replaced in the revised ICIDH with "activity" and "participation," respectively.[259] Thus, the focus has expanded from restoring functions to individuals with disabilities to recognition of the need to change public attitudes and other contextual factors that limit function. Persons with disabilities are viewed as partners in national development, rather than as a burden on the country's economy. Box 6-1 describes an example of a CBR program in Jamaica.

BOX 5-1 Community-Based Rehabilitation in Jamaica

3D Projects, Jamaica's first community-based rehabilitation (CBR) program, began in 1985. At that time, few services for people with disabilities existed outside the capital, Kingston. With continued support from its European donors, the program has gradually expanded, and it is now receiving government support amounting to about 25 percent of the annual budget. In the late 1980s, two other CBR programs, both run by nongovernmental organizations, adopted the 3D model and began providing services elsewhere in the country. By the year 2000, the whole country had CBR coverage, although not all residents with disabilities have yet been reached.

The 3D model involves several components, the majority of which are carried out by community personnel, most of whom are parents of children with disabilities. Detection occurs mainly in the community health service in Kingston and in rural hospital clinics, after which children or adults are referred to 3D clinics in the parish for identification and assessment of their disability. There a doctor or nurse practitioner works alongside the community workers using basic assessment devices that have been standardized and validated in an international epidemiological study. An individual program plan is drawn up, and the child is assigned to a community worker in the area where he or she lives.

If the child has a developmental disability, the community worker performs a developmental assessment and designs a program of training and, in some cases, physical therapy. The community worker demonstrates the chosen activities to the mother or caregiver, who is then expected to carry out the activities and exercises between weekly visits by the community worker. From time to time the child's progress is reviewed in the clinic.

The 3D program also coordinates activities designed to strengthen family and community involvement in rehabilitation, including parent orientation sessions; community workshops; and the training of health care workers, police, social workers, and teachers. An adult/adolescent program, which is mainly prevocational, and a stroke rehabilitation program are also sponsored.

The total projected (though not achieved) budget for the four parishes of the 3D program for 1999 was approximately US$500,000. This funding provided for a clientele of approximately 1,000 children and adolescents. In other words, the program costs about US$500 per child per year. Two evaluations of the program have been conducted.

Source: [40,260–262]

CBR models emerged in the 1970s, when there was increasing realization of the inadequacy of rehabilitation services in low-income countries, and of the fact that service models from developed countries would never be able to close the gap. Since 1983, WHO has produced detailed training manuals for CBR workers and has promoted CBR as the most appropriate model of rehabilitation for people with disabilities in developing countries.[258,263,264] While the WHO approach to CBR is largely home-based, model center-based approaches have also been developed.[265]

Advantages of the CBR approach are its accessibility to low-income families and reliance on low-cost and locally available resources. Disadvantages include a lack of skilled resources, funding, and time to devote to rehabilitation on the part of family members; difficulty in monitoring quality and outcomes; and isolation and lack of ongoing training and career opportunities for rehabilitation workers. Despite these drawbacks, CBR may be the most viable and cost-effective model for rehabilitative care in developing countries.

The idea that ready-made models for CBR can be implemented throughout the developing world may be naive given the complexity of the problems involved. Interventions must be flexible, sensitive to cultural beliefs, appropriate to the target country's current level of development, and compatible with local development priorities.

School-Based Models. A variety of educational options are available to some extent in developing countries, but for children with disabilities, the choices range from few to none. When available, they range from highly segregated, specialized residential and day schools, to special classes in regular schools, to full mainstreaming or inclusive education. Little information is readily available on the extent to which mainstreaming is practiced in low-income countries. Promotion of this approach began internationally following agreements such as the UNESCO Declaration of Education for All, which stipulates that all countries have a responsibility to provide equal access to education to children with disabilities as an integral part of the education system.[266] It appears likely that CBR and inclusive education are mutually reinforcing, since CBR programs need to place children in regular schools, and teachers find support from CBR workers when they accept children with disabilities.[267] Box 5-2 describes school-based programs and other activities of the Bangladesh Protibondhi Foundation.

BOX 5-2 Bangladesh Protibondhi Foundation

The Bangladesh Protibondhi Foundation (BPF), a foundation for developmentally disabled children established in 1985, has been a pioneer in the fields of service provision and research for disabled children in Bangladesh. Key activities and achievements include the following.

Kalyani Special School. The Kalyani school for children with disabilities (mainly intellectual and motor disabilities) was established in Dhaka. All children are first seen at a clinic, where they undergo a multidisciplinary assessment. Infants can also be enrolled in a mother–child early intervention program. There are special classes for children with cerebral palsy, speech and language problems, and behavioral problems such as autism. Within a sheltered workshop, adolescent boys and girls are taught carpentry, weaving, and painting. An affiliated school serving both disabled and nondisabled children was established to promote mainstreaming.

Dhamrai Rural School. In Dhamrai, a rural area 50 km north of Dhaka, the BPF runs a primary school for both normal and intellectually disabled children, who work together in class. There are services for children with motor disabilities and sensory impairments. A mother–child early intervention program is also offered. Parents of disabled children are enrolled in adult literacy programs.

Distance Training Packages. The BPF developed these packages for those families who cannot come to a center regularly. The packages consist of pictorial manuals that serve as reminders of the training mothers have received in handling or teaching their young disabled child in various aspects of care, including motor development, speech and communication, cognitive development, and activities of daily living. An evaluation revealed that use of the packages was as effective as regular attendance at a center.[268]

Community-Based Rehabilitation. The BPF runs several programs in collaboration with partner organizations, both governmental and nongovernmental, in various districts of Bangladesh. These programs use the TQ (ten questions) and two-phase method of door-to-door screening for disabilities, followed by assessment by a professional team.[269]

Institute of Special Education. A postgraduate institute was approved in 1998 by the National University. A 1-year course that leads to a B.Ed. in Special Education is administered through this institute.

Department of Special Education, Dhaka University. In 1996, the BPF team founded the first department for training teachers of intellectually, visually, and hearing disabled children within Dhaka University.

Research in Developmental Disabilities. BPF has initiated a rigorous program of research and development in the field of developmental disabilities. This program includes the following:
- Methodological research on screening and early assessment [270];
- Epidemiological studies of the prevalence of and risk factors for developmental disabilities in Bangladesh [205];
- Evaluation of the effectiveness of distance training packages using difficult-to-implement randomized controlled trial methodology [271]; and
- Development of training packages for teachers in regular schools so that disabled children can be enrolled in every class. This is a collaboration between BPF and UNESCO to promote inclusive education.[272]

Source: [271–275]

In Zimbabwe, the Ministry of Education has developed a program for disabled children focused on special-needs education, with an emphasis on integrating disabled children into mainstream schools when possible. Assessment offices, staffed by trained educational psychologists, reside in each provincial capital. The psychologist assesses students before they are in special units. The ministry supports both day and boarding special schools for children with physical, visual, and auditory disabilities. For children with mild to moderate learning difficulties, the ministry has established special classes in both primary and secondary schools. In keeping with its policy of integrating disabled children into mainstream schools, the ministry has also created resource units in both primary and secondary schools for children with moderate to severe learning disabilities and visual and hearing impairments.[273] Yet while this system provides good and expanding coverage, the program has not met the demand for places in special education.[274]

Reports from some low-income countries indicate that schools do not necessarily have the accessible facilities, trained teachers, or positive attitudes required to accommodate children with disabilities.[275] Given the already overcrowded environment of government schools in most low-income countries, a major commitment of resources will be required to accommodate these children.

Institution- and Hospital-Based Models. Institutional care and hospital-based services for children with developmental disabilities are present in many low-income countries, but serve only a small fraction of children with disabilities. There is general agreement among rehabilitation specialists that institutional care is not appropriate and should be discouraged, as it promotes psychological dependency, and prevents children from competing and interacting with their peers and from integrating into society when they eventually leave the institution. Perhaps the strongest argument against the institutional model is the cost and the limited coverage provided. The current monthly expenditure per child in an institution for disabled children in Harare, for example, is US$80, a figure that exceeds the monthly income of the majority of Zimbabwean families.

Existing institutions can, however, be adapted to play useful supporting roles in community-based approaches. Several Zimbabwean institutions, for example, have incorporated community outreach programs into their activities. Institutions that previously offered long-term residential care have been converted to boarding schools for severely disabled children, who return to their families during school vacations. Institutions can also provide short-term rehabilitation for rural children who require surgery or the fitting of appliances. Hospital rehabilitation departments that traditionally focused on the short-term rehabilitation of patients with an acute disability, particularly those at the district and provincial levels, now provide technical, administrative, and training support to community-based programs through outreach activities. Rehabilitation villages have been constructed in a number of rural hospitals, where disabled children and their caregivers can be accommodated for group activities and workshops.

Primary Health Care Models and National Strategies. There are a number of examples of primary health care models and national strategies for rehabilitation services for addressing developmental disabilities. Selected examples from two countries are given below.

In *Zimbabwe*, which has an extensive health care system, rehabilitation services have been established at all levels, including among individual communities. Four tertiary and eight provincial-level hospitals are staffed by therapists and rehabilitation technicians, while services at 55 district-level hospitals are provided by rehabilitation technicians who are supervised by therapists at the provincial level. The CBR program operates at a grassroots level and is supported by rehabilitation staff at district hospitals. The rehabilitation technicians, who have received 2 years of generic training in rehabilitation, staff rehabilitation units at the district hospitals and are actively involved in supporting the CBR program at the grassroots level. They have sufficient expertise to bridge the gap between the trained therapists at the provincial level and the village health workers responsible for implementing CBR at the village level.[276] To date, CBR has been introduced in 31 of the 55 districts in Zimbabwe, and three urban programs have been established in Harare and Bulawayo. If expansion continues at the current rate, every district will be covered by 2005.[277] The cornerstone of the Zimbabwean system of rehabilitative care for developmental disorders is the Children's Rehabilitation Unit at Harare Central Hospital (see Box 5-3), which coordinates a variety of services for children with disabilities.

BOX 5-3 Children's Rehabilitation Unit, Harare Central Hospital, Zimbabwe

The Children's Rehabilitation Unit (CRU) was established in 1986 as a joint project between the Department of Pediatrics, University of Zimbabwe, and the Department of Rehabilitation within the Ministry of Health. The CRU was intended to provide several key services, including coordination of multidisciplinary treatment for children with disabilities and their families; tertiary-level assessment, diagnostic, and treatment planning services for rehabilitation programs at the provincial and district levels, as well as for municipal clinics in urban Harare; training for medical students, therapists, rehabilitation technicians, and nurses in children's disability and rehabilitation; maintenance of a detailed computerized client register and database; and workshops intended to teach parents about their children's specific disorders and to create a sense of common purpose.

The multidisciplinary team that initially staffed the unit consisted of two physiotherapists, an occupational therapist, two speech therapists, two rehabilitation technicians, a social worker, a nursing sister, a pediatrician, and a secretary. Although the program has received some donations from nongovernmental organizations, major financial support for the unit is provided by the Ministry of Health through the Harare Central Hospital budget.

For more than a decade, the CRU has provided training in childhood disability and community-based rehabilitation (CBR) for health care and rehabilitation staff who rotate through the unit during their courses. As a result of this effort, these subjects now form part of the curricula of nurses, medical students, and postgraduate trainees in pediatrics, as well as trainee therapists. The result has been increased awareness among health professionals of the problems facing children with disabilities and their families and initiatives taking place to address them.

The main objective of the CRU is to support the development of CBR. Therefore, as a matter of policy, ongoing therapy is carried out in the community after initial assessment and training at the unit. To this end, 11 outreach groups were established in the impoverished suburbs of Harare. While providing easier access to rehabilitation services, the more important objective of the outreach program is to facilitate the formation of community-based support groups centered on the parents of disabled children. It is hoped that these groups will initiate self-help programs and lobby for disabled children at local government levels.

The initiative has led to the establishment of a number of projects, based mainly on handicrafts, that provide mothers with a source of regular income. Five groups have been able to secure funds to build small centers at which they are able to provide day care and preschool facilities for their children. The CRU continues to visit the groups on a weekly or fortnightly basis to provide rehabilitation services.

The CRU staff also organized the Zimbabwe Parents of Handicapped Children's Association, which now has 23 branches throughout the country and more than 4,500 members. The association's main objective is to serve as an advocate for children with disabilities and their families. Instead of placing high priority on the provision of rehabilitation services, however, parents have focused their attention on the social and economic problems affecting their families. Issues such as receiving priority in allocation of housing, obtaining access to special education for their children, developing income-generating projects, and addressing negative family and cultural attitudes toward people with disabilities are high on their agenda.

Although the CRU has received regular funding from external donors since its inception, the allocation of resources from the Harare Hospital administration has been sufficient to keep external donor support at a low level. To date, external support for recurrent expenditures has not exceeded US$5,000 per year. However, as support from the hospital has diminished over the last 2 years, it has become increasingly difficult to maintain the unit's activities at present levels. Initial and recurrent funding for planned expansion of the outreach program and the establishment of a resource center for children with disabilities at the unit will have to come from external donor sources, at least until there is a sustained turnaround in the national economy. As a result, service provision is vulnerable to interruptions in donor support.

Source: [278]

In *Bangladesh,* the Ministry of Social Welfare is mandated to provide services for disabled people. Presently it runs five schools for the visually impaired and seven schools for the hearing impaired. The National Centre for Special Education for children with sensory and intellectual disabilities was started a decade ago. The National Disability Foundation to support development activities for persons with disabilities has also been formed, as have the National Coordination Committee and the National Committee for Inclusive Education. The national policy on disability has been formulated and is expected to be introduced in parliament soon.

Under the Education Ministry, a Department of Special Education within the University of Dhaka was founded in 1995 to train teachers of children with sensory and intellectual disabilities (see Box 5-2). Under the Health Ministry, a Rehabilitation Institute and Hospital for the Disabled provides treatment and rehabilitation services for the physically and orthopedically disabled. The Shishu Bikash Kendro (Child Development Center) of the Dhaka Shishu hospital, an autonomous national institute, was started in 1992, and now has networks in some other major hospitals within the capital city of Dhaka and other divisional and district towns (see Box 5-4).

BOX 5-4 Shishu Bikash Kendro, Child Development and Neurology Unit, Dhaka Shishu Hospital, Bangladesh

The Child Development and Neurology Unit began operating in 1992 within the national children's acute care hospital in Dhaka city. It was the first multidisciplinary service in the health sector, with doctors, psychologists, and therapists working as a team to provide services to children presenting with a range of acute and long-standing neurological problems and developmental disabilities. The unit includes the Shishu Bikash Kendro (SBK), or Child Development Centre; an inpatient neurology ward; and the Agargaon Community Project, which provides child development and therapy services to an adjacent, economically deprived population.

Cerebral palsy, epilepsy, and developmental delay are the three major diagnoses made in the unit. To prioritize rehabilitation needs, each child is categorized for type and severity of specific functional disabilities. While motor disability is the most frequent presenting complaint, perhaps because it is so obvious to parents, other disabilities are also presented in a significant number of children.

In 1996, to overcome the problems resulting from the lack of any pediatric therapist within the country, the SBK started to train college graduates in certain aspects of the three major therapies (occupational therapy, physiotherapy, and speech and language therapy). The trainees have evolved to become developmental therapists. A diploma course in developmental therapy is now being planned in collaboration with the Institute of Special Education, Bangladesh Protibondhi Foundation (see Box 5-2).

The provision of epilepsy services has been another emphasis of the center. Certain diagnostic and treatment issues have emerged during the course of service development. While early diagnosis of treatable seizure disorders remains a problem because of the unavailability of accessible services and a lack of parental awareness, many children are being given medication for their "seizures" without a valid diagnosis. Diagnostic services have been strengthened by the development of the first pediatric electroencephalogram (EEG) services in Bangladesh by the SBK. Of 1,000 children presenting to EEG services with a diagnosis of seizure disorders (55 percent of whom were referred from other institutions and practitioners), over 50 percent did not have a seizure disorder. All these children had been on long-term medication with anti-epileptic drugs. Therefore, overmedication of very young children who may not have epilepsy is a common practice being addressed by the SBK.

The SBK also provides psychological services. Developmental psychologists see children with a range of cognitive, behavioral, and psychosocial problems. Child protection issues have emerged from this service as an aspect of children's development in which social support is required. Counseling for distressed children and families is also emerging as an important service. The SBK runs regular courses in family counseling jointly with other organizations, and also with a psychotherapist in the Psychiatric Department of Bangabandhu Sheikh Mujib Medical University. A pediatric clinical psychology service is also run biweekly by students in the Department of Clinical Psychology, Dhaka University. A range of standardized, cognitive, and developmental tests are being developed within this service.

After finding that access to services by the poorest families living close to the Shishu Hospital was limited, largely because of poor attitudes and behavior among service providers within the hospital, the SBK established the Agargaon Community Project. The project undertakes screening for childhood disability in door-to-door surveys and has led a campaign to promote optimum child development. An information booth staffed by a community health visitor and a part-time physician was constructed within the general outpatient department of the hospital. In addition to referral for rehabilitation services, the project assists with the placement of children in local schools and provides family planning and other medical and social services.

Very insignificant amounts of money have been spent on infrastructure for the services provided, such as construction of office space and equipment, because all the services were developed within well-established public health institutions at little extra cost. These modest costs are borne by each institution. Most of the necessary equipment, such as toys, assessment kits, and testing materials, has been purchased or made locally.

Human resource development was the area in which the greatest investment had to be made. The SBK has been in active collaboration with academic institutions in the United Kingdom through an Academic Link Program. Through this program, several personnel have been trained in the United Kingdom, and U.K. professionals have visited Bangladesh to provide training to others. As the field of developmental therapy has yet to be acknowledged in Bangladesh and the posts are ad hoc, funding for monthly remuneration has been obtained from local businesspeople who have been convinced about the benefits of the services provided.

Demands for SBK services have increased. Efforts are currently under way, both within Dhaka and nationally, to adapt and replicate the services.

Source: [41,135,211]

Nongovernmental organizations play a major role in developing services for disabled children in Bangladesh. The National Forum of Organizations Working with the Disabled coordinates the activities of organizations that work with all kinds of disabilities in both children and adults. At present, 80 organizations are active members of the forum. And the Bangladesh Scouts and Girls in Scouting have established open groups for disabled children so that even those children not enrolled in regular schools can form groups to become members.

Bangladesh is an active member of the South Asian CBR Network. A South Asian Assistance for Regional Cooperation (SAARC) Centre for the Disabled has also been recently established. Bangladesh has proposed a SAARC Disability Fund that has been accepted and is awaiting implementation. Bangladesh is also a member of the Special Olympics, and its participants have won several prizes in the past few years in various athletic events.

Barriers to Implementation

There are a number of barriers to the implementation of rehabilitation programs for children with developmental disabilities in low-income countries.

Lack of Program Funding. The costs of sustaining programs, failure to generate adequate government support, and a scarcity of trained or available professionals are major barriers to the expansion of rehabilitation programs for children with disabilities in low-income countries. In addition, the view is widely held that it is not worth spending money on children who, it is believed, are likely always to be dependent.

Negative Styles of Communication in Health Services. The experience of parents with health services is another major inhibiting factor. A survey in Jamaica showed that parents found the information given them by health personnel (mainly doctors and nurses) too vague or too difficult to understand. They therefore had unrealistic ideas and stopped going to clinics. Most of the problems stemmed from poor communication related to a lack of training in disability issues, lack of a sense of responsibility for the care of children with disabilities, and inappropriate communication styles.

Impact of Cultural Practices. An ethnographic study in Jamaica noted several childrearing practices that could have a negative effect on children with disabilities.[40] These included the use of corporal punishment to discipline a child and restrictions placed on the movement of children outside the home, especially girls; withdrawal of food as another form of punishment; and limited use of praise, for it is believed to make the child conceited.

Structure of Medical Services. Medically oriented paradigms, which have been followed thus far in undergraduate and postgraduate medical curricula in low-income countries to resolve all issues related to health, may be a key impediment to the provision of services for children with developmental disabilities in some countries. Most health programs are hierarchical, with the physician acting as the chief decision maker for any health team. This has been a barrier to the development of multidisciplinary teams in which each professional has a key role to play. In addition, negative attitudes and behavior on the part of health professionals have repeatedly been cited by those seeking care as barriers to their using services or seeking help in established centers.[273] Another impediment is a lack of accountability. People want service from someone they can come to repeatedly, or the same person visiting their homes. In public health institutions, where personnel are often temporary, this is not possible.

Poverty and Sparse Services Only in Major Cities. Distance from services has been cited as a key deterrent to the use of services, as money and resources are required to travel and stay overnight in a large town or city.[274] In addition, lack of pharmaceuticals at primary health care centers is cited by parents as a reason for not coming to these centers for child health and disability prevention services.[274] The cost of medicine has been given as a reason for lack of adherence to treatment for children requiring regular medication for epilepsy, while the cost of diagnostic services has been quoted as exorbitant, with public hospitals not investing in quality diagnostic services at subsidized costs.

> **Recommendation 5-3. It is apparent from the multitude of highly prevalent diseases and common environmental factors that contribute to or increase the risks for developmental disabilities, that recognition of these disabilities must become a public health priority in developing countries. Inclusive educational policies at both the national and local levels should be implemented to ensure that all children, including those with disabilities, have access to appropriate schooling. Resources must be provided in developing countries for special training and support of teachers in the recognition and teaching of children with developmental disabilities, including mental retardation and specific learning disabilities. Proven interventions detailed in the report for the prevention and treatment of causative factors for developmental disabilities should be implemented through community-based demonstration projects and subsequently adapted to meet the local needs of the communities they serve.**

Cost Analysis

Cost-effectiveness studies have been done for interventions in low-income countries that target some of the causes of developmental disabilities, interventions such as malaria prophylaxis, micronutrient supplementation and fortification, and immunization programs.[278–280] These studies have shown the interventions to be highly cost-effective in terms of their impacts on child mortality and morbidity, though they do not incorporate estimates of the number of years of disability potentially prevented.[278] Nonetheless, if an intervention is shown to be cost-effective even when the benefit of preventing long-term disability is not accounted for, the existing evidence for cost-effectiveness may be considered a lower-bound estimate of the intervention's true cost-effectiveness.

In general, when the full direct and indirect costs to individuals and society of disabilities arising early in life are considered, cost-effectiveness should be relatively easy to achieve for interventions that are effective in preventing developmental disabilities and improving children's functioning and self-sufficiency. Yet specific evidence regarding the cost-effectiveness of preventing developmental disabilities in low-income countries is lacking. Measures of the costs and benefits of rehabilitation of developmental disabilities are particularly difficult to obtain.

The cost-effectiveness of newborn screening in general is dependent on the frequency and severity of the conditions being screened for; the effectiveness of early (newborn) identification and treatment; and the availability of laboratory facilities for testing and confirmation, genetic counseling, treatment, and follow-up services. Newborn screening requires a government commitment and regulation and should include all births unless clear risk categories can be identified and subpopulations targeted. Quality control to maintain high accuracy of screening and confirmatory test results is crucial. It is usually necessary for the laboratory infrastructure and procedures for newborn screening to be centralized. A regional center for medical genetics is necessary to provide the laboratory infrastructure for newborn screening, confirmation of diagnoses, counselling, treatment, and follow-up of cases. A cost-effective strategy may be the regional development of networks of laboratories that complement each other and cover very large populations of one or more countries.[281]

The decision whether to develop a newborn screening program and for which conditions will vary from country to country. Conditions with high priority for newborn screening should be clinically severe and relatively frequent, capable of early detection and diagnosis with simple and low-cost methods, and amenable to treatment that will be most beneficial if initiated immediately after birth.

CAPACITY

Training and expertise are needed at all levels of health care, as well as in the educational and research sectors, to address the issues and recommendations included in this chapter. Training in these areas not only produces specialists who can appropriately diagnose and treat developmental disabilities, but also provides the knowledge required to train health care personnel at all levels with the skills required for intervention.[282–293] Major areas of importance include, but are not limited to, the following training programs:

Research training programs

- These programs are needed to ensure the availability of adequate numbers of researchers to carry out policy, clinical, and basic research relevant to the prevention and rehabilitation of developmental disabilities in low-income countries. Areas of training for this research would include but not be limited to immunology; medical genetics; pathology; child psychology; psychiatry and neurology; neurosciences; nutrition; pediatrics; audiology; ophthalmology; epidemiology; biostatistics; and health services management, research, and policy.

Regional rehabilitation training programs

- Such programs are necessary to produce cadres of rehabilitation workers, and to provide continuing education focused on CBR and other therapeutic interventions as well as on appropriate referrals for children with disabilities. Certificate and degree programs should be designed that are relevant to local needs and cultural contexts. Programs that might be included are developmental psychology, audiology, speech and language therapy, orthopedics, prosthetics, occupational therapy, and physical therapy.

Clinical training programs

- These programs are needed to provide expertise in areas vital to the prevention of and additional research on developmental disabilities. These programs should include pediatrics, pediatric neurology, neonatology, psychiatry, optometry, ophthalmology, obstetrics, midwifery, infectious disease control, diagnostic imaging, and nutrition.

Special education training programs

- Such programs are required to train cadres of teachers working in low-income countries in the recognition and teaching of children with special educational needs due to low cognitive abilities; specific learning disabilities; and vision, hearing, and behavioral disorders. These skills would require training in areas such as child development and special education.

Most of the immediate responsibility for prevention, early intervention, and rehabilitation occurs at the primary health care/community level. However, the range of services that can be made available, the training of health care workers, and access to more complex diagnostic and therapeutic help when needed all improve significantly when the primary care system is linked integrally to a regional or national center (see Chapter 3). Additionally, the research that is needed to further improve services often requires community participation.

While each country should develop a rehabilitation strategy suited to its own needs and development priorities, it is necessary to seek areas of convergence in which outside agencies can assist countries in the implementation of their rehabilitation programs. An obvious field for cooperation is in capacity building, particularly in the areas of training, research, and infrastructural development. This cooperation might be facilitated on a regional level through the establishment of regional training and research centers. These centers could provide training for rehabilitation staff, and assist regional governments in the development of rehabilitation programs by supporting operational research and funding infrastructure development. In the longer term, research efforts might focus on the development of strategies for prevention.

Training initiatives should be given priority to provide a foundation of skilled staff that can support the development of rehabilitation services. In establishing training courses, careful consideration should be given to the development of appropriate curricula. Consideration should also be given to reviewing the existing curricula of degree courses for therapists with a view to making them more relevant to local needs. The courses should be modified to provide broader training in rehabilitation and to include training in community development. Box 5-5 reviews some of the consequences of using a curriculum that has not been adapted to the context of developing countries.

Finally, qualified therapists are often reluctant to leave urban areas to live and work in remote rural locations. They may opt instead to leave government employment and work in the private sector, where conditions and remuneration are usually superior.

BOX 5-5 Importance of Contextually Appropriate Training

Professionals currently responsible for the delivery of rehabilitation services in the majority of African countries are graduates of Western universities or have graduated from local universities whose curricula have been adapted from Western models. This has a number of consequences.

First, Western curricula train therapists in only one aspect of rehabilitation, e.g., speech therapy. This restricts the usefulness of the curricula in the context of developing countries. Therapists are often overqualified for the tasks they are expected to perform, and the sophisticated equipment used in modern therapy is seldom available. Moreover, it is necessary to employ three therapists at each site to provide comprehensive service, and this adds considerably to costs.

Second, conventional training does not equip graduates with the skills needed to mobilize communities and develop sustainable community-based programs.

Recommendation 5-4. Training programs should be established to develop expertise in low-income countries in areas vital to the prevention and treatment of developmental disabilities and to the provision of effective rehabilitation services as detailed in the above descriptions.

Currently, disability prevention and rehabilitation specialists and workers in developing countries are isolated, and could benefit from opportunities to interact and exchange information with colleagues in similar but geographically distant contexts. The Internet could offer a low-cost means of facilitating this communication, but support is needed for the development and maintenance of the necessary information systems and for the purchase of the hardware needed to connect sites throughout the world. The Internet could serve as a relatively low-cost means of linking rehabilitation programs at multiple sites throughout the world. It could also provide information resources and continuing education, as well as opportunities for professional exchange and contact.

Recommendation 5-5. Internet capabilities should be developed and maintained to facilitate international communication among those involved in the implementation of primary prevention and rehabilitation programs for children with developmental disabilities in low-income countries.

Essential to the provision of adequate services for children and the prevention of developmental disabilities is a universal policy of adequate and sustained primary health care that will be health promotive, disease preventive, curative, and rehabilitative. Exemplary programs include under-five clinics [294–296] that provide immunization; nutrition and growth assessment; developmental, vision, and hearing screening; health education; and identification of risk factors for disabilities. Children are seen by primary health workers in these clinics regularly and frequently for monitoring and treatment. The success of these clinics requires adequate supplies of essential medications. Findings and progress are recorded on a home-based child health record, with growth charts being kept by mothers. Appropriate referrals are made for treatment and rehabilitation when indicated. This approach has been shown to be highly effective against child mortality and has also resulted in significantly accelerated motor development [282]; however, research is needed regarding its effects on other developmental parameters.

Strengthening and further development of the infrastructure and capacity of maternal and child health services are needed to ensure that the prevention of developmental disabilities is integral to the goals and activities of these services. Specific activities to be incorporated include nutritional supplementation; food fortification; immunization; antiparasitic prophylaxis; educational and counseling programs relevant to the prevention of nutritional, infectious, environmental, and genetic causes of developmental disabilities; prenatal and newborn screening for developmental disabilities, followed by relevant interventions; and referral of infants and young children with disabilities or at risk for disability to rehabilitation programs or other educational or therapeutic interventions to prevent or minimize disability. In addition, support is needed for locally relevant and appropriate rehabilitation programs, linked to primary health care, to which children with developmental disabilities and their caretakers can be referred to ensure that they achieve their potential in terms of function, independence, productivity and quality of life.

> **Recommendation 5-6. In the context of the successes of current primary health care child survival initiatives, it is essential in low-income countries that increased emphasis be placed on prevention and early identification of developmental disabilities within the primary and maternal and child health care systems. Those systems must in turn be linked to and supported by secondary and tertiary medical services. Additionally, to provide appropriate guidance to those in need of rehabilitation services for developmental disabilities, primary and maternal and child health care systems should be linked to local rehabilitation programs.**

> **Recommendation 5-7. The capacity for relevant evidence-based research should be developed. As recommended earlier in this report, national centers for training and research based in low-income countries can play an essential role in establishing this capacity (see Chapter 4). The role of these centers should include conducting clinical and community trials through demonstration projects to test the effectiveness of interventions in the prevention of developmental disabilities as well as training personnel to implement prevention and intervention strategies. The capacity of these centers should be further advanced through collaboration and communication with other centers in both the developing world and in high-income countries. For developmental disabilities, collaboration is recommended with such existing organizations as UNICEF, Save the Children, Rehabilitation International, the U.S. National Institute of Child Health and Human Development, the U.S. Centers for Disease Control and Prevention, the U.S. National Institute of Mental Health, the World Health Organization Expanded Program on Immunization, the World Health Organization Prevention of Blindness and Deafness Program, and the Commonwealth Association for Mental Handicap and Developmental Disabilities.**

Recommendation 5-8. Based on the findings of studies regarding the etiology, risk factors, and interventions for developmental disabilities presented earlier in this chapter, some specific areas of research for *national centers for training and research* might include the following:

- The cost-effectiveness of prenatal and newborn screening in specific settings.
- The reliability, validity, and feasibility of surveillance methods and information systems.
- Models for extending effective rehabilitation for children with developmental disabilities in low-income countries.
- Nervous system sequelae of cerebral malaria and their prevention.
- The cost-effectiveness of specific nutritional interventions for the prevention of developmental disabilities. These include interventions such as salt iodination; vitamin A, folate, and iron food fortification and supplementation; and education about local food sources.
- The cost-effectiveness of methods for the prevention of prevalent infections that result in developmental disabilities, including vaccination and/or prophylaxis for such diseases as congenital rubella, *Haemophilus influenzae* Type b meningitis, measles, and malaria.
- The etiology and prevention of adverse pregnancy outcomes, such as maternal morbidity and mortality, low birth weight, intrauterine growth restriction, and premature birth and birth defects with an emphasis not only on maternal and infant survival, but also on the prevention of developmental disabilities.
- The impact of maternal education, injury-prevention public awareness programs, and alleviation of poverty on the prevention of developmental disabilities.
- Methodological and prevalence studies to ensure that developmental disabilities are effectively represented by DALYs or other measures of impact so that the costs and effects of these disorders can be appropriately measured.

CONCLUSION

Epidemiological studies have provided some basic knowledge about developmental disabilities in low-income countries, including evidence of relatively high population frequencies, the contribution of various causes, and prospects for prevention. While the data are, on the whole, extremely limited, the prevalence of many of the specific causes of developmental disabilities (including genetic, nutritional, infectious, and traumatic causes) appears to be elevated in low-income countries, and many of these causes are preventable. Educational and rehabilitation interventions can help minimize disability and maximize the function of children with developmental disabilities. Nonetheless, few resources are devoted to relevant programs for children with developmental disabilities in low-income countries. The number of children with disabilities and at risk for developmental disabilities in low income countries is huge, as are the impacts of disability on national economies and quality of life. Yet the capacity for prevention, treatment, and rehabilitation is insufficient. The need to reduce the prevalence of developmental disabilities in the developing world is urgent and calls for innovative and sustained public health efforts and financial commitments.

REFERENCES

1. World Health Organization (WHO). ICD-10:International statistical classification of diseases and related health problems. 10th revision. World Health Organization: Geneva, 1992.
2. M. Procopio and P.K. Marriott. Seasonality of birth in epilepsy: A Danish study. *Acta Neurologica Scandanavica.* Nov;98(5):297–301, 1998.
3. K.L. Kwong, S.N. Wong, and K.T. So. Epilepsy in children with cerebral palsy. *Pediatric Neurology* Jul;19(1):31–36, 1998.
4. M. Procopio, P.K. Marriott, and P. Williams. Season of birth: Aetiological implications for epilepsy. *Seizure* Apr;6(2):99–105, 1997.
5. C. Garaizar and J.M. Prats-Vinas. Brain lesions of perinatal and late prenatal origin in a neuropediatric context. *Review of Neurology* Jun;26(154):934–950, 1998.
6. P. Pitche, A.D. Agbere, A.J. Gbadoe, A. Tatagan, and K. Tchangai-Walla. Bourneville's tuberous sclerosis and childhood epilepsy Apropos of 4 cases in Togo. *Bulletin of Social Pathology Exot* 91(3):235–237, 1998.
7. T.D. Cannon, I.M. Rosso, C.E. Bearden, L.E. Sanchez, and T. Hadley. A prospective cohort study of neurodevelopmental processes in the genesis and epigenesis of schizophrenia. *Developmental Psychopathology* Summer;11(3):467–485, 1999.
8. L.A. Rosenblum and M.W. Andrews. Influences of environmental demand on maternal behavior and infant development. *Acta Paediatrica* Supplement Jun;397:57–63, 1994.
9. S.E. Arnold. Neurodevelopmental abnormalities in schizophrenia: Insights from neuropathology. *Development and Psychopathology* Summer; 11 (3):439–456, 1999.
10. I.M. Sawhney, A.V. Subrahmanyan, C.P. Das, N. Khandelwal, H. Sawhney, and K. Vasishta. Neurological complications of eclampsia. *Journal of Associate Physicians of India.* Nov;47(11):1068–1071 1999.
11. D. Rice and S. Barone Jr. Critical Periods of Vulnerability for the Developing Nervous System: Evidence from Humans and Animal Models. *Environmental Health Perspectives* Jun;108(3):511–533, 2000.
12. S.A. Kirk. *Educating Exceptional Children.* Houghton Mifflin: Boston, 1962.
13. J.P. Heldt and I.F. Wessels. Community eye care 10 years after Alma Ata: Progress, problems, and priorities for private voluntary organizations in developing nations. *Ophthalmic Surgery* Jan;19(1):47–55, 1998.

14. L. Schwab and K. Kagame. Blindness in Africa: Zimbabwe schools for the blind survey. *British Journal of Ophthalmology* Jul;77(7):410–412, 1993.

15. J. Silver, C.E. Gilbert, P. Spoerer, and A. Foster. Low vision in east African blind school students: Need for optical low vision services. *British Journal of Ophthalmology* Sep;7(9):814–820, 1995.

16. N. Zerihun and D. Mabey. Blindness and low vision in Jimma Zone, Ethopia: Results of a population-based survey. *Ophthalmic Epidemiology* Mar;4(1):19–26, 1997.

17. S.N. Nwosu. Ocular problems of young adults in rural Nigeria. *International Ophthalmology* 22;(5):259–263, 1998.

18. A.D. Negrel, Z. Avognon, D. C. Minassian, M. Babegbeto, G. Oussa, and S. Bassabi. Blindness in Benin. *Marseille médical* 55(4 Pt 2):409–414, 1995.

19. N. Richman. After the flood. *American Journal of Public Health*, 83(11):1522–1524, 1993.

20. M.S.Durkin, N. Khan, L.L Davidson, S.S. Zaman, Z.A. Stein. Effects of a natural disaster on child behavior: Evidence for posttraumatic stress. *American Journal of Public Health*, 1993; 83(11):1549–1553.

21. E.B. Hook. Incidence and prevalence as measures of the frequency of birth defects. *American Journal of Epidemiology* 116: 743–747, 1982.

22. L.A. Suzuki and R.R.Valencia. Race-ethnicity and measured intelligence: Educational implications. *American Psychologist* 52(10): 1103–1114, 1997.

23. G. Altar and J.C. Riley. Frailty, sickness and death: Models of morbidity and mortality in historical populations. *Population Studies* 43:25–45, 1989.

24. M. Kramer. The rising pandemic of mental disorders and associated chronic diseases and disabilities. *Acta Psychiatrica Scandinavica* 62(supplement):282–297, 1980.

25. S.J. Olshansky, et al. Trading off longer life for worsening health: the expansion of morbidity hypothesis. *Journal of Aging and Health* 3:194–216, 1991.

26. H.G. Birch, S.A. Richardson, D. Baird et al. *Mental Subnormality in the Community: A Clinical and Epidemiologic Study*. Williams and Wilkins: Baltimore, 1970.

27. F. Diaz-Fernandez. Descriptive epidemiology of registered mentally retarded persons in Galicia (northwest Spain). *American Journal of Mental Retardation* 92(4):385–392, 1988.

28. M.S. Durkin, Z.M. Hasan, and K.Z. Hasan. Prevalence and correlates of mental retardation among children in Karachi, Pakistan. *American Journal of Epidemiology* 147(3):281–288, 1998.

29. T. Fryers and R.I. Mackay. The epidemiology of severe mental handicap. *Early Human Development* 3:277–294, 1979.

30. K.H. Gustavson, B. Hagberg, G. Hagberg, and K. Sars. Severe mental retardation in a Swedish county. I. Epidemiology, gestational age, birth weight and associated CNS handicaps in children born 1959–1970. *Acta Paediatrica Scandinavica* 66:373–279, 1977.

31. Z. Hasan and A. Hasan. Report on a population survey of mental retardation in Pakistan. *International Journal of Mental Health* 10:23–27, 1981.

32. A.D. McDonald. Severely retarded children in Quebec: Prevalence, causes and care. *American Journal of Mental Deficiency Research* 78:205–215, 1973.

33. P.C. McQueen, M.W. Spence, J.B. Garner, L.H. Pereira, and E.J.T. Winsor. Prevalence of major mental retardation and associated disabilities in the Canadian maritime provinces. *American Journal of Mental Deficiency* 91(5):460–466, 1987.

34. C.C. Murphy, M. Yeargin-Allsopp, P. Decoufle, and C.D. Drews. The administrative prevalence of mental retardation in 10-year-old children in metropolitan Atlanta, 1985 through 1987. *American Journal of Public Health* 85(3):319–323, 1995.
35. H.S. Narayanan. A study of the prevalence of mental retardation in southern India. *International Journal of Mental Health* 10:28–36, 1981.
36. C. Peckham and R. Pearson. The prevalence and nature of ascertained handicap in the National Child Development Study (1958 cohort). *Public Health* 90:111–121.
37. M. Rutter, J. Tizard, and K. Whitmore, eds. *Education, Health and Behaviour.* Longman: London, 1970.
38. Y. Shiotsuki, T. Matsuishi, K. Yoshimura, F. Yamashita, K. Yano, H. Tokimasa, et al. The prevalence of mental retardation in Kurume City. *Brain Development* 6:487–490, 1984.
39. Z.A. Stein, M.W. Susser, G. Saenger, and F. Marolla. Mental retardation in a national population of young men in The Netherlands: 1. Prevalence of severe mental retardation. *American Journal of Epidemiology* 103:477–489, 1976.
40. M. Thorburn, P. Desai, T. J. Paul, L. Malcolm, M. Durkin, and L. Davidson. Identification of childhood disability in Jamaica: The ten question screen. *International Journal of Rehabilitation Research* 15:115–127, 1992.
41. S.S. Zaman, N.Z. Khan, M.S. Durkin, and S. Islam. *Childhood Disabilities in Bangladesh.* Protibondhi Foundation: Dhaka, 1992.
42. Q.H. Zuo, X.Z. Zhang, Z. Li, Y.P. Qian, X.R. Wu, Q. Lin, et al. An epidemiological study on mental retardation among children in Chang-Qiao area of Beijing. *Chinese Medical Journal* 99(1):9–14, 1986.
43. B. Thylefors, A.D. Negrel, R. Pararajasegaram, and K.Y. Dadzie. Global data on blindness. *Bulletin of the World Health Organization* 73(1):115–121, 1995.
44. World Health Organization. Vision 2020: The Right to Sight. Program for the prevalence of blindness, 1997. Available online: www.who.int/pbd/Vision2020.
45. A. Adeoye. Survey of blindness in rural communities of south western Nigeria. *Tropical Medicine and International Health* Oct. 1(5):672–676, 1996.
46. WHO, WHA, Prevention of hearing impairment: Resolution of the 8th World Health Assembly, 48.9, 1995.
47. G.T. Mencher. Challenge of epidemiological research in the developing world: Overview. *Audiology* Jul–Aug; 39(4):178–183, 2000.
48. World Health Organization. Report of a WHO workshop in Nairobi (Octorber 1995): Prevention of hearing impairment in Africa in Nairobi, Kenya. October, 24–27, 1995 (WHO?PDH/96.3/AFR/NCD/96.1). Brazzaville, 1996.
49. S. Prasuansuk. Otological centre: Bangkok unit, prevention of hearing impairment and deafness. *Hearing International* 6(4):16–17, 1997.
50. P. Ratnesar. Surveying the prevalence of hearing impairment in school children in central Sri Lanka. *Hearing International* 4(3):11, 1995.
51. S. Kumar. Deafness and its prevention—Indian scenario. *Indian Journal of Pediatrics.* Nov–Dec;64(6):801–809, 1997.
52. People's Daily, China, October 20, 1990.
53. B. McPherson and C.A. Holborow. A study of deafness in West Africa: The Gambian hearing health project. *International Journal of Pediatrics and Otorhinolaryngology* 10, 115–135, 1985.

54. B. McPherson and S.M. Swart. Childhood hearing loss in sub-Saharan Africa; A review and recommendations. *International Journal of Pediatrics and Otorhinolaryngology* May 4;40(1):1–18, 1997.

55. D.R. Seely, S.S. Gloyd, A.D. Omope Wright, and S.J. Norton. Hearing loss prevalence and risk factors among Sierra Leonean children. *Archives of Otolaryngology— Head & Neck Surgery* 121, 853–858, 1995.

56. P. Little, A. Bridges, R. Guragain, D. Friedman, R. Prasad, and N. Weir. Hearing impairment and ear pathology in Nepal. *Journal of Laryngology and Otology* May;107(5): 395–400, 1993.

57. A.W. Smith, J. Hatcher, I.J. Mackenzie, S. Thompson, I. Bal, I. Macharia, et al. Randomized controlled trial of treatment of chronic suppurative otitis media in Kenyan schoolchildren. *Lancet* 348:1128–1133, 1996.

58. J.O. Klein. The burden of otitis media. *Vaccine* Dec8;19(supplement) I:S2–S8, 2000.

59. Prevention of Hearing Impairment from Chronic Otitis Media, Report of a WHO/CIBA Foundation Workshop. November 19–21, WHO/PDH 98.4. Geneva, 1998.

60. A.B. Chukuezi. Profound and total deafness in Owerri, Nigeria. *East African Medical Journal* Nov;68(11):905–912, 1991.

61. P.W. Alberti. The prevention of hearing loss worldwide. *Scandinavian Audiology* 25(supplement 42), 15–19, 1996.

62. A. Smith and J. Hatcher. Preventing deafness in Africa's children. *Africa Health* Nov;33–35, 1992.

63. P.O. Pharoah, T. Cooke, M.A. Johnson, R. King, and L. Mutch. Epidemiology of cerebral palsy in England and Scotland, 1984–1989. *Archives of Disease in Childhood. Fetal and Neonatal Edition.* 79(1):21–25, 1998.

64. J.M. Liu, S. Li, Q. Lin, and Z. Li. Prevalence of cerebral palsy in China. *International Journal of Epidemiology* 28(5):949–954, 1999.

65. A. Kavcic and M. V. Perat. Prevalence of cerebral palsy in Slovenia: Birth years 1981 to 1990. *Developmental Education and Child Neurology* 40(7):459–463, 1998.

66. C. Sciberras and N. Spencer. Cerebral palsy in Malta 1981 to 1990. *Developmental Medicine and Child Neurology* 41(8):508–511, 1999.

67. M.G. Rosen and J.C. Dickinson. The incidence of cerebral palsy. *American Journal of Obstetrics and Gynecology* 167:417–423, 1992.

68. S. Razdan, R. L. Kaul, A. Motta, S. Kaul, and R.K. Bhatt. Prevalence and pattern of major neurological disorders in rural Kashmir (India) in 1986. *Neuroepidemiology* 13(3):113–119, 1994.

69. Initial Demographic Study. A review of the available data on the visually disabled population. Royal National Institute for the Blind: London, 1985.

70. N. Cohen, H. Rahman, J. Sprague, M. Jahl, E. Laembujis, and M. Mitra. Prevalence and determinants of nutritional blindness in Bangladeshi children. *World Health Statistics Quarterly* 38:317–329.

71. E. Brilliant. The epidemiology of blindness in Nepal. The Seva Foundation: Berkeley, CA, 1988.

72. World Health Organization: Available data on blindness (Update 1987). WHO: Geneva, WHO/PBL/87.14, 1987.

73. H. Faal, D. Minassian, S. Sowa, and A. Foster. National survey of blindness and low vision in the Gambia: Results. *British Journal of Ophthalmology* 73:82–87, 1989.

74. World Health Organization (WHO). World Prevalence of Blindness. http//:www.who.int/pbd/Vision2020/V2020slides/sld004.htm., 2000.

75. C. Gillberg and M. Coleman. *The biology of the autistic syndromes,* 2nd edition. Mac Keith Press: London, 1992.

76. E.R. Ritvo, B. J. Freeman, C. Pingree A. Mason-Brothers, L. Jorde, W.R. Jenson, et al. The UCLA-University of Utah epidemiologic survey of autism: Prevalence. *American Journal of Psychiatry* 146:194–199, 1989.

77. I. Rapin. Austism. *New England Journal of Medicine* Jul 10;337(2):97–104, 1997.

78. P. Szatmari. The epidemiology of attention deficit hyperactivity disorder. *Child and Adolescent Clinics of North America* 1:361–371, 1992.

79. A. Adeloye. Sickle-cell anaemia. *British Medical Journal* May 5;2(861):304, 1973.

80. U. Omanga, D. Shako, M. Ntihinyurwa, and M. Mashako. [Cerebrovascular occlusion in children with sickle cell anemia seen in Kinshasa, Zaire (author's transl*)].* Annal *of Pediatrics* (Paris). May;29(5):371–374, 1982.

81. M.T. Obama, L. Dongmo, C. Nkemayim, J. Mbede, and P. Hagbe. Stroke in children in Yaounde, Cameroon. *Indian Pediatrics* Jul;31(7):791–795, 1994.

82. A. Adeloye and E.L. Odeku. The Nervous System in Sickle Cell Disease. *African Journal of Medical Sciences* Jan;1(1):33–48, 1970.

83. R.G. Steen, X. Xiong, R.K. Mulhern, J.W. Langston, and W.C. Wang. Subtle brain abnormalities in children with sickle cell disease: Relationship to blood hematocrit. *Annals of Neurology* Mar;45(3):279–286, 1999.

84. A. Drugan, Y.Yaron, R. Zamir, S.A.D. Ebrahim, M.P. Johnson, and M.I. Evans. Differential Effect of Advanced Maternal Age on Prenatal Diagnosis of Trisomies 13, 18, and 21. *Fetal Diagnosis and Therapy* 14:181–184, 1999.

85. M. Khlat and M. Khoury. Inbreeding and diseases: Demographic genetic and epidemiologic perspectives. *Epidemiology Review.* 13:28–41, 1991.

86. A. H. Bittles, W.M. Mason, J. Greene, and N.A. Rao. Reproductive behavior and health in consanguineous marriages. *Science* 252: 789–794, 1991.

87. M. Khlat. Endogamy in the Arab World. In: A.S. Teebi and T.I. Farag, eds. *Genetic Disorders Among Arab Populations.* Oxford University Press: New York, Oxford, 1997.

88. M.S. Durkin, Z.M. Hasan, and K.Z. Hasan. Prevalence and correlates of mental retardation among children in Karachi, Pakistan. *American Journal of Epidemiology* Feb 1;147(3):281–288, 1998.

89. M.M. Mokhtar, S.M. Kotb and S.R. Ismail. Autosomal recessive disorders among patients attending the genetics clinic in Alexandria. *Eastern Mediterranean Health Journal* 4(3):470–479, 1998.

90. A.R.R. Devi, N.A. Roa, A.H.Bittles. Inbreeding and the incidence of childhood genetic disorders in Karnataka, south India. *Journal of Medical Genetics* 24: 362–365, 1987.

91. S. Bundey and H. Alam. A five-year prospective study of the health of children in different ethnic groups, with particular reference to the effect of inbreeding. *European Journal of Human Genetics* 1(3): 206–219,1993.

92. L. Jaber, G. J. Halpern, and M. Shohat. The impact of consanguinity worldwide. *Community Genetics* 1:12–17, 1998.

93. World Health Organization (WHO). Report of the WHO Scientific Group. *Control of Hereditary Diseases*: WHO Technical Report Series 865, Geneva, 1996.

94. M.C. Braga, P.A. Otto, and O. Frota-Pessoa. Calculation of recurrence risks for heterogeneous genetic disorders. *American Journal of Medicine and Genetics* Nov6;95(1):36–42, 2000.

95. S.M. Zakzouk. Epidemiology and etiology of hearing impairment among infants and children in a developing country. Part I. *Journal of Otolaryngology* Oct;26(5):335–344, 1997.

96. ICMR Collaborating Centres and Central Coordinating Units, Multicentric study on genetic causes of mental retardation in India. *Indian Journal of Medical Research,* 94:161–169, 1991.

97. J.B. Familusi. Presentation at the Workshop of the IOM Committee on Neurological, Psychiatric, and Developmental Disorders: Meeting the Challenge in the Developing Countries, November 1999, Washington, D.C.

98. J.B. Familusi and J. O. Bolodeoku. Blood phenylalanine levels in mentally retarded African children: A study of 138 patients from Ibadan, Nigeria. *Tropical Geographical Medicine* Jun;28(2):96–100, 1976.

99. P. Kiepiela, A.A. Dawood, A. Moosa, H.M. Coovadia, and P. Coward. Evaluation of immunoregulatory cells in Duchenne muscular dystrophy and spinal muscular atrophy among African and Indian patients. *Journal of Neurology Science* Apr;84(2–3):247–255, 1988.

100. S.P. Lin, J.C. Chang, Y.J. Jong, T.Y. Yang, C.H. Tsai, N. M Wang, et al. . Prenatal prediction of spinal muscular atrophy in Chinese. *Prenatal Diagnosis* Jul;19(7):657–661, 1999.

101. S.P. Saha, S.K. Das, P.K.Gangopadhyay, T.N. Roy, and B. Maiti. Pattern of motor neurone disease in eastern India. *Acta Neurologica Scandanavica* Jul;96(1):14–21, 1997.

102. M.A. Salih, A.H. Malhdi, A.A. al-Jarallah, A.S. al Jarallah, M. al-Saadi, M.A. Hafeez, and S.A. Aziz. Childhood neuromuscular disorders: A decade's experience in Saudi Arabia. *Annals of Tropical Paediatrics* Dec:16(4):271–280, 1996.

103. J. B. Peiris. Spinal muscular atrophy, East and West. *Ceylon Medical Journal* Mar;38(1):9–11, 1993.

104. H. W. Hitzeroth, C. E. Niehaus, and D.C. Brill. Phenylketonuria in South Africa. *South Africa Medical Journal* Jan;85(1):33–36, 1995.

105. P.M. Jeena, A. G. Wesley, and H. M. Coovadia. Admission patterns and outcomes in a paediatric intensive care unit in South Africa over a 25-year period (1971–1995). *Intensive Care Medicine* Jan;25(1):88–94, 1999.

106. A. Tomkins. Malnutrition, morbidity, and mortality in children and their mothers. *Proceedings of the Nutritional Society* Feb;59(1):135–146, 2000.

107. B.S. Hetzel. Iodine deficiency disorders (IDD) and their eradication. *Lancet* ii: 1126–1128, 1983.

108. J.B. Stanbury, ed. *The Damaged Brain of Iodine Deficiency: Cognitive, Behavioural, Neuromotor, and Educative Aspects,* Cognizant Communications: Elmsford, NY, 1994.

109. C. Cobra, R. Kusnandi, D.Rustama, S.S. Suwardi, D. Permaesih, S. Martuti, and R.D. Semba. Infant survival is improved by oral iodine supplementation. *Journal of Nutrition,* 127:574–578, 1997.

110. S.N. Huda, S.M. Grantham-McGregor, M.R. Khan, and A. Tomkins. Biochemical hypothyroidism secondary to iodine deficiency is associated with poor school

achievement and cognition in Bangladeshi children. *Journal of Nutrition,* 129(5):908–907, 1999.

111. A. Bautista, P.A. Barker, J.T. Dunn, M. Sanchez, and D.L. Kaiser. The effects of oral iodized oil on intelligence, thyroid status, and somatic growth in school-age children from an area of endemic goiter. *American Journal of Clinical Nutrition,* 35:127–134, 1982.

112. A. Sommer and K.P. West Jr.. The duration of the effect of Vitamin A supplementation. *American Journal of Public Health* Mar; 87(3):467–469, 1997.

113. F.E. Viteri. Prevention of iron deficiency. In Institute of Medicine, *Prevention of Micronutrient Deficiencies.* National Academy Press: Washington, D.C., pp. 45–102, 1998.

114. T.O. Scholl and M.L. Hediger. Anemia and iron-deficiency anemia: compilation of data on pregnancy outcome. *American Journal of Clinical Nutrition* 59(2 Suppl):492S–500S, 1994.

115. M. Roncagliolo Mgarrido, T. Walter, P. Peirano, and B. Lozoff. Evidence of altered central nervous system development in infants with iron deficiency anemia at 6 mo: Delayed maturation of auditory brainstem responses. *American Journal of Clinical Nutrition* 68(3):683–690, 1998.

116. B. Lozoff, E. Jimenez, and A.W. Wolf. Long-term developmental outcome of infants with iron deficiency. *New England Journal of Medicine* 325(10):687–694,1991.

117. B. Lozoff , A.W. Wolf, and E. Jimenez. Iron-deficiency anemia and infant development: Effects of extended oral iron therapy. *Journal of Pediatrics* 129(3):382–389, 1996.

118. W.E. Watkins and E. Pollitt. "Stupidity or worms": Do intestinal parasites impair mental performance? *Psychological Bulletin* 121(2):171–191, 1997.

119. D.L. Wilcken. MTHFR 677C → T mutation, folate intake, neural-tube-defects, and the risk of cardiovascular disease. *Lancet* 350: 603–604, 1997.

120. N.M.J. Van der Put, F. Gabreels, E.M.B. Stevens, J.A.N. Smeitink, F. J. M. Trijbels, and T.K. A. P. Eskes, et al. A second common mutation in the methylenetetra hydrofolate reductase gene: An additional risk factor for neural-tube-defects? *American Journal of Human Genetics* 62: 1044–1051, 1998.

121. MRC Vitamin Study Group. Prevention of neural tube defects: Results of the Medical Research Council vitamin study. *Lancet* 338: 131–137, 1991.

122. J. Cravioto. [Protein-calorie malnutrition and psychological development in the child]. [article in Spanish] *Boletín de la Oficina Sanitaria Panamericana.* Oct;61(4):285–306, 1966.

123. B.O. Osuntokun. The effects of malnutrition on the development of cognitive functions of the nervous system in childhood. *Tropical Geographical Medicine* Dec;24(4):311–326, 1972.

124. J.H. French and J.B. Familusi. Cerebellar disorders in childhood. *Pediatrics Annals* Nov;12(11):825–831, 835–844, 1983.

125. M. Winick and A. Noble. Cellular responses in rats during malnutrition at various ages. *Journal of Nutrition* Jul; 89(3):300–306, 1966.

126. M.W. Susser. The challenge of causality: Human nutrition, brain development and mental performance. *Bulletin of the New York Academy of Medicine* 65(10): 1032–1049,1989.

127. M. Levav, A.F. Mirsky, P.M. Schantz, S. Castro, and M.E. Cruz. Parasitic infection in malnourished school children: Effects on behaviour and EEG. *Parasitology* Jan;110(Pt.1):103–111, 1995.

128. Z.A. Stein, M.W. Susser, G. Saenger, and F. Marolla. *Famine and Human Development: The Dutch Hunger Winter of 1944/45.* Oxford University Press: New York, 1975a.

129. H.E. Freeman, R.E. Klien, J.W. Townsend, and A. Lechtig. Nutrition and cognitive development among rural Guatemalan children. *American Journal of Public Health* 70: 1277–1285, 1980.

130. D. Rush, Z.A. Stein, M.W. Susser. A randomized controlled trial of prenatal nutritional supplementation. *Pediatrics* 65: 683–697, 1980.

131. D.P. Waber, L. Vuori-Christiansen, N. Ortiz, J.R. Clement, and N.E. Christiansen. Nutritional supplementation, maternal education and cognitive development in infants at risk of malnutrition. *American Journal of Clinical Nutrition* 34: 807–813, 1981.

132. E. Pollitt, W.E. Watkins, and M.A. Husaini. Three-month nutritional supplementation in Indonesian infants and toddlers benefits memory function 8 y later. *American Journal of Clinical Nutrition* 66(6):1357–1363, 1997.

133. E. Pollitt and R. Mathews. Breakfast and cognition: An integrative summary. *American Journal of Clinical Nutrition.* 67(4):804S–813S, 1998.

134. S. Rasheed. Major causes and consequences of childhood disability. *UNICEF* 2(4), 1999.

135. N.Z. Khan, S. Ferdous, S. Munir, S. Huq, and H. McConachie. Mortality of Urban and Rural Young Children with Cerebral Palsy in Bangladesh. *Developmental Medicine and Child Neurology,* 40: 749–753, 1998.

136. C. Holborrow, F. Martinson, and N. Anger. A study of deafness in West Africa. *International Journal of Pediatric Otorhinolaryngology* 4:107–132, 1982.

137. F.T. Cutts and E. Vynnycky. Modelling the incidence of congenital rubella syndrome in developing countries. *International Journal of Epidemiology* Dec;28(6):1176–1184, 1999.

138. M.A. St. John and S. Benjamin. An epidemic of congenital rubella in Barbados. *Annal Tropica Paediatrica* Sep;20(3):231–235, 2000.

139. J.E. Lawn, S. Reef, B. Baffoe-Bonnie, S. Adadevoh, E.O. Caul, and G.E. Griffin. Unseen blindness, unheard deafness, and unrecorded death and disability: Congenital rubella in Kumasi, Ghana. *American Journal of Public Health* Oct;90(10):1555–1561, 2000.

140. C. Hoarau, V. Ranivoharimina, M.S. Chavet-Queru, I. Rason, H. Rasatemalala, G. Rakotonirina, et al. [Congenital syphilis: update and perspectives]. [French]. *Santé* Jan-Feb;9(1):38–45, 1999.

141. P.C. van Voorst Vader. Syphilis management and treatment. *Dermatology Clinic* Oct;16(4):699–711, xi, 1998.

142. M.L. Cohen. Candidate bacterial conditions. *Bulletin of the World Health Organization* 76(supplement) 2:61–63, 1998.

143. R. Davanzo, C. Antonio, A. Pulella, O. Lincetto, and S. Schierano. Neonatal and post-neonatal onset of early congenital syphillis: A report from Mozambique. *Annal Tropica Paediatrica* 12(4):445–450, 1992.

144. P. Zuber and P. Jacquier. [Epidemiology of toxoplasmosis: worldwide status]. *Schweizerische Medizinische Wochenschrift.* Supplementum 65:S19–S22, 1995.

145. P. Sharma, I. Gupta, N.K. Ganguly, R.C. Mahajan, and N. Malla. Increasing toxoplasma seropositivity in women with bad obstetric history and in newborn. *National Medical Journal of India* Mar-Apr;10(2):65–66, 1997.

146. A. el-Nawawy, A.T. Soliman, O. el Azzouni, el-S Amer, M.A. Karim, S. Demian, et al. Maternal and neonatal prevalence of toxoplasma and cytomegalovirus (CMV) antibodies and hepatitis-B antigens in an Egyptian rural areas. *Journal of Tropical Pediatrics* Jun;42(3):154–157, 1996.

147. M.D. de Jong, G.J. Galasso, B. Gazzard, P.D. Griffiths, D.A. Jabs, E.R. Kern, et al. Summary of the II International Symposium on Cytomegalovirus. *Antiviral Research* Oct;39(3):141–162, 1998.

148. N. O'Farrell. Increasing prevalence of genital herpes in developing countries: Implications for heterosexual HIV transmission and STI control programmes. *Sexual Transmission and Infection* Dec;75(6):377–384, 1999.

149. L. Boylan and Z. Stein. The epidemiology of HIV infection in children and their mothers—vertical transmission. *Epidemiologic Reviews* 13: 143–177, 1991.

150. S.F. Davis, D.H. Rosen, S. Steinberg, P.M. Wortley, J.M. Karon, and M. Gwinn. Trends in HIV prevalence among childbearing women in the United States, 1989–1994. *JAIDS: The Journal of Acquired Immune Deficiency Syndromes* 19(2):158–164, 1998.

151. H.S. Amar, J.J. Ho, and A.J. Mohan. Human immunodeficiency virus prevalence in women at delivery using unlinked anonymous testing of newborns in the Malaysian setting. *Journal of Paediatrics and Child Health* 35(1): 63–66, 1999.

152. E.M. Connor, R.S. Sperling, R. Gelber, P. Kiselev, G. Scott, M.J. O'Sullivan, et al. Reduction of maternal-infant transmission of human immunodeficiency virus type 1 with zidovudine treatment. *New England Journal of Medicine* 331(180):1173–1180, 1994.

153. European Mode of Delivery Collaboration. Elective caesarean-section versus vaginal delivery in prevention of vertical HIV-1 transmission: A randomized clinical trial. *Lancet* 353(9158): 1030–1031, 1999.

154. International Perinatal HIV Group. The mode of delivery and the risk of vertical transmission of human immunodeficiency virus type 1: A meta-analysis of 15 prospective cohort studies. *New England Journal of Medicine* 340(13),977–987, 1999.

155. L.M. Mofenson. Short-course zidovudine for prevention of perinatal infection. *Lancet*; 353:766–767, 1999.

156. C. Chase, J. Ware, J. Hittleman, I. Blasini, R. Smith, A. Llorente et al. Early cognitive and motor development among infants born to women infected with human immunodeficiency virus. Women and Infants Transmission Study Group. *Pediatrics* Aug;106(2):E25, 2000.

157. A.L. Belman. AIDS and pediatric neurology. *Neurologic Clinics of North America.* 8(3): 571–602, 1992.

158. R.A Oberhelman, E.S. Guerrero, M.L. Fernandez, M. Silio, D. Mercado, N. Comiskey, et al. Correlations between intestinal parasitosis, physical growth, and psychomotor development among infants and children from rural Nicaragua. *American Journal of Tropical Medical Hygiene* Apr;58(4):470–475, 1998.

159. A.O. Coker, R.D. Isokpehi, B.N. Thomas, A.F. Fagbenro-Beyioku, and S.A. Omilabu. Zoonotic infections in Nigeria: Overview from a medical perspective. *Acta Tropica* Jul 21;76(1):59–63, 2000.

160. J.S. Remington, R. McLeod, and G. Desmonts. Toxoplasmosis. In: *Infectious Diseases of the Fetus and Newborn Infant, 4th edn.* Remington, J.S. and Klein, J.O., eds.W.B. Saunders: Philadelphia, pp. 140–267, 1995.

161. D. Dunn, M. Wallon, F. Peyron, E. Peterson, C. Peckham, and R. Gilbert. Mother-to-child transmission of toxoplasmosis: Risk estimates for clinical counselling. *Lancet* 353: 1929–1933, 1999.

162. J. Koppe, D. Loewer-Sieger, and H.de Roever-Bonnet. Results of 20 year follow-up of congenital toxoplasmosis. *Lancet* ii: 254–256, 1986.

163. N. Roizen, C.N. Swisher, and M. A. Stein. Neurologic and developmental outcome in treated congenital toxoplasmosis. *Pediatrics* 95: 11–20, 1995.

164. World Health Organization Haemophilus influenzae type b. Available: http://www.who.int/inf-fs/en/fact 105.html. 1998a.

165. World Health Organization. Malaria. Available: http://www.who.int/inf-fs/en/fact094.html, 1998b.

166. World Health Organization. Epidemic meningococcal disease, Fact Sheet Number 105. Available: http://www.who.org/vaccines-diseases/diseases.hib.html, 2000.

167. D. Nabarro. Roll back malaria. *Parasitologia* 41:501–504, 1999.

168. B.J. Brabin. The risks and severity of malaria in pregnant women. In: *Applied Field Research in Malaria.* Report No.1. WHO: Geneva, pp.1–34, 1991.

169. C. Menendez. Malaria during pregnancy: A priority area of malaria research and control. *Parasitologia Today* 11:178–183, 1995.

170. G. Norheim, E. Rosenqvist, P. Aavitsland, and D. A. Caugant. Meningococcal disease in Africa-Epidemiology and prevention. *Tidsskrift for den Norske Laegoforening* Jun 10;120(15):1735–1739, 2000.

171. T. Goetghebuer, T. E. West, V. Wermenbol, A. L. Cadbury, P. Milligan, N. Lloyd-Evans, and R. A. Adegbola. Outcome of meningitis caused by *Streptococcus pneumoniae* and *Haemophilus influenzae* type b in children in The Gambia. *Tropical Medicine and International Health* Mar;5(3):207–213, 2000.

172. G.O. Akpede, S.O. Dawodu, and M. E. Umoffia. Response to antimicrobial therapy in childhood bacterial meningitis in tropical Africa: report of a bi-centre experience in Nigeria, 1993–1998. *Annals of Tropical Paediatrics* Sep;19(3):237–243, 1999.

173. M. A. Bouskela, S. Grisi, and A.M. Escobar. Epidemiologic aspects of *Haemophilus influenzae* type b infection. *Review of Panama Salud Publica* May;7(5):332–339, 2000.

174. P.M. Kurkdjian, A. Bourrillon, L. Holvoet-Vermau, and E. Bingen. Pathology of Haemophilus infections: Current situation in pediatrics. *Archives of Pediatrics* Jun;7(3):S551–558, 2000.

175. K.T. Wong. Annotation: Emerging and re-emerging epidemic encephalitis: A tale of two viruses. *Neuropathology Applied Neurobiology* Aug;26(4):313–318, 2000.

176. T.J. Victoria, M. Malathi, V. Ravi, G. Palani, and N.C. Appavoo. First outbreak of Japanese encephalitis in two villages of Dharmapuri district in Tamil Nadu. *Indian Journal of Medical Research* Dec;112:193–197, 2000.

177. D. Lou, J. Song, H. Ying, R. Yao, and Z. Wang. Prognostic factors of early sequelae and fatal outcome of Japanese encephalitis. *Southeast Asian Journal of Tropical Medicine and Public Health* Dec;26(4):694–698, 1995.

178. B.V. Huy, H.C. Tu, T.V. Luan, and R. Lindqvist. Early mental and neurological sequelae after Japanese B encephalitis. *Southeast Asian Journal of Tropical Medicine and Public Health* Sep;25(3):549–553, 1994.

179. R. Kumar, A. Mathur, K.B. Singh, P. Sitholey, M. Prasad, R. Shukla, et al. Clinical sequelae of Japanese encephalitis in children. *Indian Journal of Medical Research* Jan;97:9–13, 1993

180. H.K. Hartter, O.I. Oyedele, K. Dietz, S. Kreis, J.P. Hoffman, and C.P. Muller. Placental transfer and decay of maternally acquired antimeasles antibodies in Nigerian children. *Pediatric Infectious Disease Journal* Jul;19(7):635–641, 2000.

181. P.V. Taneja and N.G. Vaidya. Infant and child mortality in Bhil tribe of Jhabua district. *Indian Journal of Pediatrics*. May-Jun;64(3):409–413, 1997.

182. M. Hodges and R.A. Williams. Registered infant and under-five deaths in Freetown, Sierra Leone from 1987–1991 and a comparison with 1969–1979. *West African Journal of Medicine* Apr-Jun;17(2):95–98, 1998.

183. P.M. Strebel. Measles. *Bulletin of the World Health Organization* 76 (Suppl. 2):154–155,1998

184. A.S. Narita and H.R. Taylor. Blindness in the tropics. *Medical Journal of Australia* Sep 29;159(6):416–420, 1993.

185. R. Whitfield, L. Schwab, D. Ross-Degnan, P. Steinkuller, and J. Swartwood. Blindness and eye disease in Kenya: ocular status survey results form the Kenya Rural Blindness Prevention Project. *British Journal of Ophthalmology* Jun;74(6):333–340, 1990.

186. S.M. Shukla. Eye diseases and control of blindness in Zambia. *Social Science and Medicine* 17(22):1781–1783, 1983.

187. World Health Organization. Global Polio Eradication Initiative. Available: http://www.who.polioeradication.org/global_status.html, 2000.

188. S. Awasthi and V.K. Pande. Cause-specific mortality in under five in the urban slums of Lucknow, north India. *Journal of Tropical Pediatrics* Dec;44(60):358–361, 1998.

189. J.A. Owa and A.I. Osinaike. Neonatal morbidity and mortality in Nigeria. *Indian Journal of Pediatrics* May–Jun;65(3):441–449, 1998.

190. K. Jamil, A. Bhuiya, K. Streatfield, and N. Chakrabarty. The immunization programme in Bangladesh: Impressive gains in coverage, but gaps remain. *Health Policy and Planning* Mar;14(1):49–58, 1999.

191. J.A. Cook. Trachoma. *Bulletin of the World Health Organization* 76(Suppl. 2):139–140, 1998.

192. P.J. Dolin, H. Faal, G.J. Johnson, D. Minassian, S. Sowa, S. Day et al. Reduction of trachoma in a sub-Saharan village in absence of a disease control programme. *Lancet* May 24;349(9064):1511–1512, 1997.

193. D. Kaimbo W.A. Kaimbo and L. Missotten. Ocular refraction in Zaire. Bulletin de la Societe Belge D'Ophtalmologie 261:101–105, 1996.

194. A. Kumar, P. K. Dey, P.N. Singla, R. S. Ambasht, and S.K. Upadhyay. Blood lead levels in children with neurological disorders. *Journal of Tropical Pediatrics* 44(6): 320–322, 1998.

195. N.Z. Khan and A.H. Khan. Lead poisoning and psychomotor delay in Bangladeshi children. *Lancet* 353:754, 1999.
196. H.L. Needleman and C.A.Gatsonis. Low-level lead exposure and the IQ of children. A meta-analysis of modern studies. *Journal of the American Medical Association* Feb 2;263(5):673–678, 1990.
197. H. L. Needleman, M.A. Schell, D. Bellinger, A. Leviton, and E.N. Allred. The long-term effects of exposure to low doses of lead in childhood: An 11-year follow-up report. *New England Journal of Medicine* 322: 83–88, 1990.
198. J.M. Burns, P. A. Baghurst, M. G. Sawyer, A. J. McMichael, and S.L. Tong. Lifetime low-level exposure to environmental lead and children's emotional and behavioral development at ages 11–13 years. The Port Pirie Cohort Study. *American Journal of Epidemiology* 149(8): 740–749, 1990.
199. E. E. Castilla, P. Ashton-Prolla, E. Barreda-Mejia, D. Brunoni, D.P. Cavalcanti, J.L. Delgadillo, et al.. Thalidomide, a current teratogen in South America. *Teratology* 54:273–277, 1996.
200. J.L. Jacobson and S.W. Jacobson. Intellectual impairment in children exposed to polychlorinated biphenyls in utero. *New England Journal of Medicine* 335:783–789, 1996.
201. M.C. Ramsey and C.R. Reynolds. Does smoking by pregnant women influence IQ, birth weight, and developmental disabilities in their infants? A methodological review and multivariate analysis. *Neuropsychology Review* 10(1):1–40, 2000
202. N. Breslau, J.E. DelDotto, and G.G. Brown. A gradient relationship between low birth weight and IQ at age 6 years. *Archives of Pediatric and Adolescent Medicine* 148: 377–383, 1994.
203. World Health Organization. Control of Major Blinding Diseases and Disorders, Fact Sheet Number 214.Available: http://www.who.int/inf-fs/en/fact214.html, 2000.
204. M.J. Wolf, B. Wolf, G. Beunen, and P. Casaer. Neurodevelopmental outcome at 1 year in Zimbabwean neonates with extreme hyperbilirubinemia. *European Journal of Pediatrics*, 158(2):111–114, 1999.
205. M.S. Durkin, N.Z. Khan, L.L. Davidson, S. Huq, S. Munir, I. Rasul, and S. S. Zaman. Prenatal and postnatal risk factors for mental retardation among children in Bangladesh. *American Journal of Epidemiology*, (in press).
206. Z. A. Stein and M. W. Susser. The epidemiology of mental retardation. In: *Stress and Disability in Childhood.* Butler, N.R. and Connor, B.D., eds.. Wright, Bristol, pp.21–46, 1984.
207. S. Islam, M. S. Durkin, and S.S. Zaman. Socioeconomic status and the prevalence of mental retardation in Bangladesh. *Mental Retardation* December; 31(6):412–417, 1993.
208. M. F. Lechat. The epidemiology of health effects of disasters. *Epidemiologic Reviews* 12:192–198, 1990.
209. G. S. Smith and P. Barss. Unintentional injuries in developing countries: The epidemiology of a neglected problem. *Epidemiologic Reviews* 13:228–266,1991.
210. P. Chabasse. The proliferation of anti-personnel landmines in developing countries: Considerable damage in human terms and a dramatically insufficient medico-social response. In: International Committee of the Red Cross. Symposium on Antipersonnel Mines. Montreux, 21–23 April, 1993. International Committee of the Red Cross Report: Geneva, pp. 85–95, 1993.

211. N.Z. Khan and M.A. Lynch. Recognizing child maltreatment in Bangladesh. *Child Abuse & Neglect* 21(8):815–818, 1997.

212. C. N. Mock, F. Abantanga, P. Cummings, and T. D. Koepsell. Incidence and outcome of injury in Ghana: A community-based survey. *Bulletin of the World Health Organization* 77(12):955–964, 1999.

213. A.A. al-Qudah. Clinical patterns of neuronal migrational disorders and parental consanguinity. *Journal of Tropical Pediatrics*. Dec;44(6):351–354, 1998.

214. A. Mutirangura, T. Norapucsunton, Y. Tannirandorn, and S. Jongpiputvanich. DNA diagnosis for clinical and prenatal diagnosis of spinal muscular atrophy in Thai patients. *Journal of the Medical Association of Thailand* Dec;79(1):S11–S14, 1996.

215. I.C. Verma. Molecular diagnosis of neurological disorders in India. *Indian Journal of Pediatrics* Sep–Oct;64(5):661–666, 1997.

216. B. Underwood. Perspectives from micronutrient malnutrition elimination/eradication programmes. *Bulletin of the World Health Organization* 76(Suppl. 2):34–37, 1998.

217. C. Bellamy. *The State of the World's Children 2001*. UNICEF: OxfordUniversity Press; Oxford, England, 2001.

218. WHO (World Health Organization). *Bulletin of the World Health Organization*. World Health Organization: Geneva 76, Suppl. 2:118–120, 1998.

219. B. Elnager, M. Eltom, F.A. Karlsson, P.P. Bourdoux, and M. Gebre-Medhin. Control of iodine deficiency using iodination of water in a goiter endemic area. *International Journal of Food Sciences and Nutrition* 48(2): 119–127, 1997.

220. UNICEF. Percent of household using iodized salt. http://www.unicef.org/statis/country_pick.cgi, 2000.

221. C.P. Howson, E.T. Kennedy, A. Horwitz, eds. *Prevention of Micronutrient Deficiencies: Tools for Policymakers and Public Health Workers*. National Academy Press: Washington, D.C., 1998.

222. WHO (World Health Organization). *Bulletin of the World Health Organization*. WHO: Geneva 76 suppl 2:156–157, 1998.

223. R.W. Steketee, J.J. Wirima, A.W. Hightower, L. Slutsker, D.L. Heymann, and J.G. Breman. The effect of malaria and malaria prevention in pregnancy on offspring birthweight, prematurity, and intrauterine growth retardation in rural Malawi. *American Journal of Tropical Medical Hygiene* 55(1):33–41, 1996.

224. M.E. Parise, J.G. Ayisi, B.L. Nahlen, L.J. Schultz, J.M. Roberts, A. Misore, et al. Efficacy of sulfadoxine-pyrimethamine for prevention of placental malaria in an area of Kenya with a high prevalence of malaria and human immunodeficiency virus infection. *American Journal of Tropical Medical Hygiene* 59:813–822, 1998.

225. O.S. Levine, B. Schwartz, N. Pierce, and M. Kane. Development, evaluation and implementation of *Haemophilus influenzae* type b vaccines for young children in developing countries: Current status and priority actions. *Pediatric Infectious Diseases* 17:95–113, 1998.

226. T. Siraprapasiri, W. Sawaddiwudhipong, and S. Rojanasuphot. Cost benefit analysis of Japanese encephalitis vaccination program in Thailand. *Southeast Asian Journal of Tropical Medicine and Public Health* 28(1):143–148, 1997.

227. P. Bonnanni. Demographic impact of vaccination: A review. *Vaccine* Oct 29;17(3):S120–125, 1999.

228. T.A. Ruff. Immunization strategies for viral diseases in developing countries. *Review of Medical Virology* Apr–Jun;9(2):121–138, 1999

229. R.B. Aylward, H.F. Hull, S.L. Cochi, R.W. Sutter, J.M. Olive and B. Melgaard. Disease eradication as a public health strategy: A case study of poliomyelitis eradication. *Bulletin of the World Health Organization* 78(3):285–297, 2000.

230. L. Kuhn and Z. Stein. Infant survival, HIV infection, and feeding alternatives in less-developed countries. *American Journal of Public Health* 87(6):926–931, 1997.

231. N.A. Wade, G.S. Birkhead, B.L. Warren, T.T. Charbonneau, P.T. French, and L. Wang. Abbreviated regimens of zidovudine prophylaxis and perinatal transmission of the human immunodeficiency virus. *New England Journal of Medicine* 339(20): 1409–1414, 1998

232. N.T. Rotta, C. Silva, L. Ohlweiler, I. Lago, R. Cabral, F. Goncalves et al. AIDS neurologic manifestations in childhood. *Review of Neurology* Aug 16–31;29(4):319–322, 1999.

233. C. Butler, J. Hittelman, and S.B. Hauger. Guidelines for the care of children and adolescents with HIV infection. Approach to neurodevelopmental and neurologic complications in pediatric HIV infection. *Journal of Pediatrics* Jul;119(1 Pt 2):S41–46, 1991.

234. H.L. Needleman. Childhood lead poisoning: A disease for the history texts. *American Journal of Public Health* 81(6): 685–687, 1991

235. A.R. Kemper, W.C. Bordley, and S.M. Downs. Cost-effectiveness analysis of lead poisoning screening strategies following the 1997 guidelines of the Centers for Disease Control and Prevention. *Archives of Pediatrics & Adolescent Medicine* 152(12): 1202–1208, 1998.

236. S.J. Rolnick, J. Nordin, and L.M. Cherney. A comparison of costs of universal versus targeted lead screening for young children. *Environmental Research* 80(1): 84–91, 1999.

237. J.S. Bajaj, A. Misra, M. Rajalakshmi, and R. Madan. Environmental release of chemicals and reproductive ecology. *Environmental Health Perspectives* 101(Suppl. 2):125–130, 1993.

238. E.E. Castilla, J.S. Lopez-Camelo, G.P. Dutra, and J.E. Paz. Birth defects monitoring in underdeveloped countries: An example from Uruguay. *International Journal of Risk & Safety in Medicine* 2:271–288, 1991.

239. M.A. Koblinsky, O. Campbell, and J. Heichelheim. Organizing delivery care: What works for safe motherhood? *Bulletin of the World Health Organization* 77(5):399–406, 1999.

240. A.T. Bang, R.A. Bang, S.B. Baitule, M.H. Reddy, and M.D. Deshmuck. Effect of home-based care and management of sepsis on neonatal mortality: Field trial in rural India. *Lancet* 354(9194):1955–1961, 1999.

241. P.M. Shah. Birth asphyxia: A crucial issue in the prevention of developmental disabilities. *Midwifery* Jun;6(2):99–107, 1990.

242. United Nations General Assembly, *Convention on the Rights of the Child*. 1989.

243. J.E. Keefe, J.E. Lovie-Kitchin, H. Maclean, and H.R. Taylor. A simplified screening test for identifying people with low vision in developing countries. *Bulletin of the World Health Organization* 74(5):525–532, 1996.

244. S.J. Hornby, S. Adolph, V.K. Gothwal, C.E. Gilbert, L. Dandona, A. Foster, et al. Requirements for optical services in children with microphthalmos, coloboma and microcornea in southern India. *Eye* Apr;14(PT 2):219–224, 2000.

245. R. Gopal, S.R. Hugo, and B. Louw. Identification and follow-up of children with hearing loss in Mauritius. *International Journal of Pediatrics and Otorhinolaryngology* Feb;57(2):99–113, 2001.

246. V.E. Newton, I.I. Macharia, P. Mugwe, B. Ototo, and S.W. Kan. Evaluation of the use of a questionnaire to detect hearing loss in Kenyan pre-school children. *International Journal of Pediatrics and Otorhinolaryngology* Mar 1;57(3):229–234, 2001.

247. B.O. Olusanya, A.A. Okolo, and G.T. Ijaduola. The hearing profile of Nigerian school children. *International Journal of Pediatrics and Otorhinolaryngology* Oct 16;55(3):173–179, 2000.

248. H. Furuta and T. Yoshino. The present situation of the use of hearing aids in rural areas of Sri Lanka: Problems and future prospects. *International Journal of Rehabilitative Research* Mar;21(1):103–107, 1998.

249. C.A. Prescott, S.S. Omoding, J. Fermor, and D. Ogilvy. An evaluation of the 'voice test' as a method for assessing hearing in children with particular reference to the situation in developing countries. *International Journal of Pediatrics and Otorhinolaryngology* Dec 15;51(3):165–170, 1999.

250. S. Ramaa. Two decades of research on learning disabilities in India. *Dyslexia* Oct-Dec;6(4):268–283, 2000.

251. B. O'Toole and R. McConkey. A training strategy for personnel working in developing countries. *International Journal of Rehabilitative Research* Sep;21(3):311–321, 1998.

252. L.M. Stough and A.R. Aguirre-Roy. Learning disabilities in Costa Rica: Challenges for an "army of teachers." *Journal of Learning Disabilities* Sep–Oct;30(50):566–571, 1997.

253. D.E. Bender, C. Auer, J. Baran, S. Rodriguez, and R. Simeonsson. Assessment of infant and early childhood development in a periurban Bolivian population. *International Journal of Rehabilitative Research* Mar;17(1):75–81, 1994.

254. M.J. Armstrong. Disability self-help organizations in the developing world: A case study from Malaysia. *International Journal of Rehabilitative Research* Sep;16(3):185–194, 1993.

255. UNESCO and the Ministry of Education and Science, Spain. The Salamanca Statement. The Final Report of the World Conference on Special Needs Education, Access and Quality. United Nations Educational, Scientific and Cultural Organization: Paris, 1994.

256. ILO, UNESCO, WHO. *Community Based Rehabilitation for and with People with Disabilities.* Joint Position Paper, World Health Organization: Geneva, 1994.

257. N.E. Groce. Disability in cross-cultural perspective: Rethinking disability. *Lancet* 354(9180):756–757, 1999.

258. World Health Organization(WHO). *International Classification of Impairments, Disabilities and Handicaps.* World Health Organization: Geneva, 1980.

259. R.J. Simeonsson, D. Lollar, J. Hollowell, and M. Adams. Revision of the International Classification of Impairments, Disabilities and Handicaps: Developmental issues. *Journal of Clinical Epidemiology* 53:113–124, 2000.

260. M.J. Thorburn. Recent developments in low-cost screening and assessment of childhood disabilities in Jamaica. Part I: Screening. *West Indian Medical Journal* Mar;42(1):10–20, 1993.

261. M.J. Thorburn , T.J. Paul, and L.M. Malcolm. Recent developments in low-cost screening and assessment of childhood disabilities in Jamaica. Part II: Assessment. *West Indian Medical Journal* Jun;42(2):46–52, 1993.

262. T. Jonsson. OMAR in rehabilitation: *A Guide on Operations Monitoring and Results*. UNDP Interregional Programme for Disabled People. United Nations Development Program: Geneva, 1994.

263. E. Helander, P. Mendis, and G. Nelson. *Training Disabled People in the Community*. World Health Organization: Geneva, 1979–1991.

264. World Health Organization (WHO). *Promoting the Development of Young Children with Cerebral Palsy: A Guide for Mid-Level Rehabilitation Workers*. World Health Organization: Geneva, 1993.

265. D. Werner. *Disabled Village Children*. Hesperian Foundation: Palo Alto, CA, 1988.

266. E. Haddad. *World Declaration of Education for All*. UNESCO: Paris, 1990.

267. M.J. Thorburn. Training of CBR personnel: Current issues and future trends. *Asia Pacific Disability Rehabilitation Journal* 11:12–17, 2000.

268. R. McConkey and B. O'Toole. Towards the new millenium. In: *Developing Countries for People with Disabilities*. O'Toole, B. and McConkey, R., eds.. Lisieux Hall Publications: Chorley, Lancs, England, p. 8, 1999.

269. S.S. Zaman, N. Khan, S. Islam, S. Banu, P. Dixit, P. Shrout, et al. Validity of the Ten Questions for screening serious childhood disability: Results from urban Bangladesh. *International Journal of Epidemiology* 19(3):613–620, 1990.

270. S.S. Zaman, N.Z. Khan, and S. Islam, eds. *From Awareness to Action: Ensuring Health, Education and Rights of Disabled*. Bangladesh Protibondhi Foundation: Dhaka, 1996.

271. H. McConachie, S. Huq, S. Munir, S. Ferdous, S. S. Zaman, and N. Z. Khan. A randomized controlled trial of alternative modes of service provision for children with cerebral palsy in Bangladesh. *Journal of Pediatrics* 137(6):769–776, 2000.

272. K.M. Munir and W.R. Beardslee. Developmental psychiatry: Is there any other kind? *Harvard Review of Psychiatry* Jan–Feb;6(5):250–262, 1999.

273. Zimbabwe Ministry of Education, Sports and Culture. *School Psychological Services and Special Needs Education*. Annual Report 1998.

274. G. Powell. *Report on Childhood Disability in Sub-Saharan Africa*. Department of Pediatrics and Child Health, University of Zimbabwe Medical School; Harare, 2000.

275. L. Mariga and L. Phachaka. *Integrating Children with Special Education Needs into Regular Schools in Lesotho. Report of a Feasibility Study.* UNICEF: Lesotho, 1993.

276. H. House et al. *Zimbabwe Steps Ahead.* Russell Publications: Nottingham, U.K., 1990.

277. S. Chidayausiku. *Community Based Rehabilitation Programme in Zimbabwe, Sida Evaluation* 15, 1998.

278. N.J. Cook and N.K. Rogers. Blindness and poverty go hand in hand. *Acta Ophthalmologica Scandinavica* Apr;74(2):204–209, 1996.

279. A. Kroeger, M. Gonzalez, and J. Ordonez-Gonzalez. Insecticide-treated materials for malaria control in Latin America: To use or not to use? *Transactions of the Royal Society of Tropical Medicine and Hygiene* Nov–Dec;93(6):565–570, 1999.

280. D.T. Jamison and W.H. Mosley. Disease control priorities in developing countries: health policy responses to epidemiological change. *American Journal of Public Health* Jan;81(1):15–22, 1991.

281. WHO-WAOPBD. *Services for the Prevention and Management of Genetic Disorders and Birth Defects in Developing Countries.* Report from Joint WHO-WAOPBD Meeting on Prevention and Care of Genetic Diseases and Birth Defects in Developing Countries. The Hague, 5–7 Jan. 1999; World Health Organization Genetics Unit: Geneva, (in press).

282. S. Hartley. Service development to meet the needs of 'people with communication disabilities' in developing countries. *Disability Rehabilitation* Aug;20(8):277–284, 1998.

283. M. Gracey. The pediatrician's role in the twenty-first century. *Acta Paediatrica Japan* Oct;40(5):393–399, 1998.

284. D. Shah, S. Shroff, and S. Sheth. Reproductive and sexual health and safe motherhood in the developing world. *European Journal of Contraception and Reproductive Health Care* Dec;4(4):217–228, 1999.

285. G.L. Stidham. Emergencies in international child health. *Current Opinon Pediatrics* Jun;9(3):254–258, 1997.

286. O.F. Fafowora. Some practical aspects of teaching medicine in Africa. *African Journal of Medicine and Medical Science* Jun;23(2):187–188, 1994.

287. P.W. Alberti. Health care economics: Impact on hearing loss prevetion in the developing world. *Scandinavian Audiology* (supplement);42:49–51, 1996.

288. P. Huguet, A. Auzemery, J.F. Ceccon, and J.F. Schemann. The Institute of Tropical Ophthalmology of Africa. [French] *MARS* 55(4 Pt 2):466–468, 1995.

289. C. Boudet, P. Bensaid, and M.S. Sanner. Ophthalmologists without borders in Northern Cameroon. [French]. *MARS* 55(4 Pt 2);415–420, 1995.

290. N. Kinabo. Eye diseases and services in Tanzania. *Social Science and Medicine* 17(22):1767–1772, 1983.

291. R.A. Mitchell, D.H. Zhou, and G.H. Watts. Emerging patterns of disability distribution in developing countries. *International Disability Studies* Oct-Dec;11(4):145–148, 1989.

292. S.L. Wirz and I. Lichtig. The use of non-specialist personnel in providing a service for children disabled by hearing impairment. *Disability Rehabilitation* May;20(5):189–194, 1998.

293. P.W. Alberti. Pediatric ear, nose and throat services' demands and resources: a global perspective. *International Journal of Pediatric Otorhinolaryngology* Oct 5(supplement);49(1):S1–S9, 1999.

294. D. Morley. The spread of comprehensive care through under-fives' clinics. *Transactions of the Royal Society of Tropical Medicine and Hygiene* 67(2):155–170, 1973.

295. D. Morley. A medical service for children under five years of age in West Africa. *Transactions of the Royal Society of Tropical Medicine and Hygiene* 57:79–88, 1963.

296. N. Cunningham. The under fives clinic. What difference does it make? *Journal of Tropical Pediatrics and Environmental Child Health* Dec;24(6):239–334, 1978.

Summary of Findings:
Epilepsy in Developing Countries

- Eighty percent of the more than 40 million people with epilepsy live in developing countries, where cultural factors frequently exacerbate the burden of disease on patients and their families. Even when assistance is sought, a treatment gap as high as 90 percent still affects some rural populations in low-income countries.

- Many risk factors for epilepsy have been identified, including birth trauma, parasitic infections (most notably cysticercosis), bacterial and viral infections, head injuries, febrile seizures, and genetic factors. Local variation in risk factors at least partly explains the marked heterogeneity in the prevalence and incidence of the disease throughout the world.

- Key preventive measures likely to significantly reduce the incidence of epilepsy include prenatal care, avoidance of labor and delivery complications, safety measures against head injuries, control of infectious and parasitic diseases, and genetic counseling for potential marriage partners who have the disease.

- Phenobarbital is recommended for the treatment of partial and generalized tonic-clonic epilepsies in developing countries due to its efficacy for a wide range of seizure types, its low cost, and its superiority to both phenytoin and carbamazepine in recent community-level studies.

- The lack of adequate drug production facilities and high prices for imported drugs restrict the availablity of anti-epileptic drugs in developing countries.

6

Epilepsy

DEFINITION

In recent epidemiological studies, epilepsy is defined by the recurrent presentation of two or more unprovoked seizures. This definition excludes single afebrile episodes, febrile seizures, and seizures that are manifestations of altered metabolic states, alcohol or drug withdrawal, and other transient cerebral insults.[1–11]

The diagnosis of epilepsy thus defined is basically clinical, because no single laboratory test can confirm the absence of the condition. The test most commonly employed for the diagnosis of epileptic abnormalities is the electroencephalogram (EEG). While the EEG is a useful tool that can assist the clinician in arriving at a diagnosis of epilepsy, however, it is not always a sensitive or specific test.[3,4]

Epilepsy manifests with several types of seizures, differing in age of onset, response to treatment, prognosis, electroencephalographic correlates, and risk factors.[12] Moreover, epilepsy that is secondary to a parasitic infestation of the brain is a disorder altogether different from genetically determined epilepsies. Nonetheless, having a single term that encompasses all of these conditions makes it possible to calculate the burden of disease from both an economic and social perspective, to estimate the demand for health services planning, and to meet other public health objectives.[13] The diagnostic classification standard currently in place for epilepsy was established by the International League Against Epilepsy in 1989 (see Box 6-1).

BOX 6-1 International Classification of Epilepsies and Epileptic Syndromes

1. Localization-related (focal, local, partial) epilepsies and syndromes.
    1.1 Idiopathic (with age-related onset)
    At present, the following syndromes are established, but more may be identified in the future:
    - Benign childhood epilepsy with centro-temporal spike;
    - Childhood epilepsy with occipital paroxysms; and
    - Primary reading epilepsy.
    1.2 Symptomatic: This category comprises syndromes of individual variability, based mainly on anatomical localization, clinical features, seizure types, and etiological factors (if known).
        1.2.1 Epilepsy is characterized by simple partial seizures with the characteristics of seizures:
        - Arising from frontal lobes;
        - Arising from parietal lobes;
        - Arising from temporal lobes;
        - Arising from occipital lobes;
        - Arising from multiple lobes; and
        - Locus of onset unknown.
        1.2.2 Characterized by complex partial seizures, that is, attacks with alteration of consciousness, often with automatisms; characterized by seizures:
        - Arising from frontal lobes;
        - Arising from parietal lobes;
        - Arising from temporal lobes;
        - Arising from occipital lobes;
        - Arising from multiple lobes; and
        - Locus of onset unknown.
        1.2.3 Characterized by secondarily generalized seizures with seizures:
        - Arising from frontal lobes;
        - Arising from parietal lobes;
        - Arising from temporal lobes;
        - Arising from occipital lobes;
        - Arising from multiple lobes; and
        - Locus of onset unknown.
    1.3 Unknown as to whether the syndrome is idiopathic or symptomatic.
2. Generalized epilepsies and syndromes
    2.1 Idiopathic (with age-related onset—listed in order of age)
        - Benign neonatal familial convulsions;
        - Benign neonatal convulsions;
        - Benign myoclonic epilepsy in infancy;
        - Childhood absence epilepsy (pyknolepsy);
        - Juvenile absence epilepsy;
        - Juvenile myoclonic epilepsy (impulsive petit mal); and
        - Epilepsy with GTCS on awakening.

    Other generalized idiopathic epilepsies, if they do not belong to one of the above syndromes, can still be classified as generalized idiopathic epilepsies.

2.2 Cryptogenic or symptomatic (in order of age)
- West syndrome (infantile spasms, Blitz-Nick-Salaam Krampfe);
- Lennox Gastaut syndrome;
- Epilepsy with myoclonic-astatic seizures; and
- Epilepsy with myoclonic absences.

2.3 Symptomatic
2.3.1 Nonspecific etiology
- Early myoclonic encephalopathy

2.3.2 Specific syndromes
- Epileptic seizures may complicate many disease states.

Under this heading are included those diseases in which seizures are a presenting or predominant feature.

3. Epilepsies and syndromes undetermined as to whether focal or generalized

3.1 With bold generalized and focal seizures
- Neonatal seizures;
- Severe myoclonic epilepsy in infancy;
- Epilepsy with continuous spike waves during slow-wave sleep; and
- Acquired epileptic aphasia (Landau-Kleffner syndrome).

3.2 Without unequivocal generalized or focal features
All cases with GTCS where clinical and EEG findings do not permit classification as clearly generalized or localization-related, such as in many cases of GTCS during sleep.

4. Special syndromes
4.1 Situation-related seizures (Gelegenheitsanfalle)
- Febrile convulsions;
- Isolated seizures or isolated status epilepticus;
- Seizures occurring only when there is an acute metabolic or toxic event due to, for example, alcohol, drugs, eclampsia, nonketotic hyperglycemia, or uremia.

Source: [14]

SCOPE OF THE PROBLEM

Among brain disorders, epilepsy stands out not only because of its high prevalence and incidence rates, but in particular because of the myths and beliefs attached to the condition in various cultures and the resulting impacts on the individual, the family, and the community.[15–19] More than 40 million people worldwide have been estimated to suffer from epilepsy, and an estimated 80 percent of those individuals live in developing countries.[5,13,19] Epilepsy commonly attacks young adults in the most productive years of their lives and frequently leads to unemployment, which often confounds the problems not only of the afflicted, but also of the family that relies on their financial support.

Stigma and Discrimination

Epilepsy remains among the most stigmatized brain disorders.[13,20] The associated stigma is more obvious in developing countries because of illiteracy and misinformation regarding the actual nature of the condition. The shame and fear associated with the disorder prevent many affected individuals from seeking treatment. As a result, their epilepsy becomes uncontrolled, with consequences for education, employment opportunities, and social acceptance.[5,21,22]

Children with epilepsy are removed from school and as adults lack the basic education needed for self-sufficiency.[22,23] Traditional medicines dispensed for epileptic seizures may be administered to children with febrile seizures with devastating consequences, such as oral burns and aspiration pneumonia.[24] Those afflicted also frequently suffer crippling malformations or death due to burns, drowning, or other accidents.[25] In Africa, for example, where open fires are used for cooking and heating, up to 30 percent of severe burns result from seizures. Because of the pervasive belief that epilepsy either is contagious or represents demonic possession, even family members may not act to pull these epilepsy sufferers from the flames.[18,26–29] Studies reveal that females with epilepsy are also less likely to marry and have children.[30] Consequently, these women are rejected by their families and often left to means of survival that include prostitution, which significantly increases their vulnerability to many sexually transmitted diseases, particularly HIV/AIDS.[18]

Treatment Gap

Even when proper medical treatment is sought and provided, patients do not recognize that long-term adherence to medications is required. The ensuing lack of adherence to treatment leads to seizure recurrences and a repetitive cycle of the social and physical burdens associated with the disorders. A treatment gap as high as 90 percent still affects many populations.[31,32] Other important factors contribute to the treatment gap, including cultural attitudes toward treatment, such as attributing the source of the illness to possession of the spirit or "the devil within." Beliefs such as these provoke individuals to seek help from traditional healers and local religious figures [33–35] and do not lead them to effective medical treatments.[27]

Epidemiological studies reveal that the prevalence of epilepsy in developing countries is higher in rural than in urban populations. Reasons for this may include inadequate medical care facilities in remote areas for pregnancy control, safe delivery methods, early detection and treatment of childhood infections, and prompt and comprehensive health care.[27] Cultural factors such as ignorance, fear, and rural illiteracy (higher than among urban populations) lead to a delay in seeking early diagnosis and treatment and compound the burden of epilepsy in these poorer regions.

In developing countries, total earnings per capita per year amount to less than what one patient with epilepsy spends on treatment annually in developed countries. It has been calculated that the gross national product per capita of most developing countries barely suffices to buy a 2-year supply of carbamazepine or valproic acid for one patient at the price at which it is sold in Europe. Therefore, monetary considerations often outweigh clinical judgment in therapeutic decisions.[34]

The availablity of anti-epileptic drugs (AEDs) in developing countries is limited because of poor drug production facilities and the inability of epilepsy sufferers to pay for the drugs. Indeed, it has been found that the developing countries, with 75 percent of the world's population, consume only 21 percent of the drugs produced globally, with drug consumption per capita being 12 times below that in the developed world.[33] Notable defects of the drug distribution systems in developing countries include a lack of suitable storage facilities, logistic coordination, and transportation, and a lack of midlevel management skills in inventorying, ordering, and stock control.[34] Poor quality control of domestically produced drugs may also be an important issue in developing countries.[33] The problems of drug supply, coupled with inadequacies in the systems for delivery of health care, prevent many from receiving the care they need.[33,34] For more information on the costs of treating epilepsy see Appendix D.

Infectious Diseases

A multitude of infectious diseases are risk factors for epilepsy. Rates of prevalence for these diseases remain high in developing countries and contribute significantly to the higher prevalence of epilepsy in these regions as compared with developed countries.[6]

Recommendation 6-1. To effectively address the needs of individuals with epilepsy and reduce the widespread stigma attached to the disease, national and local governments and health authorities of developing countries should support public education campaigns focused on the causes of epilepsy, the impact of the disease on the afflicted, and the availability of safe and effective treatments. Additionally, the rights of individuals with epilepsy under adequate treatment should be enforced to allow them equal access to employment, driving, and marriage.

PREVALENCE AND INCIDENCE

A number of recent neuroepidemiolgical studies provide fairly accurate data on the prevalence and incidence of epilepsy in various geographic regions of the world (see Tables 6-2 and 6-3).[1–4,7–11,36–41] However, the comparability of these data is limited because of the lack of consistency in diagnostic definitions and methodology. Additionally, local variations in the prevalence of risk factors and genetic factors that may predispose individuals to develop epilepsy have undoubtedly contributed to the marked heterogeneity in epilepsy prevalence and incidence throughout the world.[11,40–42]

The available community-based prevalence data on epilepsy are rather consistent for industrialized countries. The prevalence rates range from 3.3/1000 population in England to 6.6/1000 in the United States.[17] Studies in developing countries reveal much higher rates: 17/1000 in Ecuador,[1] 26–40/1000 in Liberia,[43] and 20/1000 in Tanzania.[38] The People's Republic of China (PRC) reports a rate of 4.6/1000 [2] and some areas of Uganda have recorded rates as high as 57/1000.[44]

A number of epidemiological studies have been conducted in India during the last three decades to determine the prevalence of epilepsy.[45,46] Careful scrutiny of the methodology and analysis of these studies reveals that 12 of them included house-to-house surveys with sound methodology and are comparable. The studies were conducted in various regions of India, representing populations from the north, south, east, and west of the country. They included both urban and rural populations. The prevalence rate of epilepsy was found to be 2.2–9.0/1000 population. A recent house-to-house survey included a large sample (102,557) of Bangalore urban and rural populations and showed a prevalence rate of 8.8/1000. The prevalence rate in the rural population was 11.9/1000 and in the urban population was 5.7/1000, highlighting the fact that the prevalence of epilepsy is two-fold higher in rural than in urban populations.[47] This large urban–rural difference calls for further case control studies to determine the risk factors involved, such as infections, trauma, obstetric practices, availability of health care facilities, and attitudes toward epilepsy.

TABLE 6-1 Prevalence rate of epilepsy in Africa (per 1,000 inhabitants)

Country	Inclusion Criteria	Prevalence Rate	Sampling Size	Method
Burkina-Faso [48]	RS	10.60	16,627	Community-based
Ethiopia [49, 50]		5 (urban)	3,700	Community-based
		8 (rural)		Community-based
		5.20	60,820	Community-based
Ivory Coast [48]	RS	7.60	1,176	Community-based
Liberia [51,52]	RS	28.00	4,436	Community-based
		43.00	2,733	Community-based
Nigeria [37, 53, 54]		3.01	2,592	Community-based
	RS	37.00	903	
	RS + EEG	5.30	18,951	
Senegal [55]	Generalized seizures	3.10	35,219	Community-based
South Africa [48]	RS	0.22–2.20	50,000	Community-based
			36,700	Mine workers
Tanzania [56]	RS	20.00	10,000	Community-based
Togo[57]	RS + EEG	2.30	19,241	Community-based
	RS	19.8	9,143	
Zimbabwe [58]		7.40	17,500	Community-based

TABLE 6-2 Prevalence rate of epilepsy in Latin American countries

Study	Country	Prevalence Rate[A]	Population	Year
Buenos Aires [59]	Argentina	3.7	6,194	1995
Bogota [60]	Colombia	19.5	8,970	1978
Cangahua [40]	Ecuador	14.3	72,121	1984
Changuinola [61]	Panama	57.0[B]	337	1988
Cordillera Province [62]	Bolivia	24.5	10,000	1999
Coyocan [63]	Mexico	16.0	1,013	1980
El Salvador [64]	Chile	17.7[B]	17,694	1988
Marianoa [65]	Cuba	7.5	14,445	1980
Medellin [66]	Colombia	21.4	4,549	1988
Melipilla [67]	Chile	27.6	2,085	1975
Migues [5]	Uruguay	9.1	1,975	1990
Palugillo [7]	Ecuador	22.6	221	1997
Porto Alegre [5]	Brazil	16.5		1997
Quiroga [1]	Ecuador	17.1	1,113	1985
Rural and urban population [5]	Colombia	13.2	9,800	1991
Sao Paulo [68]	Brazil	11.9		1986
Tecomatian [69]	Mexico	25.0–41.6	360	1975
Tlalpan [70]	Mexico	42.2	2,027	1976
V. del Cerro (present study) [5]	Uruguay	11.5	21,186	1993
Viacha (33)	Bolivia	26.2	1,183	1985
Z. Subtropical (23)	Ecuador	16.6	1,382	1984

[A] Per 1,000 inhabitants; includes active and nonactive epilepsy

[B] Includes only active epilepsy

The prevalence of epilepsy in developing countries increases with age, reaching a peak in the third and fourth decades. It is interesting to note that in developing countries, the prevalence rate diminishes among those aged 60 and above. This fact may be explained by the increased mortality of patients with epilepsy, spontaneous remission, and the low survival of individuals with seizure disorders due to stroke and brain tumors. Only in Rochester, Minnesota, in the United States has the population above age 60 shown an increased prevalence rate, probably reflecting the improved medical care and follow-up of such individuals.[17] As with the other age groups, the prevalence of epilepsy among children is highest in the most deprived areas of the world.[71]

Information on the incidence of epilepsy is widely available for developed countries, but the same information for developing countries is less complete. Reported figures range from 145/100,000 population per year for Japan [72,73]

to 48/100,000 per year in the United States.[28] Rates ranging from 109–190/100,000 per year have been reported for Ecuador.[12,74,75] Rates in Africa have ranged from 64/100,000 in Ethiopia [9] to 156/100,000 in Uganda.[44]

Community-based surveys have proven to be an effective method for evaluating the magnitude and distribution of the disease.[15,16] However, the results of such surveys are influenced by local cultural factors. If epilepsy carries a social stigma, which is commonly the case, patients suffering from the condition will be hidden from researchers by family members. Because of the difficulties and the expense of implementing door-to-door surveys, increased attention is being focused on the use of key community informants to identify patients suffering from epilepsy.[41,76–78] This strategy was applied success-fully, for example, in an urban marginal and rural region in Kenya.[33]

Mortality Rates

It is well known that mortality data based on the single cause of death listed on a death certificate often underrepresent the number of deaths due to predicating conditions such as epilepsy. Case fatality rates for epilepsy are low in developed countries, so that mortality statistics are not a good indicator of the frequency of the disease.[4] A community-based study done in Ethiopia revealed that 6.3 percent of patients with epilepsy had died over a 2-year period as a results of complications from the disease.[9] In Africa, epilepsy mortality has been shown to be related to status epilepticus, falls, drowning, suicide, and burns.[79] More research is needed to adequately understand this aspect of epileptic disease burden.

RISK FACTORS

Data collection on the epidemiology, etiology, and natural history of epilepsy have increased understanding of this devastating disease. Many of the risk factors for epilepsy have been identified, and understanding of their relative contribution to epilepsy incidence continues to improve.[19,80–84] It will be important for the development of efficacious and comprehensive programs for the prevention and treatment of epilepsy to further investigate and identify risk factors in developing country populations.

More recently, researchers have emphasized the importance of studying risk factors separately according to the different epilepsy types. It has also been stressed that taking into account the age of onset of epileptic disorders will increase study group homogeneity, therefore increasing the potential for identifying specific risk factors.[12,74,85,86]

Genetic

The risk of epilepsy is increased three-fold for individuals who have a first-degree relative with the condition.[87] In addition, a number of diseases that follow Mendelian patterns of inheritance may have seizures as one of their manifestations or their only manifestation. In many developing countries, consanguinity is relatively common. Such practices are likely to increase the risk of seizure disorders in any offspring. In isolated communities, specific inherited diseases may contribute to the etiology of epilepsy, as is the case in the Grand Bassa Country of Liberia and among the Wapagoro tribe in Tanzania.[43,88] However, a studied conducted in the Parsi community of Bombay showed no significant association between consanguinity and epilepsy despite the high frequency of consanguinious marriages.[81]

Pre-, Peri- and Post-Natal

In a community-based study in Ecuador,[12] significant risk factors for epilepsy starting before age 20 were found to be a positive family history (genetic factors), prematurity, perinatal hypoxia, sleep disorders in the first 3 months of life, and febrile seizures; for epilepsy starting at age 20 and above, only prematurity was found to be a significant risk factor. When the analysis was done according to seizure type, it was found that for generalized seizures, family history and febrile convulsions were significant risk factors, whereas for partial seizures, family history, prematurity, perinatal hypoxia, and sleep disorders were statistically significant factors.[12,74] Perinatal hypoxia is associated with epilepsy in developing countries as it relates to maternal and childhood malnutrition. In an Ecuadorean study, calculation of the population rate difference percentage suggested that programs aimed at controlling both prematurity and perinatal hypoxia could decrease the number of epilepsy cases by 42 percent.[12,74] In the PRC, carefully designed epidemiological studies found that the following were significant risk factors for idiopathic epilepsy: premature or difficult birth, maternal disease during pregnancy, febrile convulsions, family history for epilepsy, and maternal age above 30.[2,84] In Nigeria, the putative risk factors for epilepsy were found to be febrile convulsions, malnutrition, maternal alcohol consumption, and lack of immunizations.[37,83]

In developed countries, where acquired epilepsy constitutes about 40 percent of all cases, perinatal pathology is reported to be the cause of around 14 percent of all epilepsies.[85] In developing countries this figure should be higher, although there are no good community-based studies to provide such data. The causes of perinatal hypoxia include maternal cardiovascular disease, placental and umbilical cord disorders, prolonged labor, and airway obstruction at birth. In dystocic deliveries, the excessive reduction of fetal cranial diameter may lead to herniation of hippocampal regions through the tentorium, causing ischemia, atrophy, and subsequent gliosis of these structures (mesial sclerosis). These conditions in turn predispose to epilepsy and can now easily be visualized by magnetic resonance of the brain in individuals thus affected.[11,86,87]

In many developing countries, most deliveries in rural areas are performed by traditional birth attendants. Complications with delivery are common, and the incidence of preterm deliveries is at least twice that in developed countries.[89] Mothers in developing countries are frequently malnourished, anemic, and exposed to a variety of infections that could affect the baby in utero or at delivery and increase the risk for epilepsy.[19,86]

Parasitic Infections

Neurocysticercosis is caused by *Taenia solium* (more commonly known as tapeworm). This disease may account for up to two-thirds of late-onset epilepsy (epilepsy starting above age 20) in geographic regions in Africa, Asia, and Latin America in which this infection is endemic.[90–98] Rapid control of transmission of *T. solium* taeniosis from animal to human may be attained through a vaccine that renders pigs immune to cysticercosis.[99] (Additional information on neurocysticercosis as a risk factor for epilepsy and the implications for prevention and treatment can be found in Annex 6-1.)

Paragonomiasis, caused by the parasite *Paragonimus westermani*, is endemic to Asia, particularly Korea, Japan, the Philippines, and China, as well as some parts of Africa and South America. Epileptic seizures, usually focal motor, are a common manifestation of this condition.[11,100,101]

Schistosomiasis can also induce seizures. This is the case particularly with *S. japonicum* infections, and less commonly with *S. mansoni* and *S. haematobium* infections. Acute schistosomiasis may produce a serious encephalopathy with coma, papilledema, and partial or generalized seizures. Chronic forms of cerebral schistosomiasis, caused by embolized schistosoma eggs, are commonly manifested in epileptic attacks.[102]

Congenital toxoplasmosis, acquired during pregnancy, induces seizures in 40–60 percent of affected children, who may display mental retardation and blindness as well.[103–104] Toxoplasmosis is also a frequent opportunistic infection in patients with acquired immunodeficiency syndrome (AIDS), inducing seizures in about 25 percent of affected individuals.[105]

African trypanosomiasis, or sleeping sickness, is caused by *T. brucei*, and is widely distributed through sub-Saharan Africa. The chronic stage of the disease is characterized by progressive neurological involvement, including partial and generalized seizures.[106]

Chagas disease, caused by *T. cruzi*, is a public health problem in rural areas of Central and South America. Cerebral involvement is secondary to embolization of the parasite and manifests itself as a late-onset epilepsy, involving mainly partial seizures.[107]

Malaria is endemic to tropical Africa, Latin America, and Asia. Epilepsy is a late sequela of this common disease. Status epilepticus has been reported to occur in up to 13.6 percent of malaria cases. One-third of these occurrences are due to infection with *Plasmodium falciparum*, which produces the dreadful cerebral malaria.[87,105]

Epilepsy can also be a rare manifestation of other parasitic infections of the central nervous system, such as sparganosis [108,109] and onchocerciasis. [44,110,111]

Bacterial Infections

Tuberculous meningitis is highly prevalent in urban marginal and poor rural areas of most developing countries, but it is particularly important in Asia and certain African countries.[112–114] This infection can cause epilepsy as a late sequela in 8–14 percent of affected patients. Intracranial tuberculomas can present as space-occupying lesions and seizures.[115–117]

Pyogenic meningitis is also a common infection in the tropics, and epidemics of meningococcal meningitis occur periodically in Brazil and sub-Saharan Africa. In the United States, the overall risk for epilepsy was found to increase seven-fold among 734 survivors of intracranial infections; for individuals with a diagnosis of brain abscess, the risk was more than 40 times greater. The risk for epilepsy remains elevated in patients who have suffered from meningeal infections for at least 20 years after the illness.[118]

Viral Infections

Japanese encephalitis is perhaps the most important and best-documented form of epidemic viral encephalitis in developing countries.[119–121] Bangladesh, India, Nepal, Thailand, and Vietnam are the most affected areas. Epilepsy is a frequent manifestation, found in 1–20 percent of survivors.[122,123]

Human immunodeficiency virus (HIV) is often accompanied by seizure disorders. Up to 60 percent of patients with HIV in Africa have been diagnosed with epilepsy.[124] The rising epidemic of HIV/AIDS in Africa may soon be the leading cause of seizure disorders.

Head Injuries

In the United States severe head trauma accounted for 12 percent of epilepsy cases.[125] Annegers et al. found the risk slightly higher at 17.2 percent.[126] Head trauma related to road traffic accidents or violent assault is a very common cause of epilepsy in Brazil and Uruguay.[103,127] Occupational hazards and accidental falls due to poor safety conditions may also result in head injuries.[128–131] Head trauma is a preventable condition, and campaigns to reduce car and motorcycle accidents and other causes of these injuries may assist in reducing the occurrence of epilepsy.

Febrile Seizures

Febrile seizure is defined as an event in infancy or childhood, usually presenting between ages 3 months to 5 years, associated with fever, but without an intracranial infection or other defined cause. Febrile seizures occur in 2–4 percent of children, but rates as high as 14 percent have been reported in selected populations. Untreated fevers that lead to febrile seizures can increase the risk of developing epilepsy; however, studies show a low range of occurrence (from 1.5–7 percent) of epilepsy from febrile seizures.[81,132] The association between febrile seizures and later epilepsy are strong in studies from both developed and developing countries, however, the cause of this association remains unclear.[17,81,83] It is important to note that in areas where malaria is endemic, a child presenting with a febrile seizure may be harboring the plasmodium parasite. In some regions of Africa, 60 percent of seizure disorders seen in general hospitals in the first 6 years of life are related to malaria.[19,81–83,86]

INTERVENTIONS

Prevention

Many of the risk factors for epilepsy described in this chapter are preventable or modifiable. Such preventative measures could significantly reduce the incidence and prevalence of epilepsy in developing countries. Prevention programs that include the following components are recommended by this committee and included in WHO manuals for the primary prevention of epilepsy [133]:

- **Prenatal care**—immunization of pregnant women, improvement of mothers' nutritional status, detection of high-risk preganancies, and control of infectious diseases during pregnancy.
- **Safe delivery**—avoidance of labor and delivery complications, labor surveillance, and detection and urgent treatment of neonatal hypoxia.
- **Fever control in children**—avoidance of febrile illnesses in children, especially those prevented by vaccines; control of increases in temperature by antipyretic drugs or physical cooling agents such as baths; and neurological consultation and treatment if the child presents with recurrent febrile seizures.
- **Reduction of the causes of brain injury**—promotion and enforcement of traffic regulations and speed limits, legal punishment for drunken driving, compulsory use of seat belts and safety seats for children and of helmets for riders of bicycles and motorcycles; at work, use of helmets, safety cords, and adequate lighting; at home, elimination of angular structures located at a child's head level, safety precautions on stairs, and window safety systems;

and avoidance of neurotoxic agents, such as alcohol for pregnant mothers, lead, and pesticides.

- **Control of infectious and parasitic diseases**—extension of vaccination programs, mainly against diphtheria, pertussis, tetanus, measles, and tuberculosis, to the whole target population; environmental control of parasitic diseases, such as cysticercosis and malaria; and detection and treatment of responsible vectors.
- **Genetic counseling**—accurate medical information about the risk to offspring when one or both parents have epilepsy.

Control of environmental and genetic conditions and management of human and animal infections will continue to lead to significant reduction in the burden of epilepsy in developing countries. For example, where *T. solium* infection is endemic, up to 50 percent of all cases presenting with epilepsy are caused by cysticercosis. Strategies to reduce the impact of this condition in communities may include affordable blood tests that can be used to diagnose patients suspected of harboring these parasites, with safe and effective drugs administered to treat them along with medical and veterinary services working together to reduce the transmission of this infection from animals to humans.

Initiatives to prevent epilepsy clearly require effort from multiple sectors within local and national infrastructures. In addition to health care providers, teachers, community leaders, sanitation and transportation personnel, legislators, and the media can play an important role in implementing control measures and educating communities about the prevention of epilepsy.

Treatment

In the face of financial and organizational constraints, the choice of drug for the primary therapy of epilepsy in developing countries assumes great importance. Phenobarbital and phenytoin are the most cost-effective drugs available for the treatment of epilepsy and prove effective in 70 percent of all cases.[134–137] In India, these two drugs are the most commonly used AEDs, being administered to up to 93 percent of epilepsy patients.[138]

Phenobarbital is recommended as the first-line drug for the treatment of partial and generalized tonic-clonic epilepsies in developing countries.[31–34,76,135,139–142] Use of this old and simple drug is encouraged because of its efficacy for a wide range of seizure types and its low cost makes it suitable for use in primary health care in developing countries. Although WHO findings on the acceptability of phenobarbital were established through extensive consultation with neurologists and other specialists working in developing countries, the suitability of phenobarbital as an AED for children raised considerable concern among developed-country specialists, who contended that the drug's side effects, especially behavioral problems such as hyperactivity, might contraindicate its use.[19,143] These concerns were dismissed, however, by randomized controlled trials conducted to assess the acceptability and safety of phenobarbital for childhood epilepsy.[134–136,144] New evidence on the use of phenobarbital at the community level by primary health care personnel, compared with use of both phenytoin and carbamazepine, has established phenobarbitol as the drug of choice for initial treatment of partial and generalized epilepsies in primary health care settings.[31–34,139–141,145]

A price comparison for AEDs in six developing countries of South America showed wide variation. Phenobarbital, for example, costs only US$1.50 per monthly treatment in Colombia, and up to US$10.00 in Brazil. Similarly, phenytoin treatment costs US$1.15 per month in Venezuela and US$17.00 in Uruguay.[140] An interesting comparison conducted in Colombia, South America, demonstrated that traditional herbal treatments for epilepsy are six times more expensive than pharmacological treatment (US$2,210 vs. $364), taking into account the indirect costs of being jobless and the family expenditures required to care for epilepsy patients who continue having seizures while subjected to ineffective therapies.[140]

Primary Care. The use of primary health care workers and key community informants to identify and follow patients under treatment with either phenobarbital or phenytoin appears to be the most cost-effective intervention for reducing the treatment gap for epilepsy in developing countries. Pilot projects conducted in Asia, Africa, and Latin America using this primary health care strategy in urban marginal and rural areas have demonstrated its safety and feasibility.[31,76,113,146–148] Through use of these two inexpensive medications, up to 80 percent of patients presenting with generalized tonic-clonic seizures could be brought under control.[12,32,136,137,149]

In addition to administering and monitoring of drug treatments, trained primary care health workers can help to identify individuals with epilepsy in their communities and encourage them to seek medical attention. They can play an equally important role as health educators by providing accurate information about prevention, causes, and available treatments of epilepsy. Greater understanding of epilepsy has been shown to improve attitudes toward treatment and reduce stigma.[33,145,150–152]

Epilepsy surgery. A recent study conducted in Colombia presents evidence that surgery is a cost-effective treatment option for epilepsy patients in developing countries.[153] Twenty-six developing countries currently conduct epilepsy surgery, and available data suggest that outcomes achieved are similar to those in developed countries, but obtained at a fraction of the cost.[54] The advantages of surgery in selected cases of clinically intractable epilepsy and the possible early use of surgery to avoid more expensive, life-long pharmacotherapy may indicate that this is a cost-effective alternative for resource-poor settings capable of supporting the necessary technology and medical training.[12,154] The establishment of additional epilepsy surgery centers in developing countries will require collaborative support from research and clinical institutions.[11,155]

BOX 6-2 Model for managing epilepsy in Malawi

In Malawi, as in many developing countries, people with epilepsy travel to various traditional healers seeking treatment or a cure. These traditional healers often encourage patients to ingest a mixture of roots that precipitates purging or vomiting. Unless they are suffering from burns sustained during an epileptic seizure, patients rarely seek care at a hospital. Through community publicity and education about the availability of biomedical treatment, a program sought to encourage and promote individuals suffering from epilepsy in rural Africa to seek regular care at a hospital or health center.

After the first eight months 11 patients were attending the hospital for treatment. After an area action committee conducted a targeted information campaign, 70 more patients were receiving treatment after three months. Because many of the patients walked great distances to gain treatment, two mobile clinics were established by linking with an existing mobile health program for children under five years of age. After two years 461 patients were registered in the program. Of the 254 patients treated for epilepsy in the first 18 months, 68 percent continued treatment beyond six months. Among those same individuals, 56 percent no longer suffered seizures—showing significant improvement over the pre-treatment occurrence of one seizure per month in 88 percent of this group.

In the hospital and mobile clinics, diagnosis was based on seizure history and use of a modified form of the revised ILAE classification. Electroencephalography and CT scanning were not available. Only patients having two or more seizures in a year were treated with anticonvulsants. Simple explanatory models were used during the first visit with patients and family members. Descriptions of the disease and treatments included:

- Epilepsy is due to a scar on the brain, sometimes caused by meningitis, sometimes following cerebral malaria, sometimes inherited. Treatment aims to stop seizures from occurring in order to allow the scar to heal.
- It takes a long time for the scar to heal, and we would not consider reducing, and possibly discontinuing treatment for at least two years.
- Seizures will not stop immediately. The medicine needs time to work effectively. It may take several months to determine the dose of drugs needed for each patient. Patients should not become discouraged during this time.
- If side effects such as a rash occur the patient must stop taking the drug immediately and report to the hospital.
- Alcohol should be avoided, yet no other restrictions for diet are recommended.

Phenobarbitone and phenytoin were the only medications used because of their availability in the community and suitability for administration by trained nurses or community health workers who were familiar with their use. The population of the region was largely subsistence farmers; therefore, it was determined that medication must be provided free of charge to enable adequate treatment.

Record cards were distributed to patients to remind them of the next scheduled treatment, to track medication dosage, and to record the numbers of seizures between visits to the hospital or clinic. For the patients, the record cards clearly illustrated the number of tablets to be taken daily. The supervising physician and nurses and community health workers were able to use the information from the cards to determine any needed changes to drug treatment or dosing frequency.

Publicity in communities through widely known organizations or individuals was instrumental in the initial registration of patients and for maintaining their adherence to treatment. After an article profiling the program appeared in a national medical journal, more district and community health centers moved to establish similar models. As additional programs were developed, the following guidelines were created for the management of epilepsy in community health centers:

- publicize the availability of treatment;
- educate patients and staff;
- use simple anticonvulsant regimens with phenobarbitone or phenytoin;
- maintain adequate supplies of drugs;
- offer drugs at no charge;
- conduct monthly review clinics with a physician;
- ensure patient always sees the same health worker; and
- use mobile clinics.

As a result of the promotion of these guidelines, the number of patients seeking treatment at the hospitals and designated clinics increased significantly. These findings suggest that people with epilepsy can overcome the myths and mistaken beliefs about the disease allowing health programs for the effective treatment of epilepsy to be adopted and administered in rural areas of the developing world.

In recognizing the financial limitations and lack of medically trained professionals in the region, the program design sought to balance efficacy with simplicity of use. From 1980 to 1998 in Malawi no change in the physician to patient ratio of .05 per 1000 people was experienced. Therefore, the program relied heavily on the use of trained nurses and community health workers.

The success of the Malawi model provides a useful framework for other communities; however, limitations in the sustainability of the program must be noted. Delivery of effective care through this program greatly diminished upon the departure of the founding physician from the country. Clearly community knowledge and education about available treatments for epilepsy were essential to the program; however, future efforts would benefit from a better understanding of community attitudes toward epilepsy and health care that could be gained by engaging not only primary health care centers but also important groups such as religious, political, and social leaders. A wider community-based approach may lead to long-term, vested interest in the success and continuation of the programs.

Source: [145,152]

Recommendation 6-2. Demonstration projects for developing primary health care programs and interventions for the prevention, diagnosis, and treatment of patients suffering from generalized tonic-clonic seizures should be implemented. These projects should incorporate and evaluate the established WHO guidelines for prevention and the use of first-line anti-epileptic drugs, such as phenobarbital, phenytoin, carmabazepine, and valproic acid.

Recommendation 6-3. With the support of international, national, and local governments and non-governmental organizations, demonstration programs in 4–6 countries of Latin America, Africa and Asia, where *T. solium* teniasis and cysticercosis are endemic should be established, in order to drastically diminish active transmission of this infection and to monitor the effectiveness of such programs in the medium- and long-term on decreasing epilepsy incidence in humans and abolishing this parasitic infection in pigs.

Recommendation 6-4. Tertiary medical centers with the medical and technical expertise required for epilepsy surgery should establish such surgical centers. Assessment of the required surgical training and medical equipment should be in collaboration with surgical centers already established in developing countries and centers in developed countries. Financial and technical support from developed country institutions will be important.

The range of social, economic, and medical consequences associated with epilepsy, along with the availability of cost-effective methods of treatment that are efficacious in up to 70 percent of treated patients, is the most compelling reason for this disease to receive high priority in public health planning and education.

CAPACITY

Training

An important strategy for control of epilepsy in developing countries may be training PHCWs (see Box 6-3).[40,150,152] In developing countries, trained neurologists are scarce and cannot cope with the huge tasks of diagnosis, treatment, and surveillance of patients with epilepsy, especially in rural areas.[149,157,158] Even general medical practitioners are often unavailable in rural regions that contain communities of less than 1,000 inhabitants each, separated by long distances and poor road conditions. The role of medical specialists and general practitioners will be essential for conducting appropriate training, developing safe and cost-effective protocols for pharmacotherapy, confirming diagnosis, initiating treatment, and overseeing the operation of general medical clinics and community health care centers (see Box 6-3).[12,76,136]

Nurses, medical technicians, and trained primary health care workers have proven to be very helpful in managing patients with epilepsy. When provided with appropriate training and supervision, they are able to oversee the course of treatment for patients in remote areas, which includes the monitoring of blood levels for toxicity during pharmacotherapy and attention to other possible drug side effects.[76,149,157,160,161] Community mental health and social workers can often assist patients and families in coping with the social, financial, and psychological consequences of the disease.[162]

BOX 6-3 An Epilepsy Treatment Program for Primary Health Care Workers in Ecuador

In 1987 the government of Ecuador agreed to sponsor a pilot project to study the feasibility of using an informal health system, comprising a community and its primary health care workers (PHCWs), to identify, treat, and control patients suffering from tonic-clonic seizures, the most frequent and easy-to-treat epilepsy type. The PHCW was a member of the community who had received 6 months of training in basic skills needed to diagnose and treat the most common medical illnesses in his/her community. A 3-day course presented by trained neurologists enabled the PHCWs to detect cases of epilepsy and to use phenobarbital for their control, following strict algorithms developed by specialists in the urban university hospital center.[140,141,144] In one community, the PHCW identified and treated 16 patients with generalized tonic-clonic epilepsy. In a control community, 12 patients were treated by a fully trained neurologist. Eight patients in the first group and 7 in the second completed the 12-month study. Compliance and side effects were comparable in the two groups. No difference was seen among patients treated by the PHCW and the neurologist. The PHCW was able to use the protocols for epilepsy detection. Although the diagnosis was confirmed by a physician, the PHCW was capable of administering the phenobarbital and managing its side effects. Moreover, the PHCW was able to obtain the patients' confidence throughout the treatment period and to help them adjust within the community.[141]

Results of this study and others indicate that the use of PHCWs for the identification, treatment with low-dose phenobarbital, and surveillance of patients with generalized tonic-clonic epilepsy is feasible and practical in remote communities where medical expertise is difficult to obtain or nonexistent. This strategy may help millions of patients with epilepsy in rural areas of developing countries who currently receive no treatment.

BOX 6-4 Use of District-Level Doctors (India)

A review of neuroepidemiological surveys conducted in different regions of India indicates that nearly 8 to 10 million people have epilepsy. With the wide gap between available trained neurologists (550) and the projected minimum required (5,000), alternative strategies to provide care for people with epilepsy need to be developed. WHO has promoted care of persons with epilepsy as part of primary health care in developing countries since 1975.[159]

In India, integration of mental health care with primary health care has included epilepsy as one of the prorities, along with psychoses, depression, and mental retardation, since 1975. Training manuals and materials have also been developed and evaluated.[163,164] Pilot programs covering populations of 40,000 to 2 million have shown the feasibility of care of epilepsy by primary care doctors. A concept for a national Epilepsy Control Programme has been developed following a series of workshops funded by WHO. One of the key elements is to train district medical officers (physicians and pediatricians) in the diagnosis and management of epilepsy.

In the 25 states of the country, there are nearly 500 districts, with an average population of 1.5 to 2 million in a district. District-level medical officers and administrative staff are responsible for implementing, executing, and monitoring various health programs at the level of primary health centers and taluks (regional governments) under their jurisdiction.

District medical officers are given training on indentification, diagnosis, and drug treatment. They are also provided insight into psychosocial issues, such as education, marriage, and employment, related to epilepsy. The importance of compliance by patients and continuous availability of a free supply of commonly used anti-epileptic drugs has been emphasized. The district medical officers have also been motivated to conduct outreach epilepsy clinics involving the primary health center (PHC) doctors and to train PHC doctors in the diagnosis and treatment of epilepsy. This strategy will facilitate networking of epilepsy. The training program was conducted as a 2-day workshop.

Neurologists with special interest and expertise in epilepsy formed the resource faculty. Fifty-seven district medical officers drawn from 10 states have already completed the programs. During the training a standardized validated questionnaire covering the various elements of the training were administered to the district medical officers. Pre- and post-training analysis has shown that the training program had significant impact (70–80%) on the knowledge and skills in the management of epilepsy.

It is planned to extend this program to cover all the districts in the country by identifying nodal neurologists in the different states who in turn would supervise the epilepsy control program.

Source: [164]

Research

Despite the difficulties in gathering data on epilepsy discussed earlier in this chapter, WHO has been successful in sponsoring a worldwide initiative to obtain epidemiological data on epilepsy, specifically from developing countries where such information was incomplete or lacking.[1–3] Use of the Protocol for the Epidemiological Investigation of Neurological Disorders in Developing Countries, developed by WHO more than 15 years ago, made it possible to gather data on the disease from Africa, Latin America, and Asia, and to compare it with data from Europe and North America.[15] The results made clear to the world that epilepsy was a significant public health problem in the majority of the investigated geographic areas and prompted the World Health Assembly to sponsor the Initiative To Help People with Epilepsy.[165]

The full picture of the epidemiology of epilepsy remains inconclusive. Research is needed to ascertain specific risk factors for the development of the disease, particularly in developing-country environments. Genetic causes should be explored in various geographic locations and among different ethnic groups. Such research would improve the cost-effectiveness of efforts for prevention and treatment. The findings from such efforts could have an impact in both developed and developing countries.

In 1997, three international organizations—WHO, the International League Against Epilepsy (ILAE), and the International Bureau for Epilepsy (IBE)—joined forces to initiate the Global Campaign Against Epilepsy (GCAE). The strategy of the GCAE includes two parallel and simultaneous tracks: (1) raising of general awareness and understanding of epilepsy, and (2) support for departments of health in identifying needs and promoting education, training, treatment, services, research, and prevention nationally. One of the main activities within the second track of the GCAE is development of demonstration projects, being carried out in a number of countries in Africa, Asia, and Latin America. The objectives of the demonstration projects are:

- To reduce the treatment gap and the physical and social morbidity of people suffering from epilepsy through intervention at the community level;
- To train and educate health professionals;
- To dispel stigma and promote a positive attitude toward people with epilepsy in the community;
- To identify and assess the potential for prevention of epilepsy; and
- To develop a model for promotion of epilepsy control worldwide and for its integration into the health systems of participating countries.

Through this program a questionnaire designed to standardize data collection methodologies has been developed in collaboration with the Institute of Neurological Epidemiology and Tropical Neurology of Limoge (France) and the

Pan-African Association of Neurological Sciences.[166] The estimated duration of this project is 5 years.

The availability of human and technical resources for medical assessment of patients with epilepsy differs widely among developing countries, as well as between urban and rural areas within a country. Training of personnel at all levels of intervention for patients with epilepsy is a principal requirement for the success of any initiative aimed at helping these individuals.[147] Educational programs for professionals and patients must be based on perceived local needs and differing social and cultural conditions. Multiple levels of international, governmental, and nongovernmental organizations could assume an important role in this effort, as could national centers for training and research that included epilepsy as a priority disease on their research and planning agendas (see Chapters 3 and 4 for more information on nationals centers for training and research).[19,80–84,147,167]

In this context, it is important that GCAE be enlisted by all national governments and local communities in developing countries attempting to address the burden of epilepsy to accomplish the following objectives:

- To increase public and professional awareness of epilepsy as a universal, treatable brain disorder;
- To raise epilepsy to a new plane of acceptability in the public domain;
- To promote public and professional education about epilepsy;
- To identify the needs of people with epilepsy on a national and regional basis; and
- To encourage governments and departments of health to address the needs of people with epilepsy, including awareness, education, diagnosis, treatment, care, services, and prevention.

Recommendation 6-5. Guidelines for training and treatment protocols should be established by national centers of training and research. Where possible, these centers should work in conjunction with the WHO/ILEA/IBE Global Campaign Against Epilepsy. These centers should be informed by local epidemiological research and should reflect the needs of the population.

Specific programs of operational research for implementing training, prevention, and treatment should include the following:

- Specialists and general practitioners who are well-informed about current knowledge on the management and prevention of epilepsy and sensitized to the cultural attitudes within their societies that will impact the training they provide to other levels of health care personnel.

- Training of nurses who can appropriately supervise PHCWs and monitor the treatment outcome of patients in community-based, primary health care centers.
- Training of primary health care personnel and key community informants that will enable them to counsel their communities on methods of preventing epilepsy and to identify and administer the treatment of patients with epilepsy at the community level.
- Training surgery teams to function in selected major cities of developing countries where the necessary equipment can be maintained.
- Adequate drug supplies and means of distribution
- Methods for surveillance that provide data collection for:
  - Cost-outcome analyses that provide government officials and funding agencies the information needed for health planning and continued program development;
  - Quality-of-life and disease burden measurements for epileptic patients; and
  - Socioeconomic determinants of the outcome measures that could best reflect optimal care for epilepsy patients in developing countries.

Recommendation 6-6. Research on the causes of epilepsy and the outcomes of treatment are needed in developing countries. Collaborative research between national centers and research centers in developed countries should be supported.

Collaborative research should include but not be limited to the following investigations:

- Risk factors for epilepsy related to infectious diseases that remain common and endemic in most developing countries;
- Exploration of genetic risk factors for epilepsy among different geographic and ethnic populations;
- Nutritional status, genetic factors, and dietary factors that will affect dosage recommendations for AEDs; and
- Immunological research directed at developing a cost-effective vaccine against porcine and, eventually, human cysticercosis.

ANNEX 6-1
Neurocysticercosis

The parasitosis produced by *Taenia solium*, the pork tapeworm, is recognized as one of the leading causes of epilepsy in the developing world. When the larval stages of this parasite, cysticerci, invade the human brain, the resulting neurocysticercosis (NCC) induces epilepsy in a high proportion of cases, and is now being diagnosed in numerous countries throughout Africa, Asia, and Latin America, where this zoonosis still constitutes a serious public health problem.[79,80,90,97] In these studies, up to 50 percent of epilepsy cases have been shown to have cysticercosis as a putative factor.

NCC is highly prevalent in communities with poor sanitation, the crowded coexistence of humans and animals, and a lack of adequate water and sewage systems. Recently, NCC has been recognized in industrialized countries with increasing frequency, the result of both migrant infected populations and locally acquired cases.[168–172]

BIOLOGICAL CYCLE

The biological cycle of this parasite involves an intermediary host, the pig, which becomes contaminated with *Taenia solium* eggs contained in feces of infected humans. These eggs then invade the pig's tissues, hatching into larvae known as cysticerci. In endemic areas, up to 25 percent of roaming pigs may be infected at any one time, and local slaughterhouses diagnose cysticercosis in 5–11 percent of pigs.[173]

The parasite is transmitted to humans when they eat poorly cooked meat. The cysticercus attaches to the intestinal mucosa and develops into the adult taenia, a flat worm that my be several meters long and live for up to 20 years. The distal portions of the parasite (proglotids) contain several thousand eggs, which are immediately infectious when released to the environment. In addition to environmental contamination, infected humans can contaminate other humans, directly, who then acquire cysticercosis.[174] When the larvae reach the nervous system (NCC) they can produce serious symptomatology, often manifested as epileptic fits and intracable headaches.[173]

The clinical manifestations of NCC are present in only 40 percent of individuals with proven larval invasion to the brain.[97] The symptomatology depends on the number of invading cysts and their localization in the central nervous system. A few cysts localized in the cerebral cortex may be responsible for focal neurological signs and symptoms, such as aphasia, hemiparesis, or partial seizures, whereas a single cyst placed within the ventricular system may produce increased intracranial pressure and sudden death.

EPIDEMIOLOGY

Data on the epidemiology of NCC have been elusive because of its clinical characteristics, with a wide array of manifestations; the variable period of incubation, from a few months to more than 20 years; the lack of adequate diagnostic methods; and the low reporting rates for the disease. Recently, with the advent of newer immunological techniques—notably enzyme-linked immunoelectrotransfer blot (EITB) and the wider use of brain computed tomography (CT)—a clearer picture of the distribution and extent of the disease has emerged. The prevalence of NCC has been estimated to be from 3 percent (based on autopsy studies) to 9 percent (based on immunological studies).[93,97,175]

To assess cysticercosis as a significant risk factor for epilepsy, researchers from Ecuador conducted an epidemiological study in the village of San Pablo del Lago, 80 miles north of Quito, the capital city, where *T. solium* taeniosis/cysticercosis had been shown to be endemic.[93] The study used the WHO Protocol for the Epidemiological Investigation of Neurological Disorders in Developing Countries. This protocol is based on a structured interview and a task-based selective neurological examination. For the Ecuadoran study, a third step was added, which consisted of confirming the clinical diagnosis by immunological (EITB) and CT testing. The CT criteria for the diagnosis of NCC were based on the extensive descriptions of the condition in the literature. A symptom-free control sample population was studied to assess the statistical significance of the presence or absence of *T. solium* NCC for the etiology of cases presenting with seizure disorders. This approach strengthened the specificity of the protocol for the detection of *T. solium* infection.[93]

Complete information was collected for 2,723 individuals living in the urban nucleus of San Pablo del Lago. Thirty-one individuals were confirmed to suffer from active epilepsy, as defined in previous community-based studies. Thus, the point prevalence ratio was 1.4/1000 (confidence interval [C.I.] 7.7–15.4).

In the general group of patients confirmed with epilepsy, 16 (51.6 percent) were classified as having generalized seizures and 15 (48.4 percent) as having partial seizures. In the 14 patients with positive CT findings for NCC, 5 (35.7 percent) had generalized seizures, and 9 (64.3 percent) had partial seizures.

All patients with confirmed active epilepsy were invited to undergo further examination at the clinical center in Quito for completion of ancillary investigations for epilepsy, but 5 refused CT examinations, and 3 of these refused to have blood drawn for immunological testing. In 14 of the 26 subjects (53.8 percent) with epilepsy who agreed to be examined, there was CT evidence of past or recent NCC infection. In 11 of these 26 patients, epilepsy had first started when they were above age 20. In this group of late-onset epilepsy cases, NCC was found in 7 cases (64 percent).

Three of 6 men (50 percent) and 2 of 8 females (25 percent) for whom CT findings were consistent with a diagnosis of NCC also had EITB positivity for this infection. In total, only one-third of epilepsy patients with NCC diagnosed by CT had a concomitant positive EITB (5/14, or 35.7 percent). Four of 5 individuals studied by CT and showing single or multiple viable cysts had a positive EITB (80 percent), whereas only 1 of 9 who displayed single or multiple calcifications had a positive EITB (11 percent). One other patient with epilepsy had a positive EITB with a negative CT.

In the seizure-free random sample of the population, 118 CTs were completed. Of these, 17 were positive for NCC, for a prevalence ratio of 144/1000 (CI of 85–212). In the same sample, it was possible to have serum taken for EITB in 96 cases, 10 of which were positive for cysticercal infection, for a prevalence ratio of 104/1000 (CI of 52–167).

Chi square analysis was performed to compare the epilepsy-free random sample of the population with the epilepsy cases associated with cysticercal infection proven by either of the two clinical tests used—CT scanning or EITB testing. Among the epilepsy cases, a statistically significant difference was found for the CT diagnosis of NCC OR 6.93, CI 2.7–17.5, $p < 0.001$), but not the EITB diagnosis (OR 2.75, CI 0.8–7.1, $p < 0.12$, NS), using Mantel-Haenzel statistics. This discrepancy between the CT and EITB results may be explained on the basis of a long-standing chronic condition, in which early antibody disappearance occurs.

The results of this study indicate that the prevalence of NCC in communities in which this infection is endemic may be as high as 14 percent, when CT scanning is used as the diagnostic standard. The results also confirm that NCC is a major risk factor for epilepsy in these areas.[93] The evidence suggests that up to two-thirds of late-onset epilepsy cases may be due to this infection in such endemic regions.

It is possible to confirm the high prevalence figures for epilepsy reported in developing countries using the WHO protocol. If the epilepsy ratio found in the Ecuadoran study is corrected by eliminating those cases linked to cysticercal infection, the remaining figure (17 patients, or 6.2/1000) is almost identical to that reported for Rochester, Minnesota (6 per 1,000).

PREVENTION

T. solium taeniosis/cysticercosis can be prevented by a long-term approach involving appropriate legislation, health education, modernization of pig husbandry practices, improved meat inspection, provision of adequate sanitary facilities, and measures to detect and treat human tapeworm carriers. However, modernization of sanitary infrastructure is expensive and beyond the current capabilities of most rural populations. Moreover, changing attitudes, beliefs, and behaviors is a difficult task that can be accomplished only after years of community health education.[162] Given political and economic realities in countries where NCC is endemic, there is little hope that all these measures can be implemented in the near future. To achieve more rapid progress in reducing active transmission of the disease, community-based interventions for the detection and mass treatment of endemic foci with taenicidal drugs have been proposed and implemented successfully in Ecuador and Mexico.[176] Progress in control can be attained by integrating these activities within primary health care systems. *T. solium* taeniosis/cysticercosis is, therefore, a potentially eradicable condition, although the concerted political action of involved governments will be needed to achieve this goal.[98,176,177]

TREATMENT

Fifteen years ago, treatment of patients with NCC was confined to excision of surgically accessible cysts and the use of steroids for the treatment of parasitic-induced inflammation. In recent years, the development of safe and effective chemotherapeutic agents has changed the prognosis for this condition.[97,98] Praziquantel and albendazole, given orally, have proven to be active against intracerebral cysts. Praziquantel is used in doses of 50 mg/kg/day, divided into three intakes, for 15 days.[178] Albendazole is usually given in doses of 800 mg/day for 8 days.[179,180] Higher daily dosages and longer treatment periods are sometimes needed for severe cases, or when the cysts are located within the ventricular system. Oral or intravenous steroids are now widely used, in various therapeutic schemes, to counteract the inflammatory reactions associated with both the presence of the parasite and the therapy itself. Anticonvulsants are indicated when seizures are the main manifestation of the disease. Intestinal taeniosis is usually cured with a single dose of praziquantel, as low as 5 mg/kg [176].

Patients with parenchymal NCC typically present with seizures. In the Ecuadoran study, two of three patients with epilepsy secondary to NCC presented with partial seizures. Although anticonvulsants are routinely prescribed, Latin American researchers advocate the concomitant use of antiparasitic drugs and steroids where there is evidence of active NCC [179–181]. In fact, there appears to be a decrease in seizure frequency in patients thus treated [182,183].

The Ecuadoran study and others in Africa and Asia [90,94,184,185] revealed that individuals suffering from the consequences of NCC are subject to limiting illnesses such as intractable headaches and seizures that hamper their well-being and limit their productivity as active community members. NCC is a preventable and treatable infection. Programs and research designed to eradicate NCC in developing countries would lead to the elimination of a sizable number of epilepsy cases and the associated human suffering.

REFERENCES

1. M.E. Cruz, B.S. Schoenberg, R. Ruales, P. Barberis, J. Proano, F. Bossano, et al. Pilot study to detect neurologic disease in Ecuador among a population with a high prevalence of endemic goiter. *Neuroepidemiology* 4:108–116, 1985.

2. S.C. Li, B.S. Schoenberg, C.C. Wang, X.M. Cheng, S.S. Zhou, and C.L. Bolis. Epidemiology of epilepsy in the urban population of the People's Republic of China. *Epilepsia* 26:391–394, 1985.

3. B.O. Osuntokun, B.S. Schoenberg, V.A. Nottidge et al. Research protocol for measuring the prevalence of neurologic disorders in developing countries. *Neuroepidemiology* 1:143–153, 1982.

4. M.E. Cruz, P. Barberis, and B.S. Schoenberg. Epidemiology of Epilepsy. In: *Neurology*, Poeck, K., Freund, H.J. and Ganshirt, H. eds. Springer-Verlag: Berlin-Heidelberg, pp.229–239, 1986.

5. P. Jallon. Epilepsy in developing countries. *Epilepsia* 38(10): 1143–1151, 1997.

6. P. R. M. de Bittencourt, B. Adamolekum, N. Bharucha, A. Carpio, O.H. Cassio, M.A. Dumas, et al. Epilepsy in the Tropics: I. Epidemiology, Socioeconomic Risk Factors, and Etiology. *Epilepsia* 37(11):1121–1127, 1996.

7. E. M. Basch, M.E. Cruz, D. Tapia, and A. Cruz. Prevalence of epilepsy in a migrant population near Quito, Ecuador. *Neuroepidemiology* 16: 94–98, 1997.

8. N. Karaagac. S.N. Yeni, M. Senocak, M. Bozluolcay, F.K. Savrun, H. Ozdemir, et al. Prevalence of epilepsy in Silivri, a rural area of Turkey. *Epilepsia* 40(5): 637–642, 1999.

9. R. Tekle-Haimanot, L. Forsgreen, and J. Ekstedt. Incidence of epilepsy in rural central Ethiopia. *Epilepsia* 38 (5): 541–546, 1997.

10. H. Aziz, S.M. Ali, P. Frances, M. I. Khan, and K.Z. Hasan. Epilepsy in Pakistan: A population-based epidemiologic study. *Epilepsia* 35(5): 950–958, 1994.

11. N. Senanayake and G.C. Roman. Epidemiology of epilepsy in developing countries. *Bulletin of the World Health Organization* 71(2): 247–258, 1993.

12. I. Cruz, F. Bossano, and M.E. Cruz. Factores de riesgo para la epilepsia en una comunidad andina del Ecuador. In: Academia Ecuatoriana de Neurociencias, Cruz, M.E., Ed., *Control Comunitario de la Epilepsia.* Quito, 1991.
13. J. M. Bertolote. Epilepsy as a public health problem. *Tropical and Geographical Medicine* 46(3): 28–30, 1994.
14. Commission on Classification and Terminology of the International League Against Epilepsy, Proposal for revised classification of epilepsies and epileptic syndromes. *Epilepsia* 30: 389-399, 1989.
15. B.S. Schoenberg. Recent studies of the epidemiology of epilepsy in developing countries: A coordinated program for prevention and control. *Epilepsia* 28(6):721–722, 1987.
16. D.W. Anderson, F.A. Bryan, B.S.H. Harris, J.T. Lessler, and J.P. Gagnon. A survey approach for finding cases of epilepsy. *Public Health Report* Jul–Aug;100(4):386–393, 1985.
17. W.A. Jaiser and L.T. Kurland. The epidemiology of epilepsy in Rochester, Minnesota, 1935 Through 1967. *Epilepsia* 16:1–66, 1975.
18. L. Jilek-Aall, W. Jilek, J. Kaaya, L. Mkombachepa, and K. Hilliary. Psychosocial study of epilepsy in Africa. *Social Science and Medicine* 45:783–795, 1997.
19. S.D. Shorvon, and P.J. Farmer. Epilepsy in developing countries: A review of epidemiological, sociocultural, and treatment aspects. *Epilepsia* 29(1): S36–S54, 1988.
20. A. Awaritefe, A.C. Longe, and M. Awaritefe. Epilepsy and psychosis: A comparison of societal attitudes. *Epilepsia* Jan–Feb;26(1):1–9, 1985.
21. G. Scambler and A. Hopkins. Being epileptic; coming to terms with stigma. *Social Health and Illness* 8:26–43, 1986.
22. G. L. Bribeck. Barriers to care for patients with neurologic disease in rural Zambia. *Archives of Neurology* 57:41414–41417, 2000.
23. W.B. Matuja and H.T. Rwiza. Knowledge, attitude and practice (KAP) towards epilepsy in secondary school students in Tanzania. *Central African Journal of Medicine* Jan;40(1):13–18, 1994.
24. K. K. Hampton, R. C. Peatfield, T. Pullar, H. J. Bodansky, C. Walton, and M. Feely. Burns because of epilepsy. *British Medical Journal* 296(11): 16–17, 1988.
25. H. T. Rwiza, I. Mtega, and W. B. P. Matiya. The clinical and social characteristics of epilepsy patients in the Ulanga Districi, Tanzania. *Journal of Epilepsy* 5:162–169, 1993.
26. D.C. Gadjusek. Introduction of *Taenia solium* into West New Guinea with a note on an epidemic of burns from cysticercus epilepsy in the Ekari people of the Wissel Lakes area. *Papua New Guinea Medical Journal* 21:329–342, 1978.
27. W.A. Hauser and D.C. Hesdorffer. *Epilepsy Frequency, Causes and Consequences.* Demos Publications: New York, 1990.
28. T. Wandra, R. Subahar, G.M. Simanjuntak, S.S. Margano, T. Suroso, M. Okamoto, et al. Resurgence of cases of epileptic seizures and burns associated with cysticercosis in Assologaima, Jayawijaya, Irian Jaya, Indonesia, 1991–1995. *Transactions of the Royal Society of Tropical Medicine and Hygiene* Jan–Feb;94(1):46–50, 2000.
29. M. Berrocal. Burns and epilepsy. *Acta Chirurgiae Plasticae* 39(1):22–27, 1997.
30. D. Nag. Gender and Epilepsy: A Clinician's Experience. *Neurologic Society of India* Jun;48:99–104, 2000.

31. C. Kaiser, G, Asaba, C. Mugisa, W. Kipp, S. Kasoro, T. Rubaale, et al. Antiepileptic drug treatment in rural Africa: Involving the community. *Tropical Doctor* 28:73–77, 1998.

32. H. Meinardi, R.A. Scott, R. Reis, and J.W. Sander. The treatment gap in epilepsy: The current situation and ways forward. *Epilepsia* Jan;42(1):136–149, 2001.

33. A.T. Feksi, J. Kaamugisha, J.W.A.S. Sander, S. Gatiti, and S.D. Shorvon. Comprehensive primary health care antiepileptic drug treatment programme in rural and semi-urban Kenya. *Lancet* 337:406–409, 1991.

34. B. Adamolekun and H. Meinardi. Problems of drug therapy of epilepsy in developing countries. *Tropical and Geographical Medicine* 42:178–181, 1990.

35. T. Banerjee, and G. Banerjee. Determinants of help-seeking behavior in cases of epilepsy attending a teaching hospital in India: An indigenous explanatory model. *International Journal of Social Psychiatry* 41(3): 217–230, 1995.

36. A. Kleinman, W. Z. Wang, S. Li, X. Cheng, X. D, K. Tun, and J. Kleinman. The Social Course of Epilepsy: Chronic Illness as Social Experience in Interior China. *Social Science and Medicine* 40(10):1319–1330, 1995.

37. B.O. Osuntokun, A.O. Adeuja, B.S. Schoenberg, O. Bademosi, V.A. Nottidge, A.O. Olumide, et al. Neurological disorders in Nigerian Africans: A community-based study. *Acta Neurologica Scandinavica* Jan;75(10):13–21, 1987.

38. H.T. Rwiza, G.P. Kolonzo, J. Haule, W.B. Matuja, I. Mteza, P. Mbena, et al. Prevalence and incidence of epilepsy in Ulanga, a rural Tanzanian district: A community-based study. *Epilepsia* 33(6): 1051–1056, 1992.

39. J. E. Mendizabal and L.F. Salguero. Prevalence of epilepsy in a rural community of Guatemala. *Epilepsia* 37(4): 373–376, 1996.

40. M. Placencia, J. Suarez, F. Crespo, D.S. Shorvon, J.W.A.S. Sander, and R. H. Ellison. A large-scale study of epilepsy in Ecuador: Methodological aspects. *Neuroepidemiology* 11:74–84, 1992.

41. J.W.A.S. Sander and S.D. Shorvon. Incidence and prevalence studies in epilepsy and their methodological problems: A review. *Journal of Neurology, Neurosurgery, and Psychiatry* 50:829–839, 1987.

42. B.S. Schoenberg. Clinical neuroepidemiology in developing countries. Neurology for few neurologists. *Neuroepidemiology* 1:137–142, 1982.

43. J. Goudsmit, F.W. Van der Waals, and D.C. Gajdusek. Epilepsy in the Gbawein and Wroughbarh clan of Grand Bassa country, Liberia: the endemic occurrence of "see-ee" in the native population. *Neuroepidemiology* 2: 24–34, 1983.

44. C. Kaiser, C. Benninger, G. Asaba, C. Mugisa, G. Kabagambe, W. Kipp, et al. Clinical and electro-clinical classification of epileptic seizure in west Uganda. *Bulletin de la Société de Pathologie Exotique* 93(4):255–259, 2000.

45. R. Sridharan and B.N. Murthy. Prevalence and Pattern of Epilepsy in India. *Epilepsia* May;40(5):631–636, 1999.

46. D.K. Pal. Methodologic issues in assessing risk factors for epilepsy in an epidemiologica study in India. *Neurology* Dec 10;53(9), 2058–2063, 1999.

47. K. S. Mani, G. Rangan, H. V. Srinivas, S. Kalyanasundaram, S. Narendran, and A.K. Reddy. The Yelandur study: A community-based approach to epilepsy in rural South India-Epidemiological aspects. *Seizure* Aug;7(4):281–288, 1998.

48. B. Kouassi. Presentation at the Workshop of the IOM Committee on Nervous System Disorders in Developing Countries, November 8–9, Washington, D.C., 1999.

49. R. Giel. The problem of epilepsy in Ethiopia. *Tropical and Geographic Medicine* Dec;22(4):439–442, 1970.
50. R. Tekle-Haimanot, M. Abebe, A. Gebre-Mariam, L. Forsgren, J. Heijbel, G. Holmgren, et al. Community-based study of neurological disorders in rural central Ethiopia. *Neuroepidemiology* 9(5):263–277, 1990.
51. J. Goudsmit and F.W. van der Waals. Endemic epilepsy in an isolated region of Liberia. *Lancet* Mar5;1(8323):528–529, 1983.
52. C. Gerrits. A West African epilepsy focus. *Lancet* Feb 12;1(8320):358, 1983.
53. T.O. Dada. Epilepsy in Lagos, Nigeria. *African Journal of Medical Science* Apr;1(2):161–184, 1970.
54. B.O. Osuntokun, B.S. Schoenberg, V.A. Nottidge, A. Adeuja, O. Kale, A. Adeyefa, O. Bademosi, A. Olumide, A.B.O. Oyediran, C.A. Pearson, and C.L. Bolis. Research protocol for measuring the prevalence of neurologic disorders in developing countries: Results of a pilot study in Nigeria, *Neuroepidemiology* 1:143–153, 1982.
55. H. Collomb, M. Dumas, P.L. Girard, and I.P. N'Diaye. [Neurology in Senegal (10-year report)]. *Bulletin de la Société Médicale d'Afrique Noire de Langue Française* [French]16(4):575–580, 1971.
56. W.G. Jilek, and L.M. Jilek-Aall. The problem of epilepsy in a rural Tanzanian tribe. *The African Journal of Medical Sciences* 1: 305–307, 1970.
57. M. Dumas, K. Grunitzky, M. Belo, F. Dabis, M. Deniau, B.Bouteille, et al. [Cysticercosis and neurocysticercosis in Togo]. *La Presse Médicale* [French] Feb 2;20(4):179–180, 1991.
58. L. F. Levy. Epilepsy in Rhodesia, Zambia, and Malawi. *African Journal of Medical Science* Jul;1(3):291–303, 1970.
59. D. W. Anderson, M.O. Melcon, and R.H. Vergara. Methods for a prevalence survey of neurological disorders in Junin, Buenos Aires, Argentina. *Neuroepidemiology* 14(3):110–122, 1995.
60. J.C. Gomez, E. Arciniegas, and J. Torres. Prevalence of epilepsy in Bogota, Colombia. *Neurology* Jan;28(1):90–94, 1978.
61. F. Gracia, S.L. de Lao, L. Castillo, M. Larreategui, C. Archbold, M.M. Brenes, et al. Epidemiology of epilepsy in Guaymi Indians from Bocase del Toro, Province, Republic of Panama. *Epilepsia* Nov-Dec;31(6):718–723, 1990.
62. A. Nicoletti, A. Reggio, A. Bartoloni, G. Failla, G. Sofia, F. Bartalesi, et al. Prevalence of epilepsy in rural Bolivia: A door-to-door survey. *Neurology* Dec 10;53(9):2064–2069, 1999.
63. L. Ramirez de Lara and H. Lara Tapia. [Neurologic epidemiology in Mexico. A complete study]. *Salud Publica de México* Sep-Oct;22(5):501–511, 1980.
64. J. Lavados, L. Germain, A. Morales, M. Campero, and P. Lavados. A descriptive study of epilepsy in the district of El Salvador, Chile, 1984–1988. *Acta Neurologica Scandinavica* Apr;85(4):249–256, 1992.
65. M.A. Pascual Lopez, J. Pascual Gispert, L. Rodrgiuez Rivera, F. Rojas Ocho, and A. Tejeiros. [Epilepsy: empidemiological study in a child population]. *Boletín Médico del Hospital Infantil de México* Jul-Aug;37(4):811–821, 1980.
66. L. Zuloaga, C. Soto, D. Jaramillo, O. Mora, C. Betaneur, and R. Londono. [Prevalence of epilepsy in Medellin, Colombia, 1983]. *Boletín de la Oficina Sanitaria Panamericana* Apr;104(4):231–244, 1988.

67. N. Chiofalo, A. Kirschbaum, A. Fuentes, M.L. Cordero, and J. Madsen. Prevalence of epilepsy in children of Melipilla, Chile. *Epilepsia* Jun;20(3):261–266, 1979.

68. R. Marino Junior, A. Cukiert, and E. Pinho. [Epidemiological aspects of epilepsy in Sao Paulo: A prevalence study]. *Arquivos de Neuro-Psiquiatria* Sep;44(3):243–254, 1986.

69. L. Marquez and L. Olivares. [Epilepsy in Mexico. Epidemiologic study of a rural community]. *Salud Publica de México* Sep–Oct;21(5):487–495, 1979.

70. L. Olivare. [Neurological epidemiology in Mexico. Study of an urban population sample]. *Salud Publica de México* [Spanish] Jul–Aug;18(4):665–672, 1976.

71. J.L. Deen, T. Vos, S. R.A. Hutty, and J. Tulloch. Injuries and noncommunicable diseases: Emerging health problems of children in developing countries. *Bulletin of the World Health Organization* 77(6):518–524, 1999.

72. Ministry of Health and Welfare. Patients' survey. Tokyo:Kousei Toukei Kyokai, 1992.

73. S. Ohtahara and S. Ishida. *Epidemiology of epilepsy*. In: *Epileptology*, Akimoto H. and Yamauchi, T., eds. Iwasaki Gakujut su Shuppan: Tokyo, 38–53, 1984.

74. I. Cruz, F. Bossano, and M.E. Cruz. Population-based case control study of epilepsy in an Andean community (abstract). Proceedings, Annual Scientific Meeting of the WFN Research Committee on Neuroepidemiology, Chicago, 1989.

75. M. Placencia, S.D. Shorvon, V. Paredes, C. Bimos, J.W.A.S. Sander, J. Suarez, et al. Epileptic seizures in an Andean region of Ecuador: Incidence and prevalence and regional variation. *Brain* 115:771–782, 1992.

76. P. Desai, M.V. Padma, S. Jain, and M.C. Maheshwari. Knowledge, attitudes and practice of epilepsy: Experience at a comprehensive rural health services project. *Seizure* 7:133–138, 1998.

77. M. Gourie-Devi, G. Gururaj, and P. Satishchandra. Neuroepidcmiology in India. A perspective. In: *Recent Advances in Tropical Neurology*, Rose, F.C., ed. Elsevier: Oxfordshire, U.K., 1995.

78. S.S. Gorin. Cost-outcome analysis and service planning in a CMHC. *Hospital and Community Psychiatry* 37(7):697–671, 1986.

79. L. Jilek-Aall and H.T. Rwiza. Prognosis of epilepsy in a rural African community: A 30-year old follow-up of 164 patients in an outpatient clinic in rural Tanzania. *Epilepsia* 33(4):645–650, 1992.

80. A. Carpio and A. Hauser. The distribution and etiology of epilepsy in the tropics of America. *Review of Ecuadorian Neurology* 2:137–145, 1993.

81. N.E. Bharucha, E.P. Bharucha, A.E. Bharucha, A.V. Bhise, and B. S. Schoenberg. Case-control study of epilepsy in the Parsi community of Bombay: A population-based study. *Neurology* 38:312, 1988.

82. H.H. Garcia, R. Gilman, M. Martinez, V.C. Tsang, J.B. Pilcher, G. Herrera, et al. Cysticercosis as a major cause of epilepsy in Peru. The Cysticercosis Working Group in Peru (CWG). *Lancet* Jan 23;341(8839):197–200, 1993.

83. A. Ogunniya, B.O. Osuntokun, O. Bademosi, A.O.G. Adeuja, and B.S. Schoenberg. Risk factors for epilepsy: Case control study in Nigerians. *Epilepsia* 28:280–285, 1987.

84. S.C. Li and B.S. Schoenberg. Risk factors for epilepsy in China and other developing countries. *Chinese Medical Journal* (English) Oct;100(10):813–815, 1987.

85. J. F. Annegers, W.A. Rocca, and W. A. Hauser. Causes of Epilepsy: Contributions of the Rochester Epidemiology Project. *Mayo Clinic Proceedings* Jun;71(6):570–575, 1996.

86. P.M. Leary, G. Riordan, B. Schlegel, and S. Morris. Childhood secondary (symptomatic) epilepsy, seizure control, and intellectual handicap in a nontropical region of South Africa. *Epilepsia* 40 (8):1110–1113, 1999.

87. P. Senga, H.F. Mayanda, and S. Nzingoula. Profile of seizures in infants and young children in Brazzaville (Congo). *Annales de Pediatrie* 32:477–480, 1985.

88. H.T. Rwiza, G.P. Kilonzo, J. Haule, W.B. Matuja, I. Mteza, P. Mbena, P.M. Kilima, G. Mwaluko, R. Mwang'ombola, F. Mwaijande, et al. Prevalence and indicence of epilepsy in Ulanga, a rural Tanzanian district: A community-based study. *Epilepsia* Nov–Dec;33(6):1051–1056, 1992.

89. J. V. Gulmezoglu, A.Metin, and M. de Onis. Nutritional and Antimicrobial Interventions to Prevent Preterm Birth: An Overview of Randomized Controlled Trials. *Obstetrical and Gynecological Survey* Sep;53(9):575–585, 1998.

90. P. M. Preux, Z. Melaku, M. Druet-Cabanac et al. Cysticercosis and neurocysticercosis in Africa: Current status. *Neurological Infections and Epidemiology* 1:63–68, 1996.

91. I. Cruz, M.E. Cruz, P. Schantz, and C.L. Bolis. The WHO protocol for epidemiological investigation of neurological disorders applied to *T. solium* taeniasis/cysticercosis research (abstract). *Journal of Neurological Sciences* 150 (supp): 256, 1997.

92. M.E. Cruz, P.M. Preux, C. Debrock, I. Cruz, P.M. Schantz, V.C. Shantz, et al. Epidemiologie de la cysticercose cérébrale dans une communauté des Andes en Equateur. *Bulletin de la Societe de Pathologie Exotique* 92 (1):38–41, 1999.

93. M.E. Cruz, P. M. Schantz, I. Cruz, et al. Epilepsy and Neurocysticercosis in an Andean community. *International Journal of Epidemiology* 28:799–803, 1999.

94. M. E. Cruz, J. Culebras-Fernandez, P. Canelos, et al. Epilepsia y neurocisticercosis en niños y adolescentes de una comunidad andina del Ecuador. *Pediatrica Baca Ortiz* 5(1): 17–22, 1999.

95. C. Bern, H.H. Garcia, C. Evans, A. E. Gonzalez, M. Verastegui, V.C. Tsang, and R.H. Gilman. Magnitude of the disease burden from neurocysticercosis in a developing country. *Clinical Infectious Diseases* 29:1203–1209, 1999.

96. D.K. Pal, A. Carpio, and J.W.A.S. Sander. Neurocysticercosis and epilepsy in developing countries. *Journal of Neurology, Neurosurgery and Psychiatry* 68:137–143, 2000.

97. H.H. Garcia, R.H. Gilman, V.C.W. Tsang, and A.E. Gonzalez. Clinical significance of neurocysticercosis in endemic villages. *Transactions of the Royal Society of Tropical Medicine and Hygiene* Mar–Apr; 91(2):176–178, 1997.

98. A.C. White Jr. Neurocysticercosis: Updates on epidemiology, pathogenesis, diagnosis, and management. *Annual Review of Medicine* 51:187–206, 2000.

99. M.W. Lightowlers. Eradication of *Taenia solium* cysticercosis: A role for vaccination of pigs. *International Journal of Parasitology* Jun;29(6):811–8117, 1999.

100. S. J. Oh. Cerebral paragonimiasis. *Journal of the Neurological Sciences* 8:27–48, 1968.

101. S. Toyonaga, M. Kurisaka, K. Mori, and N. Suzuki. Cerebral paragonimiasis: Report of five cases. *Neurologica Medico-Chirurgica* 32:157–162, 1992.

102. Z.S. Yi. Clinical analysis and follow-up study of 92 cases of cerebral schistosomiasis. *Zhonghua Shen Jing Jing Shen Ke Za Zhi* Jun;21(3):156–159, 189, 1988.

103. P.R.M. Bittencourt and M. Turner. Latin American Aspects. In: *Comprehensive Epileptology*, Dam, M. and Gram, L., eds. Raven Press: New York, 807–819, 1991.

104. A. Carpio, H. Calle, J. Torres, and B. Sheperd. Retardo mental epilepsia: Aspectos clincos e pronostico. *Revista de la Facultad e Ciencias Medicas de la Universidad de Cuenca* 16:29–43, 1987.

105. P.R.M. Bittencourt, C.M. Garcia, and P. Lorenzana. Epilepsy and parasitosis of the central nervous system. In: *Recent Advances in Epilepsy.* Pedley, T.A. and Meldrum, B.S., eds. Churchill Livingstone: Edinburgh, vol. 4:pp.123–159, 1988.

106. World Health Organization (WHO). *Control and Surveillance of African Trypanosomiasis.* Report of a WHO Expert Committee, WHO Technical Report Series, 881. World Health Organization: Geneva, 1998.

107. E. Jardim and O. M. Takayanagui. Epilepsy and chronic Chagas disease. *Arquivos de Neuro-Psiquiatria* 39:32–41, 1981.

108. N.E. Bharucha, S.N. Bhagwati, and M.M. Kanphade. Epilepsy and solitary lesions. *Surgical Neurology* Aug;52(2):208–209, 1999.

109. Y. Kong, S.Y. Cho, and W.S. Kang. Sparganum infections in normal adult population and epileptic patients in Korea: A seroepidemiologic observation. *Kisaengchunghak Chapchi* Jun;32(2):85–92, 1994.

110. C. Kaiser, G. Asaba, M. Leichsenring, and G. Kabagambe. High incidence of epilepsy related to onchocerciasis in West Uganda. *Epilepsy Research* May;30(3):247–251, 1998.

111. M. Druet-Cabanac, P.M. Preux, B. Bouteille, P. Bernet-Bernady, J. Dunand, A. Hopkins, et al. Onchocerciasis and epilepsy: A matched case-control study in the Central African Republic. *American Journal of Epidemiology* Mar 15;149(6):565–570, 1999.

112. W. Mak. Tuberculosis meningitis in Hong Kong: Experience in a regional hospital. *International Journal of Tuberculosis and Lung Disease* Dec;2(12):1040–1043, 1998.

113. R.T. Danaya, F.A. Johnson, and U. Ambihaipahar. Childhood epilepsy in Papua, New Guinea. *Papua New Guinea Medical Journal* Mar;37(1):3–6, 1994.

114. A.S. Karstaedt, S. Valtchanova, R. Barriere, and H.H. Crewe-Brown. Tuberculosis meningitis in South African urban adults. *QJM* Nov;91(11):743–747, 1998.

115. J. Lorber. Long-term follow-up of 100 children who recovered from tuberculous meningitis. *Pediatrics* 28:778–782, 1961.

116. M. Donner and O. Wasz-Hockert. Late neurological sequelae of tuberculous meningitis. *Acta Paediatrica* 51:34–38, 1962.

117. M. Bahemuka and H. Murungi. Tuberculosis of the nervous system: A clinical, radiological and pathological study of 39 consecutive cases in Riyadh, Saudi Arabia. *Journal of the Neurological Sciences* 90:67–76, 1989.

118. J.F. Annegers, W.A. Hauser, E. Beghi, A. Nicolosi, and L.T. Kurland. The risk of unprovoked seizures after encephalitis and meningitis. *Neurology* 38:1407–1410, 1988.

119. D. Lou, J. Song, H. Ying, R. Yao, and Z. Wang. Prognostic factors of early sequelae and fatal outcome of Japanese encephalitis. *Southeast Asian Journal of Tropical Medicine and Public Health* Dec;26(4):694–698, 1995.

120. B.V. Huy, H.C. Tu, T.V. Luan, and R. Lindqvist. Early mental and neurological sequelae after Japanese B encephalitis. *Southeast Asian Journal of Tropical Medicine and Public Health* Sep;25(3):549–553, 1994.

121. R. Kumar, A. Mathur, K.B. Singh, P. Sitholey, M. Prasad, R. Shukla, et al. Clinical sequelae of Japanese encephalitis in children. *Indian Journal of Medical Research* Jan;97:9–13, 1993.

122. M. Gourie-Devi and D.H. Deshpande. Japanese encephalitis. In: *Paediatric problems.* Prasad, L.S. and Kulczycki, L.L. eds. S. Chand: New Delhi, 340–356, 1982.

123. B. Poneprasert. Japanese encephalitis in children in northern Thailand. *South-East Asian Journal of Tropical Medicine and Public Health* 20:599–603, 1989.

124. H.G. Wieser, J. Wang, P. Panyiotou, et al. Incidence of epileptic seizures in AIDS patients. *Epilepsia* 34(S2):36, 1993.

125. W.A. Hauser, J.F. Annegers, and L.T. Kurland. Incidence of epilepsy and unprovoked seizures in Rochester, Minnesota: 1935–1984. *Epilepsia* 34:453–468, 1993.

126. J.F. Annegers and S. P. Coan. The risks of epilepsy after traumatic brain injury. *Seizure* Oct 9(7):453–457, 2000.

127. E.G. de Pasquet, M. Pietra, S. Bonnevaure, et al. Estudio epidemiologico de 500 epilepticos adultos procedentes de una poblaciones hopitalaria. *Acta Neurologica Latinoamericana* 22:50–65, 1976.

128. D.R.W. Haddock. An attempt to assess the prevalence of epilepsy in Accra. *Ghana Medical Journal* 6:140, 1967.

129. B.V. Tellang and E.S.G. Hettiaratchi. Patterns of epilepsy in Kenya—A clinical analysis of 115 cases. *East African Medical Journal* 58:437–444, 1981.

130. J. E. Cosnett. Neurological disorders in the Zulu. *Neurology* (Minneap.), 14:443–454, 1964.

131. P.R.M. Bittencourt and M. Turner. Epilepsy in the third world: Latin American aspects. In: *Comprehensive Epileptology,* Dam, M. and Gram, L., eds. Raven Press: New York, pp.807–820, 1991.

132. T. Tsuboi and S.H.Endo. Febrile convulsions followed by nonfebrile convulsions: A clinical, electroencephalographic and follow-up study. *Neuropaediatriae* 8:209–223,1977.

133. WHO (World Health Organization). *Primary Prevention of Mental, Neurological and Psychosocial Disorders.* WHO:Geneva pp.54–74, 1998.

134. S. Ismael. The efficacy of phenobarbital in controlling epilepsy in children. *Paediatrica Indonesiana* Mar-Apr;30(3-4):97–110, 1990.

135. D. K. Pal, T. Das, G. Chaudhury, A. L. Johnson, and B. G. Neville. Randomized controlled trial to assess acceptibility of phenobarbital for childhood epilepsy in rural India. *Lancet* Jan3;351(9095):19–23, 1998.

136. I.M. Sawhney, O.P. Lekhra, J.S. Shashi, A. Prabhakar, and J.S. Chopra. Evaluation of epilepsy management in a developing country: A prospective study of 407 patients. *Acta Neurologica Scandinavica* 94: 19–23, 1996.

137. R.D. Elwes, A.L. Johnson, S.D. Shorvon, and E.H. Reynolds. The prognosis for seizure control in newly diagnosed epilepsy. *New England Journal of Medicine* Oct 11;311(15):944–947, 1984.

138. K.S. Mani. Collaborative epidemiological study on epilepsy in India. Final report of the Bangalore Centre. Department of Neurology, National Institute of Mental Health and Neurosciences: Bangalore, 1987.

139. S.A. Al-Shammari, T.A. Khoja, and S.A. Rajeh. Role of primary care physicians in the care of epileptic patients. *Public Health* 110:47–48, 1996.

140. M.E. Cruz, B.S. Schoenberg, F. Sevilla, and R. Echeverria. Protocolo para el desarrollo de una estrategia para el control comunitario de la epilepsia. In: *Control Comunitario de la Epilepsia,* Cruz, M.E., ed. Publimpress: Quito, 1991, pp. 159–168.

141. F. Bossano, D. Tapia, J. Castro Luna, and M.E. Cruz. Plan piloto de control comunitario de la epilepsia en dos comunidades rurales andinas del Ecuador. In: *Control Comunitario de la Epilepsia,* Cruz, M.E., ed. Publimpress: Quito, 1991, pp. 169–178.

142. B. Adamolekun, J.K. Mielke, and D.E. Ball. An evaluation of the impact of health worker and patient education on the care and compliance of patients with epilepsy in Zimbabwe. *Epilepsia* 40 (4): 507–511, 1999.

143. M.J. Brodie, and M.A. Dichter. Antiepileptic drugs. *The New England Journal of Medicine* 334(3): 168–175, 1996.

144. M. Placencia, J.W.A.S. Sander, S.D. Shorvon, M. Roman, F. Alarcon, C. Bimos, et al. Antiepileptic drug treatment in a community health-care setting in northern Ecuador: A prospective 12-month assessment. *Epilepsy Research* 14:237–244, 1993.

145. A.E. Watts. A model for managing epilepsy in a rural community in Africa. *British Medical Journal* 298:805–807, 1989.

146. P.M. Preux, F. Tiemagni, L. Fodzo, P. Kandem, P. Ngouafong, F. Ndonko, et al. Antiepileptic Therapies in the Mifi Province in Cameroon. *Epilepsia* 41(4):432–439, 2000.

147. H.T. Rwiza. The Muhimbili epilepsy project, a three-pronged approach: Assessment of the size of the problem, organization of an epilepsy care system and research on risk factors. *Tropical and Geographical Medicine* 46(3):S22–S24, 1994.

148. D.E. Ball, J. Mielke, B. Adamolekun, T. Mundanda, and J. McLean. Community leader education to increase epilepsy attendance at clinics in Epworth, Zimbabwe. *Epilepsia* Aug;41(8):1044–1045, 2000.

149. S. C. Li. [A report on a feasibility test of "community control of epilepsy" proposed by WHO]. *Zhonghua Shen Jing Jing Shen Ke Zu Zhi* [Chinese]. Jun;22(3):144–147, 190, 1989.

150. S.D. Shorvon, Y.M. Hart, J.W.A.S. Sander, and F. van Andel. *The Management of Epilepsy in Developing Countries: an ICBERG Manual.* Royal Sociey of Medicine Services: London, ICSS 175, 1991.

151. J.T. De Jong. A comprehensive public mental programme in Guinea-Bissau: A useful model for African, Asian, and Latin American countries. *Psychological Medicine* 26:97–108, 1996.

152. R.A. Scott, S.D. Lhatoo, and J.W.A.S. Sander. The treatment of epilepsy in developing countries: Where do we go from here? *Bulletin of the World Health Organization* 79(4), 2001.

153. I.E. Tureczek, J. Fandino-Franky, and H.G. Wieser. Comparison of the epilepsy surgery programs in Cartagena, Colombia, and Zurich, Switzerland. *Epilepsia* 41(Supplement 4):S35–S40, 2000.

154. H.G. Wieser and H. Silfvenius. Overview: Epilepsy surgery in developing countries. *Epilepsia* 41(4):S3–S9, 2000.

155. M.B. Rao and K. Radhakrishnan. Is epilepsy surgery possible in countries with limited resources? *Epilepsia* (supplement) 4:S31–S34, 2000.

156. P.D. Williamson and B.C. Jobst. Epilepsy surgery in developing countries. *Epilepsia* 41(supplement) 4:S45–S50, 2000.

157. J. Kaamugisha and A.T. Feksi. Determining the prevalence of epilepsy in the semi-urban population of Nakuru, Kenya, comparing two independent methods not apparently used before in epilepsy studies. *Neuroepidemiology* 7:115–121, 1988.

158. B. Adamolekun, J. Meilke, D. Ball, and T. Mundanda. An evaluation of the management of epilepsy by primary health care nurse in Chitungwiza, Zimbabwe. *Epilepsy Research* May;39(3):177–181, 2000.

159. WHO (World Health Organization). *International Classification of Impairments, Disabilities, and Handicaps.* World Health Organization: Geneva, 1980.

160. L. Risdale, I. Kwan, and C. Cryer. Newly diagnosed epilepsy: can nurse specialists help? A randomized controlled trial. Epilepsy Care Evaluation Group. *Epilepsia* Aug;41(8):1014–1019, 2000.

161. R. Coleman, G. Gill, and D. Wilkinson. Noncommunicable disease management in resource-poor settings: A primary care model from rural South Africa. *Bulletin of the World Health Organization* 76(6):633–640, 1998.

162. L. Jilek-Aall. Morbus sacer in Africa: Some religious aspects of epilepsy in traditional cultures. *Epilepsia* Mar;40(3):382–386, 1999.

163. R. S. Murthy and N. N. Wig. The WHO collaborative study on strategies for extending mental health care, IV: A training approach to enhancing the availability of mental health manpower in a developing country. *American Journal of Psychiatry* Nov;140(11):1486–1490, 1983.

164. M. Gourie-Devi, G. Gururaj, P. Satishchandra, and D.K. Subbakrishna. Neuro-epidemiological pilot survey of an urban population in a developing country. A study in Bangalore, south India. *Neuroepidemiology* 15(6):313–320, 1996.

165. Initiative of support to people with epilepsy. Geneva, World Health Organization, 1990 (unpublished document WHO/MNH/MND/90.3; available in English, French, Portuguese and Spanish from Mental Disorders Control, World Health Organization, 1211 Geneva 27, Switzerland).

166. P.M. Preux. [Questionnaire in a study of epilepsy in tropical countries]. *Bulletin de la Société de Pathologie Exotique* [French] 93(4):276–278, 2000.

167. N.K. Leidy, A.M. Rentz, and E.M. Grace. Evaluating health-related quality of life outcomes in clinical trials of antiepileptic drug therapy. *Epilesia* 39(9):965–977,1998.

168. E. Dietrichs, T. Tyssvang, N.O. Aanonsen, and S. J. Bakke. Cerebral cysticercosis in Norway. *Acta Neurologica Scandinavica* Oct;88(4):296–298, 1993.

169. J. L. Yong and B.A. Warren. Neurocysticercosis: A report of four cases. *Pathology* Jul;26(3):244–249, 1994.

170. J. Walker, S. Chen, D. Packham, and P. McIntyre. Five cases of neurocysticercosis diagnosed in Sydney. *Southeast Asian Journal of Tropical Medicine and Public Health* Dec;22 (supplement): 242–244, 1991.

171. M. Buitrago, B. Edwards, and F. Rosner. Neurocysticercosis: Report of fifteen cases. *Mt. Sinai Journal of Medicine* Nov;62(6):439–444, 1995.

172. P.M. Schantz, A.C. Moore, J.L. Munoz, B.J. Hartman, J. A. Schaefer, A.M. Aron, et al. Neurocysticercosis in an Orthodox Jewish community in New York City. *New England Journal of Medicine* Sep 3;327(10):692–695, 1992.

173. J. Proano, A.L. Alarcon, and R. Sempertegui. Ecuadorian program for control and surveillance of *Taenia solium*, taeniasis/cysticercosis, 19th International Epilepsy congress, Internatinal League Against Epilepsy, Rio de Janeiro, 1991.

174. J.F. Bale Jr. Cysticercosis. *Current Treatment Options in Neurology* Jul;2(4):355–360, 2000.

175. S. Antoniuk. [Epidemiology of neurocysticercosis]. *Review of Neurology* [Spanish] Aug 16-31;29(4):331–334, 1999.

176. P.M. Schantz, M. Cruz, and Z. Pawlowski. Potential eradicability of taeniasis and cysticercosis. *Bulletin of the Pan American Health Organization* 27(4):397–403, 1993.

177. M.T. Medina, P. Genton, M.C. Montova, S. Cordova, C. Dravet, and J. Sotelo. Effect of anticysticercal treatment on the prognosis of epilepsy in neurocysticercosis: A pilot trial. *Epilepsia* 34:1024–1027, 1993.

178. M.E. Cruz. Praziquantel no tratamento ambulatorial da neurocysticercose. *Journal Brasileiro de Medicina* (supp), 79–84, 1983.

179. M. Cruz, I. Cruz, and J. Horton. Albendazole vs Praziquantel in the treatment of cerebral cysticercosis: Clinical evaluation. *Transactions of the Royal Society of Tropical Medicine and Hygiene* 85 (2):224–247, 1991.

180. I. Cruz, M.E. Cruz, F. Carrasco, and J. Horton. Neurocysticercosis: Optimum dose treatment with albendazole. *Journal of the Neurological Sciences* 133:152–154, 1995

181. L.D. De Ghetaldi, R.M. Norman, and A.W. Couville. Cerebral cysticercosis treated biphasically with dexamethazone and praziquantel. *Annals of Internal Medicine* 99:179–181, 1983.

182. V. Vasquez and J. Sotelo. The course of seizures after treatment of cerebral cysticercosis. *The New England Journal of Medicine* 327:696–701, 1992.

183. O.H. Del Brutto. Prognostic factors for seizure recurrence after withdrawal of antiepileptic drugs in patients with neurocysticercosis. *Neurology* 44:1706–1709, 1994.

184. P.S. Craig, M.T. Rogan, and J.C. Allan. Detection, screening and community epidemiology of taeniid cestode zooneses: Cystic echinococcosis, almeolar echinococcosis and neurocysticercosis. *Advanced Parasitology* 38:169–250, 1996.

185. J.M. Murthy and R. Yangala. Acute symptomatic seizures-incidence and etiological spectrum: A hospital-based study from South India. *Seizure* May;8(3):162–165, 1999.

Summary of Findings:
Schizophrenia in Developing Countries

- The average lifetime risk of schizophrenia is about 1 percent. Compared to its incidence and prevalence, the social and economic costs of schizophrenia are disproportionately high. The condition causes greater chronic disability than any other mental disorder, in part because of its early age of onset and the stigma of "insanity."

- In both developed and developing countries, schizophrenia is associated with excess mortality from a variety of causes associated with poor self-care, inadequate nutrition, heavy smoking, and medical neglect. At least part of this excess mortality is preventable.

- A high proportion of better outcomes for schizophrenia in developing countries has been reported by numerous investigators. The reasons for this are unknown, but may involve interactions between specific genetic and environmental factors. Research on this topic could have fundamental implications for the management and treatment of schizophrenia in both developing and developed countries.

- Schizophrenia and other psychotic illnesses can be controlled with a variety of treatments that offer significant returns in terms of symptom improvement, quality of life, and reintegration into the community. The choice of an antipsychotic therapeutic agent, however, must involve a balance between several potentially conflicting factors: clinical efficacy, profile and incidence of adverse effects, acceptability and likelihood of treatment adherence, and cost-effectiveness.

7

Schizophrenia

DEFINITION

Although schizophrenia is likely to have originated early in the evolution of man, it was identified as a disease only about 100 years ago by Kraepelin [1] under the name *dementia praecox* (early "mental enfeeblement"). In 1911, Bleuler [2] renamed the condition *schizophrenia*, suggesting that its salient characteristic was the "splitting" of mental functions. Whereas Kraepelin emphasized the deteriorating long-term course of the illness, Bleuler highlighted its fundamental symptoms: the inability to maintain coherence of ideas (loosening of associations); blunting or incongruity of affect; loss of the capacity for goal-directed action or coexistence of incompatible volitional impulses (ambivalence); and withdrawal into an inner world populated by private fantasies (autism). These symptoms were thought to be more closely related to the neurobiological substrate of the disease than its more conspicuous accessory phenomena, such as hallucinations, delusions, and bizarre behavior. At present, the manifestations of schizophrenia are commonly classified into "positive" symptoms and signs, including hallucinations, delusions, and disorganized thought, and "negative" disorders, such as blunted affect, amotivation, poverty of speech, and social withdrawal.[3]

Current diagnostic concepts of schizophrenia are descendants of Kraepelin's and Bleuler's ideas. Since the 1970s, the World Health Organization (WHO) and the American Psychiatric Association (APA) have been instrumental in promoting standard rules and criteria designed to improve the reliability of diagnostic assessment and enhance the comparability of mental health statistics and research data worldwide. The products of this work, the *Tenth Revision of the*

International Classification of Diseases (ICD-10) [4] and the APA *Diagnostic and Statistical Manual, fourth edition, DSM-IV,*[5] now serve as a common language for psychiatry and mental health care worldwide. The two systems identify schizophrenia in a broadly similar manner (see Table 7-1).

Notwithstanding international agreement on diagnosis, it is important to bear in mind that schizophrenia remains a clinical syndrome and that the neurobiology underlying its manifestations is not yet fully understood. There is at present no biological test or marker that can identify the disease (or a predisposition to it) independently of clinical assessment. Furthermore, the clinical

TABLE 7-1 Overview of the ICD-10 and DSM-IV Criteria for Diagnosis of Schizophrenia

ICD-10 Schizophrenia (F20)	DSM-IV Schizophrenia (295)
One month or more of at least one of the following symptoms:	*A. One month or more of at least two of the following symptoms:*
(a) thought echo, withdrawal, insertion, broadcasting	(a) delusions
(b) delusions of control and passivity	(b) hallucinations
(c) voices; 3rd person, commentary, coming from part of body	(c) disorganized speech
(d) persistent delusions	(d) grossly disorganized or catatonic behavior
	(e) negative symptoms
or at least two of the following:	
	B. Social and occupational dysfunction
(e) persistent hallucinations accompanied by delusions	One or more areas affected
(f) incoherence, irrelevant speech, neologisms	(work, relationships, self-care)
(g) catatonic signs	
(h) negative symptoms	*C. Duration*
(i) significant consistent change in personal behavior	Continuous symptoms and signs for $\geq$ 6 months
	These 6 months must include:
	• At least 1 month of symptoms meeting criterion A
	• Various combinations of prodromal and residual symptoms
Exclude:	*Exclude:*
Full manic or depressive episode preceding the onset of schizophrenic symptoms	Schizoaffective and mood disorder
Organic brain disease	Substance use or a medical condition
Alcohol or drug intoxication or withdrawal	Autism or pervasive developmental disorder

Source: [4,5]

concept of schizophrenia does not tell us whether one or several pathological processes are involved or whether the causes of schizophrenia are the same in all cases. These gaps in the biological characterization of schizophrenia reflect the complexity of the disease, as well as our incomplete understanding of the basic neurobiology underlying psychological functions—such as memory, multimodal sensory integration, self-monitoring, and goal-directed action—that are impaired in those with schizophrenia. Neuroscience research in the next decade is likely to contribute substantial new insights into the causes of the disorder.

The question of whether cases clinically diagnosed as schizophrenia in developing countries are homologous with similarly diagnosed cases in Western cultures is of critical importance, considering that the biological basis of the disorder still eludes reliable identification. To accept that schizophrenia is universal implies that its essential features can be reliably identified in different populations; that the constellation of symptoms is coherent and replicable; that consistent associations with age and gender are present; and that the course, outcome, and response to treatment show a common pattern.

Cross-cultural similarities in the clinical presentation of disorders broadly corresponding to the diagnostic entity of schizophrenia have been reported by numerous researchers.[6] Yet until recently, the belief has been widespread that schizophrenia is a Western disease with no counterpart in indigenous populations untouched by modern technology and lifestyles.[7] That such beliefs are mistaken has been demonstrated by the fact that no human group has yet been found to be free of schizophrenia, provided that the size of the population is sufficient for a disorder of low incidence to become manifest. Research systematically addressing these issues was conducted within the WHO program of schizophrenia studies in some 27 developing and developed countries over the last three decades.[8–13] The results of these studies support the clinical validity of the diagnostic concept of schizophrenia in diverse populations, and reveal that the symptoms and syndromes accepted as characteristic of schizophrenia can be found in patients in all cultures and geographical areas covered by the research.

Although no single symptom can be pinpointed as characteristic of schizophrenia in all patients and all settings, the overall pattern of the clinical presentation of the disorder is remarkably invariant across cultures. For example, acutely ill patients in very different cultural settings describe strikingly similar positive symptoms, such as hallucinatory voices commenting on their every thought and action, the experience of their thoughts being taken away by some alien agency or broadcast at large, or their surroundings being imbued with special meaning. Negative symptoms, such as psychomotor poverty, social withdrawal, and amotivation, are found to occur in varying proportions of patients irrespective of the cultural setting.

The conclusion that patients diagnosed with schizophrenia in different cultures suffer from the same disorder is further supported by the similarity in the age- and sex-specific distribution of the onset of symptoms, which in all settings has a high peak in early adulthood (in both males and females) and a second, lower peak at age 35 and over (females only). Considering the variety of social norms, attitudes, and beliefs about illness across cultures, the similarity of the subjective experience of core schizophrenic symptoms and of the age at which they first occur in males and females is striking. The findings suggest that the disorders of perception, thought, and self-awareness characteristic of schizophrenia are likely to have a common pathophysiological basis across various cultures.

Notwithstanding such overall similarity, there are variations in the clinical presentation of schizophrenia in different cultures that may influence recognition and treatment of the disease. Lambo [13] described a characteristic symptom complex in Nigeria consisting of anxiety, depression, vague hypochondriacal symptoms, bizarre magico-mystical ideas, episodic twilight or confusional states, atypical depersonalization, emotional lability, and retrospective falsification of memory based on hallucinations or delusions. Pfeiffer,[14] drawing on observations in Indonesia, concluded that the disease pictures are essentially the same as in Central Europe, but he also described several local characteristics, such as frequent confusion, an admixture of manic features, and rarity of systematized delusions.

Certain subtypes of schizophrenia, such as the acute onset form and the catatonic subtype (characterized by bizarre movement disorders) are more common in developing countries than in the West. In the WHO 10-country study.[11] acute onset characterized 40.3 percent and catatonic schizophrenia 10.3 percent of the cases in developing countries, compared with 10.9 and 1.2 percent, respectively, in the developed world. In isolated groups, such as island, highlands, or tribal populations, schizophrenic psychoses may present with certain atypical features, most likely as a result of ancestral founder effects and genetic drift. A more common clinical problem in developing countries may be the differentiation of schizophrenia from psychoses due to infectious or parasitic diseases. Lambo [13] has drawn attention to the observation that in Africa, psychosis associated with trypanosomiasis often has a slow, insidious onset and may mimic "Western" schizophrenia, whereas acute schizophrenia in Africa, often characterized by confusion and agitation, may resemble "European" psychoses accompanying physical disease.

Since a variety of infectious, parasitic, and nutritional diseases are endemic in the developing world, it has been suggested that a high proportion of the cases of schizophrenia in those populations may in fact be symptomatic psychoses accompanying physical diseases such as malaria or typhoid fever.[15] The available evidence does not support this view. In the WHO 10-country study,[11] only 11.7 percent of a large number of individuals with psychotic symptoms who were screened for inclusion in India and Nigeria were excluded on the grounds of having an acute or chronic physical disease that might explain their psychotic symptoms. On the other hand, common febrile illnesses may be among the factors precipitating the onset of acute, brief transient psychoses that are relatively frequent in developing countries, but bear no relationship to schizophrenia.[16] A more likely brain pathology contributing to cases of psychosis with schizophrenia-like features is epilepsy. The association between temporal lobe epilepsy and a chronic, interictal psychosis that is difficult to distinguish from schizophrenia has been well documented clinically.[17] Recent epidemiological studies in Europe point to a tenfold increase in the risk of schizophrenia-like psychosis among people suffering from epilepsy.[18,19] No comparable data are available from developing countries, but considering that epilepsy is a frequent disorder in many regions of the developing world, it is to be expected that undiagnosed and untreated epilepsy may account for some cases of schizophrenia-like psychoses, especially in areas where epilepsy is endemic (see Chapter 6).

SCOPE OF THE PROBLEM

Mortality

In both developing and developed countries, schizophrenia is associated with excess mortality from a variety of causes. In Taiwan, data collected over a 15-year period indicate that of all mental disorders followed up, schizophrenia was associated with the highest mortality, representing an 80 percent increase over the mortality of the general population.[20] In the WHO International Pilot Study of Schizophrenia (IPSS),[21] the percentages of patients in Agra and Ibadan who died during the 5-year follow-up were 9.0 and 7.1, respectively, and were higher than the percentage (4.9) for the total study cohort.

Whereas in the past, the excess mortality among individuals with schizophrenia was due mainly to communicable diseases such as tuberculosis, the leading causes of premature death among patients with schizophrenia at present are suicide, accidents, and common physical diseases. In developed countries, the suicide risk associated with schizophrenia is now nearly as high as that associated with major depression (4–6 percent lifetime risk).[22] In persons with schizophrenia, suicide may occur at any stage of the progression of the disorder, but the risk is particularly high in the first 6 months after the first psychotic episode, as well as following periods of frequent hospital admission and discharge.[23] Although depressive symptoms often underlie suicide in people with schizophrenia, a sense of hopelessness, negative assessment of the future, and heavy alcohol use may drive suicidal behavior in the absence of marked mood disorder.[24,25] In the developing world, suicide-related mortality is a problem as well, but the majority of deaths among those suffering from schizophrenia are due to physical illness and accidents. In both developed and developing countries, schizophrenia is associated with excess mortality from respiratory, gastrointestinal, and cardiovascular diseases, which are likely to be caused or exacerbated by poor self-care, inadequate nutrition, heavy smoking (common in schizophrenia patients), and medical neglect. At least part of this excess mortality is preventable.[26]

Social and Economic Costs

Schizophrenia is associated with greater chronic disability than any other mental disorder. Both the positive and negative symptoms of the disease interfere seriously with a person's capacity to cope with the demands of daily living. Patients with schizophrenia experience particular difficulty in dealing with complex demands and environments, especially those that involve social interaction and decoding of social communication.[27] Moreover, the onset is usually at a developmental stage of incomplete social maturation, educational attainment, and acquisition of occupational skills. The intervention of schizophrenia at this stage results in a severely truncated repertoire of social skills and lifelong socioeconomic disadvantage. These factors are exacerbated by the societal reaction to individuals manifesting the behavior associated with "insanity," which generally involves stigma and social exclusion.[28]

The above adverse factors interact to cause a "social breakdown syndrome" [29] that results in the loss of social support networks and a greatly diminished quality of life for a substantial proportion of those affected by schizophrenia.[30] Many schizophrenic patients end up on the streets or in the criminal justice system and are exposed to abuse, even in psychiatric hospitals. Such outcomes are not uncommon in either developed or developing countries, although in the latter settings, traditional family and community structures are still capable of providing a protective environment, and probably fewer patients are marginalized by society.[31]

The social and economic costs of schizophrenia are disproportionately high relative to its incidence and prevalence. According to tentative estimates by WHO and the World Bank, in 1990 schizophrenia accounted for 2.3 percent of the burden of disease (disability adjusted life years [DALYs]) in established market economies and 0.8 percent in demographically developing regions. The projections for 2020 are 2.0 and 1.2 percent, respectively. In terms of DALYs, predicted demographic trends include more than a 50 percent increase in the disease burden attributable to schizophrenia in developing countries, a burden approaching that of malaria and nutritional deficiency.

The total cost of illness for schizophrenia is disproportionately high relative to the population point prevalence of the disease (on average, 5 per 1000) or lifetime morbid risk (on average, 1 percent). In developed market economies, the direct costs of schizophrenia, incurred by hospital or community-based treatment, supervised accommodation, and related services, amount to 1.4 to 2.8

percent of the national health care expenditure and up to one-fifth of the direct costs of all mental disorders.[32–34] Although estimates of the indirect costs of schizophrenia vary greatly depending on the method of analysis and the underlying assumptions, these costs are likely to be comparable in scale to the direct costs, considering lost productivity and employment, the economically devastating long-term impact of the illness on the patient's family, other caregivers' opportunity costs, the increased mortality of people with schizophrenia, the costs to the criminal justice system, and other issues related to public concerns about safety. Estimates based on the Epidemiological Catchment Areas study in the United States put the direct costs of schizophrenia in 1990 at $17.3 billion and the indirect costs at $15.2 billion.[35]

An important aspect of the economics of schizophrenia is the so-called funding imbalance effect: studies indicate that 97 percent of the total lifetime costs of schizophrenia are incurred by fewer than 50 percent of the patients diagnosed with the disorder.[32] While this finding points to a hard-core subset of cases with severe chronic illness, multiple disabilities, and excessive dependence on services and other support, it also suggests that in more than 50 percent of those with schizophrenia, the disorder is less disabling or treatment more effective.

Most of the economic evidence on schizophrenia comes from studies conducted in the Western market economies. However, mental health economics is a young discipline. Thus evidence on the costs of schizophrenia even in developed countries is at present limited, and such data are quite scarce for the majority of developing countries, although individual studies provide some insight into the likely economic impact of the disease.[36] Since both the direct and indirect costs of schizophrenia are context-bound, extrapolations not only from the developed to the developing world but also across countries at comparable levels of gross domestic product (GDP) per capita must be made with caution, given the diversity of cultures, social structures, and health care systems.

Thus although the generic cost-driving factors associated with schizophrenia are likely to be similar around the world (management of the chronic or relapsing symptoms and impairments, provision of inpatient and outpatient care and medication, mortality, lost productivity and unemployability, impact on the family, and impact on the community), their relative weight and hence the structure of the direct and indirect costs of the illness are likely to vary considerably. Hospital or other residential care, which generates more than 75 percent of the direct costs of schizophrenia in high-income countries,[33,34] is likely to account for a smaller fraction in developing countries because of lower staffing and equipment costs. On the other hand, the proportion of direct costs attributable to dispensing of antipsychotic medication, which is less than 5 percent of the total direct costs in developed countries,[33] is likely to be higher in developing countries.

It is difficult to estimate the economic impact of schizophrenia on families in developing countries. A study conducted in Nigeria [37] revealed that caregiver opportunity costs (e.g., family members' lost productivity or income) were not of a different order from those in the developed world. Yet the aggregate family costs in developing countries may, in fact, be substantially higher since (1) a larger proportion of schizophrenic patients live with their families as compared to patients in Western societies; (2) the family, not mental health services, is likely to be the first line of treatment and management of psychotic episodes; and (3) the cost of purchasing prescribed maintenance medication is usually borne by the family. Additional direct costs may be incurred by the necessity to travel, often long distances, to the nearest hospital or clinic, as well as by payment for the services of traditional healers. In many traditional communities, the stigma associated with mental illness may affect the family as a whole and restrict, for instance, marital opportunities for younger family members. While lost educational opportunities are likely to be a problem, lost paid employment is more difficult to quantify, and therefore less likely to appear prominently in estimates of the indirect illness burden in developing countries. On the other hand, reintegration of a family member who has suffered a psychotic episode into the domestic economy may be much easier to achieve than formal employment, and this may be one factor in the better and longer remissions of patients with schizophrenia observed in developing countries.[11]

Another aspect of the social and economic costs of schizophrenia is the commonly perceived association between the disease and criminal behavior alluded to above. Crimes committed by persons with schizophrenia tend to receive wide media coverage and to reinforce popular ideas about dangerousness associated with mental illness. It is important to dispel such prejudicial attitudes.[38] Carefully designed studies in Europe and elsewhere indicate that a small proportion of patients with schizophrenia tend to be overrepresented among the perpetrators of violent offenses, including homicide. However, the population-attributable fraction of such offenses committed by persons with schizophrenia is negligibly small compared with the total number of offenses in the community. Moreover, the rate of apprehension and incarceration is likely to be high among patients with schizophrenia because of their conspicuous behavior and appearance, rather than the seriousness of the offense. Issues of protecting patients' rights must therefore be an important part of anti-stigma campaigns in both developing and developed countries.

Recommendation 7-1. Governments, development agencies, and other sponsoring bodies should be made aware of the fact that schizophrenia and other psychotic illnesses are treatable conditions, and that significant returns in terms of symptom control, quality of life, and reintegration into the community can be achieved if increased funding is provided for local and regional programs that incorporate best-practice procedures and criteria.

PREVALENCE AND INCIDENCE

Epidemiological research reveals that schizophrenia is a disorder of low population incidence (2–4 new cases per 10,000 population per year), relatively high point prevalence (5 per 1000), and a very high disablement rate (in Western societies up to 70 percent of patients become severely disabled). The average lifetime risk of schizophrenia is about 1 percent and is approximately the same for males and females. Although a proportion of cases (estimated at 15 to 20 percent) do recover or improve, in the majority the disorder runs a chronic or recurrent course.

Prevalence

The availability of epidemiological data on schizophrenia in developing countries is uneven. While the prevalence of schizophrenia has been explored by numerous surveys in regions such as the Indian subcontinent, China, and Southeast Asia, the data on Africa and parts of Latin America are limited. Results of prevalence studies carried out in developing countries since the 1960s are presented in Table 7-2. For comparison, the table also includes selected studies from developed countries. The majority are point prevalence surveys in which case finding and enumeration are likely to have been fairly complete. However, some of the communities studied are small, and the rates may be unstable since they are based on only a few cases of schizophrenia. Where larger populations have been studied, as in India and China, it appears possible to discern certain trends.

Indian psychiatrists have carried out an impressive number of epidemiological investigations that include a large-scale study sponsored by the Indian Council of Medical Research,[39] covering a total population of 146,380. Given a methodological caveat about direct comparisons across studies, the survey data from India and Sri Lanka indicate a prevalence of schizophrenia ranging from 1.1 per 1000 [40] to 5.9 per 1000.[41] Since these two studies deal with relatively small populations, a range of 2.2–2.5 per 1000, supported by the two large-scale surveys, is more likely to be consistent and representative for the population of the Indian subcontinent as a whole. This range is similar to that obtained in the majority of European surveys.[42] However, if the lower life expectancy in India, as compared with European populations, is taken into account, the true age-standardized Indian prevalence rates are likely to be higher than the European rates.

In 1981–1982, a comprehensive survey was carried out across several provinces of China in which a sample of 51,982 individuals were interviewed with standardized instruments.[43] The study revealed a point prevalence of 6.1 per 1000 in urban areas and 3.4 per 1000 in rural settings. Given that two-thirds of China's population was living in rural areas, it was estimated that there were more than 4.5 million persons with schizophrenia nationwide. In 1993, another multisite epidemiological study showed a prevalence rate of 6.6 per 1000. With a population of 1.3 billion, this meant there were as many as 7.8 million schizophrenic patients in China.[44] According to the Chinese studies, of all patients with mental disorders, 49 percent were diagnosed with schizophrenia, making it the most prevalent disorder, responsible for an estimated 80 percent of all disability attributed to mental illness (mental disorders in their entirety were estimated to account for 18 percent of the total burden of disease in China).

Few systematic surveys of psychoses have been carried out in Africa, although there is no dearth of clinical, service-based descriptive studies. An exception is a recent well-designed community survey in an area of Ethiopia with a population of 100,000 in the age range 15–49 years. The results of this survey indicated a point prevalence of schizophrenia of 4.8 per 1000; with adjustment for underascertainment, the estimated "true" prevalence was 7.1 per 1000.[45]

In conclusion, the reported point prevalence of schizophrenia in most areas of the developing world where epidemiological surveys have been conducted is comparable to that in the developed world. Taking into account factors such as higher mortality among people with serious mental disorders and incomplete ascertainment of a proportion of cases, it is likely that the reported rates are underestimates of the true prevalence of the disorder.

Incidence

Data on the incidence of schizophrenia (new cases per 10,000 population ascertained over a defined period, usually a year) in developing countries are scarce. Table 7-3 lists the results of several such studies, along with findings on the incidence of schizophrenia in developed countries.

To date, the only direct comparison of incidence rates across geographically defined areas in developing countries and areas in developed countries is provided by the WHO 10-country study.[11] Standardized procedures and diagnostic instruments were applied in each area by well-trained local psychiatrists, and inter-center reliability of data collection was monitored. A total of 1379 persons who met criteria for schizophrenia and related disorders were identified at their first contact with any medical or nonmedical "helping agency" (which included indigenous healers in developing countries). A 15-year follow-up has now been completed.[12]

The highest rates for ICD-9 schizophrenia (0.35 and 0.42 per 1000) across the study sites were found in two Indian areas. However, when the comparison was restricted to cases manifesting "first-rank" symptoms (see ICD-10 criteria, Table 7-1), there were no significant differences in incidence rates among various settings. In recent years, replications of the design of the WHO 10-country study, including its research instruments and procedures, have been carried out with very similar results by investigators in India,[46] the Caribbean,[47,48] and the United Kingdom.[49,50]

RISK FACTORS

Genetic

There is strong evidence that genetic vulnerability plays an important role in the causation of schizophrenia.[51,52] A person's risk of developing the disorder increases steeply with the degree of genetic relatedness to an individual with the disease.

Follow-up studies of children adopted away early in life have shown that their risk of developing schizophrenia as adults is predicted solely by having a biological parent with the disorder and not by the characteristics of the adoptive family. However, the pattern of occurrence of schizophrenia in families is not compatible with the transmission of a single gene; rather, it indicates that multiple genes are involved, each having a relatively small effect on the probability of developing the disease.[53,54] Furthermore, the evidence indicates that having the predisposing genes is not sufficient for the development of clinical disease. Such genes may remain unexpressed unless some other factor, most likely an environmental one, triggers their activity.

Environmental

Many environmental influences have been examined as possible risk factors for the development of schizophrenia.[55,56] These range from complications of pregnancy and birth to early viral infection, urban birth, malnutrition, head injury, toxic effects of psychoactive substances such as cannabis, and psychosocial adversity (see Table 7-4). None of these putative risk factors has been unequivocally validated, and it is possible that different environmental exposures may interact with the predisposing genes at different developmental stages.[57]

Few risk factors have been specifically identified or validated in developing countries, although obstetric complications and early brain injury due to neuroinfection, toxic effects, other trauma, or maternal malnutrition during gestation are likely to be involved in a greater proportion of cases of adult schizophrenia in the developing than in the developed world. Among the potential psychosocial risk factors, migration stress has been suggested by studies in India [58] and Taiwan [59] in which refugees or migrants were found to be overrepresented among schizophrenic patients. Some support for a role of psychosocial adversity in the causation or precipitation of schizophrenia is provided by studies that have highlighted an unusually high incidence of the disorder among the offspring of Afro-Caribbean migrants in the United Kingdom. Since the excess schizophrenia morbidity is limited to the U.K.-born second generation, loss of traditional social support systems and demoralization stress linked to societal stereotyping and prejudice are being explored as possible risk factors interacting

TABLE 7-2 Selected prevalence studies of schizophrenia

Country	Population	Method	Prevalence per 1000 population at risk
Surveys in developed countries			
Germany [60]	Area in Thuringia (n = 37,561); age >10	Census	2.4
Denmark [61,62]	Island population (n = 50,000)	Repeat census	3.9 → 3.3
USA [63]	Household sample	Census	2.9
Sweden [64,65]	Community in southern Sweden	Repeat census	6.7 → 4.5
Croatia [66]	Sample of 9,201 households	Census	5.9
Russia [67]	Population sample (n = 35,590)	Census	3.8
USA [68]	Aggregated data across 5 ECA sites	Sample survey	7.0 (point) 15.0 (lifetime)
United Kingdom [69]	London health district (n = 112,127)	Census; interviews of a sample (n = 172)	5.1
Australia [70]	4 urban areas (n = 1,084,978)	Census; interviews of a sample (n = 980)	3.1–5.9 (point)[A] 3.9–6.9 (one year)[B]
Surveys in developing countries			
Taiwan [59,71]	Population sample	Repeat census	2.1 → 1.4
Iran [72]	Rural area (n = 11,585)	Census	2.1
India [73]	4 areas in Agra (n = 29,468)	Census	2.6
India [73]	Rural area (n = 46,380)	Census	2.2 (point)
India [74]	Urban (n = 101,229)	Census	2.5 (point)
Indonesia [75]	Slum area in West Jakarta (n = 100,107)	Two-stage survey: (a) key informants (b) interview	1.4 (point)
Korea [76]	Urban and rural	Census	Lifetime: 3.0 (urban) 4.0 (rural)
Hong Kong [77]	Community sample (n = 7,229)	DIS interviews	Lifetime: 1.2 (males) 1.3 (females)
Kosrae (Micronesia) [78]	Island population (n = 5,500)	Key informants & clinic records; some interviews	6.8 (point), age > 15
Ethiopia [79]	District (n = 227,135) south of Addis Ababa; mixed urban & rural	Two-stage survey: (a) door-to-door & key informants; (b) SCAN interviews	7.1 (point), age 15–49

[A] All psychoses
[B] Schizophrenia and other non-affective psychoses

TABLE 7-3 Selected incidence studies of schizophrenia

Country	Population	Method	Rate per 1000
A. Europe and North America			
Norway [80]	Total population	First admissions 1926–1935 (n = 14,231)	0.24
Germany [81]	City of Mannheim (n = 330,000)	Case register	0.54
Russia [82]	Moscow district (n = 248,000)	Follow-back of prevalent cases	0.20 (male) 0.19 (female)
Iceland [83]	Total population	First admissions 1966–1967 (n = 2,388)	0.27
UK [84]	London (Camberwell)	Case register	0.25 (ICD) 0.17 (RDC) 0.08 (DSM-III)
Canada [85]	Area in Quebec (n = 338,300)	First admissions	0.31 (ICD) 0.09 (DSM-III)
UK [86]	London health district (n = 112,127)	2 censuses, 5 years apart	0.21 (DSM-IIIR)
UK [87]	Nottingham	2 cohorts of first contacts (1978–1980 and 1992–1994)	0.25 → 0.29 (all psychoses) 0.14 → 0.09 (ICD-10 schizo-phrenia)
B. Asia and the Caribbean			
Mauritius[88]	Total population (n = 257,000)	First admissions	0.24 (Africans) 0.14 (Indian Hindus) 0.09 (Indian Moslems)
Taiwan[71]	3 communities (n = 39,024)	Household survey	0.17
India [46]	Area in Madras (n = 43,097)	Door-to-door survey and key informants	0.41
Jamaica [47]	Total population (n = 2,46 mln)	First contacts	0.24 ('broad') 0.21 ('restrictive')
Barbados [48]	Total population (n = 262,000)	First contacts	0.32 ('broad') 0.28 ('restrictive')

with genetic vulnerability.[89,90] No systematic studies have been carried out on the possible contribution of widespread tropical diseases to psychiatric morbidity in the developing countries.

Urban birth has been shown as a risk factor for later schizophrenia in several developed country studies.[57,91,92] Studies in developing countries confirming similar findings have yet to be conducted. Such evidence coupled with the growing urbanization of developing countries would suggest a projected increase in schizophrenia prevalence. Additional research is needed to determine how such environmental risk factors interact with genetic risk factors. Understanding these could lead to better treatments and possible intervention strategies.[57]

Brain Pathology

No unique pattern of brain pathology has been found in those suffering from schizophrenia. However, multiple abnormalities that distinguish the brains of people with schizophrenia from those of control subjects have been identified and confirmed by meta-analysis.[93] Important findings have resulted from the new brain imaging technologies (computed tomography, magnetic resonance imaging) that have supplemented classical postmortem studies. Generally, the structural anomalies that have been found in schizophrenic brains involve (1) reductions in gray matter volume, (2) enlargement of the cerebral ventricles, and (3) attenuation of the normal brain asymmetry along the antero-posterior axis. It remains controversial whether these abnormalities are progressive or static, and whether they precede or follow the onset of the disease.[93]

Neurochemistry

At the level of central nervous system neurotransmission, excessive production of the neurotransmitter dopamine and excessive density and sensitivity of certain subtypes of dopaminergic receptors have long been suspected of mediating some of the symptoms and behavioral abnormalities that characterize schizophrenia. Most of the pharmacological agents that have proven effective in controlling the positive symptoms of schizophrenia target dopaminergic receptors. However, recent research suggests a much more complex picture of neurotransmission dysregulation in schizophrenia involving multiple systems, notably serotonin and glutamate, as well as a host of other modulating molecules. Since none of the known genetic variants of the proteins building the neuroreceptor sites or transporting neurotransmitter molecules has thus far been found to be linked specifically to schizophrenia, it is uncertain whether neurotransmission dysregulation is a primary cause of the disorder or a secondary complication.[94]

Functional Neuroimaging and Cognitive Deficits

Findings indicate that in patients with schizophrenia, the activation response to stimuli engaging the so-called executive functions (planning and self-monitoring) is attenuated and that, in comparison with controls, the brains of these patients process information less efficiently.[95] Functional brain imaging involving measurement of the brain's hemodynamic, metabolic, or electrical response to cognitive challenges provides a window to brain function in real time. At the level of neurocognitive task performance, a multifaceted dysfunction involving vigilance and sustained attention, working memory, the ability to inhibit inappropriate responses, and the volitional retrieval of lexical information has repeatedly been identified in patients with schizophrenia.[96,97] Some of these deficits can also be found in clinically normal biological relatives of patients with schizophrenia, suggesting that they may be markers of genetic vulnerability to the disorder.[98,99]

Neurodevelopmental

Abnormalities in brain structure and neurocognitive functioning may be present long before the first outbreak of schizophrenia. Minor physical anomalies that originate in fetal development (such as cleft palate or fingerprint anomalies) tend to be more frequent in patients with schizophrenia than in normal controls. Such findings have given rise to the hypothesis that schizophrenia is a neurodevelopmental disorder that begins in utero or early in life and becomes clinically manifest when a certain level of central nervous system maturation is reached in late adolescence or early adulthood.[100] Indirect support for this view is provided by prospective studies that have documented a number of behavioral peculiarities, such as poor social skills, 'schizoid' traits, and low IQ in children who later develop schizophrenia. Although such neurodevelopmental features can be found in a subset of cases of schizophrenia, they are absent in the histories of a substantial proportion of cases, including those of late onset, suggesting that there may be more than one etiological pathway to the disorder. [101,102]

Associations with Age and Gender

Incidence and prevalence data from developing countries suggest a clustering of onset of schizophrenia in early adulthood, similar to that observed in developed countries. The onset tends to be earlier in males than in females.[103] In both sexes, however, it tends to occur at an earlier age in developing countries.[11] An important difference between developing and developed countries is that the male/female ratio of cases of schizophrenia, which in the majority of

TABLE 7-4 Risk Factors and Antecedents of Schizophrenia

Risk Factor or Antecedent	Estimated Effect Size (odds ratio or relative risk)
Familial (family member with schizophrenia)	
Biological parent	7.0–10.0
Two parents	37.0
MZ twin	45.0–50.0
DZ twin	14.0
Nontwin sibling	9.0–12.0
Second-degree relative	1.1
Social and demographic	
Low socioeconomic status	3.0
Single marital status	4.0
Stressful life events	1.5
Migrant/minority status (e.g., Afro-Caribbeans in U.K.)	1.7–10.7
Urban birth	1.4
Pregnancy and birth-related	
Obstetric complications	2.0–4.4
Birth weight < 2000 g	6.2
Birth weight < 2500 g	3.4
Perinatal brain damage	6.9
Neurodevelopmental	
Early central nervous system infection	4.8
Epilepsy	2.3
Low IQ (< 74)	8.6
Social adjustment difficulty in childhood and adolescence	30.7

Source: [12]

developed countries indicates a higher morbidity in males, is attenuated or inverted in some developing countries (higher rates in women than in men have been reported from prevalence studies in India, Sri Lanka, and China). Given that in many developing countries, women have higher mortality than men, this finding suggests that if adjustment for mortality could be made, the risk of schizophrenia for women in developing countries would be even higher. Causes of such higher risk of schizophrenia among women in developing countries may involve both biological and psychosocial factors, and require further research. The specific stresses associated with the female role in traditional societies have already been related to the reported high risk of female suicide and reactive psychosis.[104] Whether role-related stress in women can be pathogenic with regard to schizophrenia remains to be investigated (see the discussion of the role of gender in Chapter 2.)

Substance Abuse Comorbidity

High prevalence of substance use by patients with schizophrenia has been reported in many studies conducted in developed countries.[105] Apart from tobacco and alcohol, drugs commonly abused include cannabis, amphetamines, and cocaine. Use of tobacco and cannabis far exceeds that of other substances.[30] Heavy use of street drugs may be a predisposing factor to violent behavior, although the evidence for this link is mainly circumstantial.[106] There is, however, adequate evidence that heavy cannabis use can precipitate psychotic relapse in patients with schizophrenia who have achieved remission.[107] In contrast, there is little evidence that cannabis intoxication can cause a chronic, schizophrenia-like "cannabis psychosis".[108] Although use of psychoactive substances is not uncommon,[58] there is at present almost no evidence that substance abuse by patients with schizophrenia in developing countries is a comorbidity problem on a scale comparable to that in many developed countries.

Factors Affecting Course and Outcome

Perhaps the most important difference between schizophrenia in the developed and developing worlds concerns the course and outcome of the condition. Earlier reports based on small clinical samples pointed to a less disabling course and a high rate of recovery from schizophrenic psychoses in developing countries such as Mauritius [88] and Sri Lanka,[109] even for cases manifesting symptoms of potentially severe schizophrenia according to Western prognostic criteria. However, selection bias could not be ruled out since the studies were based on hospital admissions; standard assessment procedures and explicit diagnostic criteria were not used; and clinical improvement could have been confounded with the social adjustment many patients achieve in a comparatively undemanding environment.

These methodological issues were addressed in the WHO multicenter studies by employing standardized assessment and more refined measures of course and outcome than in previous research. The 2- and 5-year follow-up assessments of patients in the IPSS [8,9,21] indicated that significantly higher proportions of patients in India, Colombia, and Nigeria had better outcomes on all measures than patients in the developed countries. The IPSS may not have been free of bias, however, since patients were recruited from hospitals. Bed availability and admission policies could have led to overselection of chronic cases in developed countries and acute cases in developing countries. Such bias was practically eliminated in the subsequent WHO 10-country study,[11] in which potential cases were assessed upon their first contact with community services. The 2-year follow-up confirmed the finding that the outcome of schizophrenia was generally better in developing than in developed countries.

Analysis of the data led to the important conclusion that the better overall pattern of course and outcome in developing countries was due mainly to a significantly greater percentage of patients remaining in stable remission of symptoms over longer periods after recovery from acute psychotic illness, not to fewer or shorter psychotic episodes. The pattern was significantly predicted by setting (developing country), acute onset, being married or cohabiting with a partner, and having a supportive network (close friends). Being female was generally associated with a more favorable outcome as well. The length of remission was unrelated to pharmacological maintenance treatment, which was administered only to a small proportion of patients in developing countries. Independently of the WHO studies, a high proportion of better outcomes for schizophrenia in developing countries has been reported by numerous investigators.[110–113]

Although the possible factors underlying the better outcome for schizophrenia in developing countries have been the subject of much speculation, the causes remain essentially unknown. Differences in the course and outcome of a disease may be related to genetic variations across and within populations, yet nothing specific can be said at present about the role of such variations in the course and outcome of schizophrenia. A diagnostic bias resulting from inclusion as "schizophrenia" of a substantial proportion of benign, acute psychotic illnesses of good prognosis, or of psychoses due to transient acute physical illness, can be practically ruled out in the WHO studies, where such cases were carefully screened out. All factors considered, it is entirely plausible that the psychosocial environment plays a central role in the course and outcome of schizophrenia, given the contrasts between developing and developed countries with regard to social support systems, kinship networks, beliefs and expectations about mental disease, and the attributes of the "sick role".[114,115] In the end, the reality may involve interactions between genetic factors and specific aspects of the environment, and the better outcome for schizophrenia in developing countries should be seen as a compelling subject for research that could lead to the discovery of fundamental implications for the management and treatment of schizophrenia in both developing and developed countries.

Recommendation 7-2. **Research into the genetic epidemiology, neurobiology, prognosis, and outcome of schizophrenia and related disorders in developing countries offers great potential to enhance global knowledge about the nature of these conditions and to provide novel insights into their causes and possible prevention. Collaborative research into these disorders, involving consortia of centers and investigators in developing and developed countries, should be a special focus for program development and funding by the U.S. National Institutes of Health, the research funding bodies of the European Union, other industrialized nations, and international agencies such as WHO.**

INTERVENTIONS

It is estimated that in 1990, over 67 percent of all persons with schizophrenia in developing countries (estimated at 17.2 million) were not receiving any treatment,[116] and there is no evidence that the proportion of treated patients is increasing. This finding raises important ethical and economic questions of equity and waste of human potential, considering that the introduction of antipsychotic pharmacotherapy, the shift from institutional to community care, and other advances introduced in recent decades have profoundly altered the treatment and management of schizophrenia. Developing countries have benefited disproportionately little from these developments.

It is of overriding importance to recognize that the symptoms and behavioral impairments associated with schizophrenia are shaped by interactions between intrinsic vulnerabilities caused by the disease and the psychosocial environment. Good practice in the management and treatment of schizophrenia requires addressing both sides of this interaction, as well as the significant individual variation in the course of the disorder. In about 10–15 percent of cases in developed countries and more than 30 percent of cases in developing countries, the disorder is limited to a single psychotic episode that often resolves in a stable remission with little residual impairment. The majority of cases, however, involve recurrent episodes with partial remissions and progressive development of disabling deficits. In another 10–15 percent of cases, the course is unremitting, resulting in a profound impairment in all spheres of mental life.[11] For the majority of patients in developed countries and for a substantial proportion of patients in developing countries, treatment and care need to be provided on a lifelong basis, with periodic reviews of outcome and adjustment of the mix of interventions according to need and the phase of the illness.

Recommendation 7.3. Current knowledge about schizophrenia suggests that biological vulnerability affecting brain development and function and environmental influences, including psychosocial factors, interact and potentiate each other at every stage of the disorder—preclinical, acute, and residual. Programs aiming at early treatment, stabilization, and rehabilitation of those afflicted should be cognizant of this essential feature of schizophrenia and engage the interactive system as a whole—the patient, the family, and the community.

Prevention

At present, there is no proven method of primary prevention of schizophrenia, that is, of intervening at a presymptomatic stage with a view to removing or blocking the causes of subsequent illness—even in individuals known to be at increased risk by virtue of having a first-degree relative with the disorder. None of the known risk factors or putative disease markers, and no combination of such risk factors or markers, is sufficiently sensitive and specific to ensure the minimum of positive predictive value required of a screening test for preclinical disease.[117] Nor is there any intervention available that is known to result in a guaranteed high rate of prevention success should preclinical disease be identifiable. Nevertheless, research into presymptomatic detection of schizophrenia is important,[118] and the prospect of prevention is likely to become increasingly realistic with advances in knowledge about the genetic basis for the disorder and its neurodevelopmental pathophysiology.

Treatment

In contrast to prevention, there is sufficient knowledge of interventions that can substantially ameliorate the course of schizophrenia and reduce the resulting impairments and disabilities.

Early Treatment

Evidence suggests that even in countries with well-developed services, treatment of the majority of patients with schizophrenia is initiated after, on average, 1 year of presence of psychotic symptoms and up to 5 years of prodromal manifestations.[119] Yet there is good evidence that correct diagnosis and initiation of treatment as early as possible can have a positive impact on the subsequent course of the disorder.[120]

Pharmacotherapy

Antipsychotic medication is the mainstay of treatment of schizophrenia and is indicated for the majority of patients over prolonged periods with no fixed limit to duration.[121] Two classes of pharmacological agents are available. The two offer approximately equal efficacy in controlling the positive symptoms of the disorder, but differ considerably in their side effects and tolerability, as well as cost.

The *conventional antipsychotics* (e.g., phenothiazines, butyrophenones, and thioxanthenes), which block the dopamine D2 receptor in the brain, are effective in producing clinical improvement in an average of 60 percent of patients within 6 weeks. However, they have multiple side effects, including extrapyramidal symptoms (muscle rigidity and tremor), akathisia (inner tension and motor restlessness), dystonia (cramp-like contractions of muscles), sedation (drowsiness), and anticholinergic effects (dryness of mouth, blurring of vision). Although such side effects can be alleviated by adjusting the dosage or administering antiparkinsonian drugs, they cause many patients to discontinue therapy and risk relapse. Moreover, prolonged use of conventional antipsychotics may be a contributing factor to tardive dyskinesia—a difficult-to-treat movement disorder that affects an average of 1 in 10 patients with schizophrenia.

The *atypical antipsychotics* (clozapine, risperidone, olanzapine, quetiapine, and sertindole) have a different pharmacological profile in that they have a lower affinity for dopaminergic receptors, but target a wider range of brain neurotransmitter systems. Clozapine has been demonstrated to be highly effective in controlling symptoms in patients who have proven resistant to other antipsychotics, and there is also some evidence that the atypicals ameliorate negative symptoms and cognitive disturbances that are uninfluenced by conventional antipsychotics. Moreover, the atypicals are considerably better tolerated, being less likely to produce the subjectively unpleasant side effects referred to above, although sedation is quite marked with clozapine, and weight gain is associated with olanzapine. In a small proportion (less than 1 percent) of patients, clozapine can induce agranulocytosis (impaired production of white blood cells), which is potentially dangerous and may necessitate withdrawal of the drug. For this reason, clozapine administration necessitates white blood cell monitoring on a weekly basis, a requirement that is likely to restrict the applicability of clozapine in developing-country settings. Such safety restrictions do not apply to the other atypical antipsychotics. However, the current unavailability of injectable depot forms of these newer drugs and their significantly higher cost may contribute to their limited use in developing countries.

In this context, any recommendation about the choice of an antipsychotic therapeutic agent of wide applicability in developing countries must balance several considerations that are, at least in part, conflicting: clinical efficacy, adverse effects profile and incidence, acceptability and likelihood of treatment adherence, and cost-effectiveness. While evidence on the clinical efficacy of conventional and atypical antipsychotic drugs is generally consistent and indicates a fair amount of comparability between the two classes in terms of broad clinical outcomes, evaluations to date of their adverse effects, acceptability, and treatment adherence clearly favor the newer atypical drugs.[122] A caveat, however, is that the atypical antipsychotics are increasingly being seen as not entirely free of adverse effects, and longer observation time is needed for a final verdict on their side-effects profile.

It is in the area of cost-effectiveness that the current evidence on the antipsychotics is conflicting. For example, a study using pharmacoeconomic modeling that estimated a superior 2-year cost-effectiveness of risperidone as compared with haloperidol [123] can be contrasted with a recent naturalistic 1-year follow-up study in which it was found that the high cost of risperidone was not offset by a reduction in readmission rates as compared with conventional antipsychotics.[124] In another study,[125] substantial cost savings with clozapine were observed only for the minority of patients with a very high rate of hospital use prior to initiation of treatment.

In practical terms, almost the entire body of information on the comparative efficacy, safety, and cost-effectiveness of atypical antispychotics versus conventional neuroleptics originates in research in the developed countries. Conclusions and recommendations that are heavily weighted by such evidence may fail to take into account some important factors. First, there are population differences in the therapeutic response and occurrence of side effects of antipsychotic treatments in developed and developing countries.[126] Whatever the ultimate explanation, a high proportion of patients with schizophrenia in developing countries tends to have a more favorable natural history of the disorder (as discussed earlier). There also is some evidence that the same therapeutic effect is achieved with considerably lower doses of haloperidol in Asian patients as compared with Caucasians.[127] If such observations were to be confirmed by more systematic research, one could conclude that very different standard protocols for antipsychotic treatment need to be formulated for developed and developing countries. Second, considering that an estimated three-quarters of all patients with schizophrenia in developing countries are not treated at all, any antipsychotic drug of choice must be made widely available and affordable. Cost, therefore, is a consideration of much higher priority for developing than for developed countries.

For these reasons, it may be both unrealistic and unnecessary to apply to developing countries the clinical and economic considerations that have been advanced to promote the wider use of atypical antipsychotics in therapeutic settings in developed countries. If universal availability at low cost is the ultimate objective, conventional antipsychotic drugs such as chlorpromazine and haloperidol are clearly to be preferred at present, although the situation may eventually be reassessed when some of the current atypicals come off-patent, and inexpensive generics become widely available.

The Primary Health Care Model

The generic primary health care model (see Chapter 3) is probably the single most important vehicle for providing essential care within the community to the majority of patients with schizophrenic disorders in the developing world. The model is well adapted to the acute shortage of medical staff in rural areas and redefines the role of psychiatrists and other mental health professionals as being focused primarily on providing training; designing methodological tools, such as problem detection and treatment guidelines; and offering tertiary consultation.[128–131]

The primary health care model has been implemented in a number of developing countries.[128–131] The lack of systematic data collection and exchange of information across the developing world, however, makes it impossible at present to estimate the number and percentage of patients with schizophrenia who are receiving care within the primary health care system. One evaluation of the model was carried out in two pilot regions in Tanzania in the 1980s, with fieldwork participation by epidemiologists and social scientists.[131] The Tanzanian model, in which five generic mental health and neurological problems (acute psychosis, chronic psychosis, depression, epilepsy, and severe anxiety) were targeted for identification and treatment at the primary health care level, was shown to be highly effective in dramatically reducing referrals to mental hospitals, increasing the number of people receiving treatment for mental disorders, and decreasing overall direct costs.

Recommendation 7-4. A feasible and affordable community-based management program for those with schizophrenia should have five specific aims:
- **Reduce the frequency of psychotic relapses.**
- **Reduce the risk of the "social breakdown syndrome" and subsequent social withdrawal and isolation.**
- **Reduce the risk of premature mortality due to suicide, accidents, or physical disease.**
- **Reduce the risk of criminal or offending behavior.**
- **Reduce stigma and protect the patient's human rights.**
- **Such a program should involve at least three operational components:**

  1.   Pharmacological treatment with specific guidelines for symptom control in acute episodes, maintenance of stabilization and prevention of relapse, and means of ensuring adherence to the treatment protocol.

  2.   Mobilization of family and community support, including providing education about the nature of the disorder and its treatment, involving the family in simple problem-

solving skills training, and involving the local community in providing a supportive and nonstigmatizing environment.

3. Provision of local rehabilitation opportunities, such as maintaining the patient in appropriate work and social roles within the community, and creating opportunities for occupational and social skills retraining.

Family Interventions

Since the majority of schizophrenic patients in developing countries live with their families, evidence-supported interventions at the level of the family group should be a high priority. Family psychoeducation about the nature and course of the disorder, its treatment, and the patient's needs has been shown to increase the family's capacity for coping with abnormal behavior and to reduce the need for hospitalization.[132–134] Psychoeducation can be delivered in group sessions with families and is cost-effective in low-income settings.

A family-based intervention for schizophrenic patients in China, evaluated in a randomized controlled trial, was found to be significantly more effective than standard posthospital management in reducing rehospitalization and the family burden.[132] In the Centro de Atencion Psicosocial in Leon (Nicaragua), where 80 percent of all care is delivered on a group basis, a 1-year follow-up of a sample of patients showed statistically significant functional improvement and family satisfaction.[133] Another well-evaluated intervention that can be linked to psychoeducation is the reduction of family "expressed emotion." Patients with schizophrenia are particularly vulnerable to criticism and signs of hostility on the part of emotionally overinvolved, close members of their daily living environment.[134] Such emotional overinvolvement was shown in the WHO 10-country study [11] to be a critical factor contributing to psychotic relapse, and its reduction through targeted psychoeducation results in fewer relapses and hospital readmissions. Additional studies have shown varying results when critical comments were analyzed separately from emotional overinvolvement—critical comments remain a contributing factor to relapse; however, emotional overinvolvement has been associated with better social outcomes in some cases.[135]

Group Interventions Focused on the Patient

Several well-established models for patient-focused group interventions can be effective in urban agglomerations in developing countries. The *clubhouse* model, whose prototype is Fountain House, established in New York City in 1948, provides a family-like rehabilitative environment for patients with chronic impairments. The aim is to meet on a daily basis patients' needs for social communication in a nonstressful environment and assist them in obtaining jobs in the community. This generic model has been implemented successfully in

Fountain House Lahore (Pakistan), which has been in existence for more than 25 years and has attained wide recognition.[136,137] Various forms of community-based day programs, drop-in centers, patient cooperatives, and self-help groups have emerged in many developing countries, with apparent success as regards their acceptance by patients, communities, and families, although few of these programs have been formally evaluated. More structured interventions—incorporating elements of models such as the University of California-Los Angeles modular program of living skills training,[138] the Pittsburgh social skills program,[139] case management, or assertive community treatment—are problematic with regard to their feasibility in most developing-country settings, except in a small number of well-staffed university or research centers.

Therapeutic Communities

The hospital-based therapeutic community model, which gained considerable popularity in Europe and North America in the 1950s and 1960s, has been largely superseded in developed countries by decentralized, community-based forms of care. In developing countries, however, similar models have evolved without a hospital base or as an alternative to the hospital. An example is the Aro Village in Ibadan (Nigeria), where patients with psychoses are admitted for up to several months together with one or more members of their families, who act as caregivers or cotherapists. Treatment, including pharmacotherapy and occupational therapy (involving traditional crafts, music, and dance), is provided under the supervision of a psychiatrist, skilled nurses, and social workers in a typical Nigerian village environment in which family and social roles are recreated and maintained.[140] Another model is the rehabilitation villages in Tanzania, where the emphasis is on communal living and relearning simple skills in agricultural work (see Box 4-5 in Chapter 4).

Recommendation 7-5. Special attention should be drawn to the large number of people with schizophrenia who have lost their supportive network and are homeless, vagrant, or in prison. Appropriate programs and community-based facilities (such as the rehabilitation villages in Tanzania) should be established with government and local community support to improve the quality of life and safeguard the physical health and survival of these patients.

Role of the Hospital

Although some mental hospitals designed on the Western institutional model may once have played a useful role, at present their adverse effects on mental health care provision outweigh any benefits. These negative effects have become particularly visible in the postindependence era, when many governments have found themselves unable to support and maintain such institutions, allowing them to deteriorate into squalid, essentially antitherapeutic environments. In countries, such as Tanzania, that have introduced primary health care, it has been possible to close the old hospitals fully or partially with no detriment to mental health care.[131]

Even if the needs of the majority of people with severe mental illness can be met within the community, brief admission to a sheltered environment may be of benefit to a small proportion of patients. The experience of some developing countries shows that such limited inpatient care is best provided in small units within regional or district general hospitals.[130,131]

It must also be noted that rapid economic development and modernization in certain developing countries may weaken the family and community support structures that are prerequisite for models, such as primary health care, that are aimed at reintegration of schizophrenia sufferers into community life. Thus, governments and private agencies may be tempted to build new mental hospitals that could become long-term receptacles for patients whose families are no longer willing or able to retain them.[141] Raising the awareness of politicians, community leaders, and health professionals regarding the possible adverse consequences of inappropriately managed and maintained institutions for the treatment of mental illness should be an important priority.

> **Recommendation 7-6. Inpatient hospital care has a well-defined, albeit limited, place in the treatment and management of schizophrenia. It is indicated, for example, when (1) a state of acute, severe agitation or stupor potentially leading to life-threatening complications cannot be safely managed on an ambulatory basis; (2) in the presence of acute psychotic symptoms there is a significant risk of suicide, self-mutilation, or aggression towards others; or (3) there is a need for diagnostic investigations that cannot be conducted on an outpatient basis. Inpatient admissions should be brief, carried out with the least restraint appropriate to the situation and with utmost respect for the patient's dignity, and in accordance with the legal provisions of the country and the ethical guidelines issued by international bodies such as the World Health Organization and the World Psychiatric Association. Such admissions are best managed in small inpatient units within general hospitals. Under no circumstances should hospital admission be undertaken with the aim of removing people with psychotic illness from public places or facilities, or otherwise restricting their freedom.**

CAPACITY

The vast majority of people whose lives are profoundly affected by schizophrenia reside in developing countries. As indicated earlier, the incidence and prevalence of schizophrenia in developing countries at best are no different from what is found in the developed world, and at worst may be higher. Although a greater proportion of people with schizophrenia in developing countries experience longer periods of symptomatic recovery as compared with patients in the West, the burden of illness is severe and affects the productivity and quality of life of many families. The predicament of patients and families is likely to worsen as many of these countries experience the pressures of economic restructuring, increasing income inequality, unemployment, and cuts in public spending on health care. The traditional economic and psychosocial resources of the family, which in the past have been capable of absorbing much of the impact of severe mental illness, may quickly become eroded. The dilemmas facing health care planners in the People's Republic of China and the difficulties facing patients, families, and mental health workers as economic reform unfolds are described in Box 7-1.

Developing countries differ greatly in the structure, underlying philosophy, and methods of funding of their health services. By and large, the correlation between GDP and the extent of population coverage with essential health care appears to be weak. This observation applies also to mental health care. For example, some countries with scarce economic resources, such as Cuba and Tanzania, have in place systems of health care delivery that continue to provide basic treatment and social assistance to the majority of people with severe mental disorders. In other countries with developing market economies, equitable provision of mental health care has ceased to be an imperative for governments, and some of these countries have experienced a net reduction in programs designed to ensure affordable treatment for people with serious mental illnesses.

Recommendation 7-7. Sponsoring organizations at the regional, national, and global levels (including WHO, the World Bank, and industry) should collaborate to identify, across various developing countries, successful schizophrenia management models that meet the criteria outlined in recommendation 7-4 above, promote and support their role as demonstration projects, establish simple evaluation projects, and disseminate good-practice experiences internationally.

BOX 7-1 Treatment and Rehabilitation of Patients with Schizophrenia in China

In November 1999, the Chinese Ministry of Health acknowledged that the biggest problem facing the chronically mentally ill was that most have no access to psychiatric treatment. The Ministry reported that there were 575 psychiatric treatment and rehabilitation facilities (i.e., hospitals) with more than 110,000 dedicated psychiatric beds. To serve the patients in those beds, more than 80 percent of whom are diagnosed with schizophrenia, there are 13,000 physicians (a much smaller number of whom are fully trained psychiatrists), as well as about 64,000 nurses and other health workers.

The era of economic reforms has brought great pressure to bear on the mentally ill and their families. Social services and health care financing in rural areas have withered. Most rural patients with mental illness have no health insurance and no access to care; hence, they go without psychiatric treatment. Pronounced stigma, poverty, and the absence of professional services place an enormous burden of care on families. In China, 90 percent of patients with schizophrenia live with their families, compared with 40 percent in the United States. Those families are held legally responsible for the actions of their psychotic members. It is not uncommon in urban areas for parents to retire from work to care full time for adult children with schizophrenia.

The Chinese mental hospital system is divided under two ministries: Health and Civil Affairs. The latter is responsible for social welfare support of those in deep poverty or without families. Civil Affairs hospitals are low level with minimally trained staff, limited material resources, and only a few rehabilitation programs that work. There are also psychiatric hospitals under police authority and in railroad and military administrations. Hence there is a fragmented, overlapping, inefficient system of care. In contrast, a number of China's largest cities offer innovative psychoeducational and rehabilitation programs. The latter include factory and family intervention programs. There are also a few model rural rehabilitation programs that use guardianship networks and home beds to help monitor and care for patients in the community.

One of the more innovative models of treatment and rehabilitation for schizophrenic patients was developed over a 40-year period in Shanghai, China's largest city. Since 1956 a Municipal Coordinating Committee has operated in Shanghai's 20 districts/counties and 297 neighborhood/township-level administrative zones. The three-level delivery system includes the municipal level, the district/county level, and neighborhood/township units that range from specialized psychiatric hospitals to local clinics and rehabilitation settings. Hundreds of psychiatrists and psychiatric nurses, more than 1,000 primary care physicians, and over 100,000 community volunteers participate. There are welfare factories, occupational therapy stations, guardianship networks, walk-in clinics, psychological counseling facilities, and telephone hotlines. Research has demonstrated that the factory and family methods have reduced symptoms, dysfunction, and hospitalization, and are cost-effective. A parallel family program in Hubei Province has demonstrated in a clinical trial that if it were generalized to the nation as a whole, it would save as much money as is currently spent on all mental health services for the chronically mentally ill in China.

Yet these model local demonstration projects have never been generalized to China as a whole. And in the current era of economic reforms, it is uncertain whether these programs can survive. Failing state industries are reluctant to accept rehabilitated patients back to their work site; psychiatric hospitals, now faced with declining occupancy owing to prices that patients and work units can no longer afford, are less interested in rehabilitating patients; and funding is drying up for community services. Because the Shanghai and other programs have proven so successful that they are models for other developing societies, their decline as an unintended consequence of China's return to the market would represent a terrible loss.

Source: [142–152]

A common denominator in the great variety of situations and systems of care for people afflicted with psychotic illnesses in the developing world is that the modest successes achieved in many countries are increasingly vulnerable to the local repercussions of economic globalization. In all societies, including developing countries, the stigma surrounding mental illness is likely to mean that people with severe mental disorders are the first and most seriously disadvantaged by shrinking government health expenditures. Thus it is imperative to initiate on an international scale proactive measures designed to forestall such developments.

REFERENCES

1. E. Kraepelin. *Psychiatrie.* 5 Auflage. Barth: Leipzig, 1896.
2. E. Bleuler. *Dementia praecox oder die Gruppe der Schizophrenien.* Deuticke: Leipzig, 1911.
3. N.C. Andreasen and M. Flaum. Schizophrenia: The characteristic symptoms. *Schizophrenia Bulletin* 17, 27–49, 1991.
4. World Health Organization. *The ICD-10 Classification of Mental and Behavioural Disorders. Clinical descriptions and diagnostic gudelines.* World Health Organization: Geneva, 1992.
5. American Psychiatric Association. *Diagnostic and Statistical Manual of Mental Disorders, Fourth Edition.* American Psychiatric Association, Washington D.C., 1994.
6. H.B.M. Murphy. *Comparative Psychiatry.* Springer: Berlin, pp. 63–90, 1982.

7. G. Devereux. *Basic Problems in Ethnopsychiatry.* University of Chicago Press: Chicago, 1980.
8. World Health Organization. *Report of the International Pilot Study of Schizophrenia,* vol.1. World Health Organization: Geneva, 1973.
9. World Health Organization. *Schizophrenia. An International Follow-Up Study.* Wiley & Sons: Chichester, 1979.
10. A. Jablensky, R. Schwarz and T. Tomov. WHO collaborative study of impairments and disabilities associated with schizophrenic disorders. *Acta Psychiatrica Scandinavica* Supplement 285, 152–163, 1980.
11. A. Jablensky, N. Sartorius, G. Ernberg, M. Anker, A. Korten, J. E. Cooper, et al. Schizophrenia: Manifestations, Incidence and Course in Different Cultures. A World Health Organization Ten-Country Study. *Psychological Medicine,* Monograph Supplement 20, Cambridge University Press: Cambridge, 1992.
12. N. Sartorius, W. Gulbinat, G. Harrison, E. Laska, and C. Siegel. Long-term follow-up of schizophrenia in 16 countries. A description of the International Study of Schizophrenia conducted by the World Health Organization. *Social Psychiatry and Psychiatric Epidemiology* 31: 249–258, 1996.
13. T.A. Lambo. *Schizophrenia and borderline states.* In *Transcultural Psychiatry,* A.V. De Reuck and S.R. Porter, eds. CIBA Foundation Symposium. Churchill: London, 1965.
14. W.M. Pfeiffer. Psychiatrische Besonderheiten in Indonesien. *In Beiträge zur vergleichenden Psychiatrie,* N. Petrilowitsch, ed.. Karger: Basel, pp.102–142, 1967.
15. B.O. Osuntokun, O. Bademosi, K. Ogunremi and S.G. Wright. Neuropsychiatric manifestations of typhoid fever in 959 patients. *Archives of Neurology* 27: 7–13, 1972.
16. P.Y. Collins, V.K. Varma, N.N. Wig, R. Mojtabai, R. Dat, and E. Susser. Fever and acute brief psychosis in urban and rural settings in north India. *British Journal of Psychiatry* 174: 520–524, 1999.
17. J.D.C. Mellers, B.K. Toone, and W.A. Lishman. A neuropsychological comparison of schizophrenia and schizophrenia-like psychosis of epilepsy. *Psychological Medicine* 30:325–335, 2000.
18. T. Makikyro, J.T. Karvonen, H. Hakko, P. Mieminen, M. Joukamaa, M. Isohanni and M.R. Jarvelin. Comorbidity of hospital-treated psychiatric and physical disorders with special reference to schizophrenia: A 28 year follow-up of the 1966 Northern Finland general population birth cohort. *Public Health* 112:221–228, 1998.
19. S.R. Bredkjaer, P.B. Mortensen, and J. Parnas. Epilepsy and non-organic non-affective psychosis. National epidemiologic study *British Journal of Psychiatry* 172:235–238, 1998.
20. T.Y. Lin, H.M. Chu, H. Rin, C. Hsu, E.K.Yeh, and C. Chen. Effects of social change on mental disorders in Taiwan: Observations based on a 15-year follow-up survey of general populations in three communities. *Acta Psychiatrica Scandinavica* 79, Supplement. 348, 11–34, 1989.
21. J. Leff, N. Sartorius, A. Jablensky, A. Korten, and G. Ernberg. The International Pilot Study of Schizophrenia: Five-year follow-up findings. *Psychological Medicine* 22, 131–145,1992.
22. H.M. Inskip, E.C. Harris, and B. Barraclough. Lifetime risk of suicide for affective disorder, alcoholism and schizophrenia. *British Journal of Psychiatry* 172:35–37, 1998.

23. C.D. Rossau and P.B. Mortensen. Risk factors for suicide in patients with schizophrenia: Nested case-control study. *British Journal of Psychiatry* 171:355–359, 1997.

24. C.B. Caldwell and I.I. Gottesman. Schizophrenics kill themselves too: A review of risk factors for suicide. *Schizophrenia Bulletin* 16:571–589, 1990.

25. H. Heilar, E.T. Isometsa, M.M. Henriksson, M.E. Heikkinen, M.J. Marttunen, and J. K. Lonnqvist. Suicide and schizophrenia: A nationwide psychological autopsy study on age-and sex-specific clinical characteristics of 92 suicide victims with schizophrenia. *American Journal of Psychiatry* 154:1235–1242, 1997.

26. S. Brown. Excess mortality of schizophrenia. A meta-analysis. *British Journal of Psychiatry* 171:502–508, 1997.

27. H.B.M. Murphy. The schizophrenia-evoking role of complex social demands. In Kaplan, A.R., ed. *Genetic Factors in Schizophrenia.* Charles C. Thomas: Springfield, IL, 1972.

28. R. Cancro and A.T. Meyerson. Prevention of disability and stigma related to schizophrenia: A review. In *Schizophrenia*, Maj, M. and Sartorius, N., eds.,vol 2, WPA Series Evidence and Experience in Psychiatry, Wiley: Chichester, pp.243–278,1999.

29. E.M. Gruenberg. The epidemiology of schizophrenia. In Arieti, S., ed. *American Handbook of Psychiatry*, Second Edition, vol. 2. Basic Books: New York, pp.448–463, 1974.

30. A. Jablensky, J. McGrath, H. Herrman, D. Castle, O. Gureje, M. Evans, et al. Psychotic disorders in urban areas: An overview of the Study on Low Prevalence Disorders. *Australian and New Zealand Journal of Psychiatry* 34: 221–236, 2000.

31. R.S. Murthy, K. Kumar, and S. Chatterji. Schizophrenia: Epidemiology and community aspects. In *Schizophrenia: the Indian Scene*, Kulhara, P., Avasthi, A. and Verma, S., eds. Postgraduate Institute of Medical Education & Research: Chandigarh, pp.39–65, 1997.

32. L.M. Davies and M.F. Drummond. Economics and schizophrenia: The real cost. *British Journal of Psychiatry* 165, Suppl 25: 18–21, 1994.

33. M. Knapp, S. Almond, M. Percudani. Costs of schizophrenia: A review. In *Schizophrenia*, Maj, M. and Sartorius, N., eds. vol 2, WPA Series Evidence and Experience in Psychiatry, Wiley: Chichester, pp.407–453, 1999.

34. P.J. Weiden and M. Olfson. Cost of relapse in schizophrenia. *Schizophrenia Bulletin* 21: 419–429, 1995.

35. S.J. Keith, D.A. Regier, and D.S. Rae. Schizophrenic disorders. In: *Psychiatric Disorders in America, The Epidemiologic Catchment Area Study*. Robins, L.N. and Regier, D.A.,eds., The Free Press: New York, 1991.

36. A. Shah and R. Jenkins R. Mental health economic studies from developing countries reviewed in the context of those from developed countries. *Acta Psychiatrica Scandinavica* 100: 1–18, 1999.

37. I.S. Martyns-Yellowe. The burden of schizophrenia on the family: A study from Nigeria. *British Journal of Psychiatry* 161: 779–782, 1992.

38. P.J. Taylor and J. Gunn. Homicides by people with mental illness: Myth and reality. *British Journal of Psychiatry* 174: 9–14, 1999.

39. Indian Council of Medical Research. *Multi-Centered Collaborative Study of Factors Associated with Course and Outcome of Schizophrenia.* ICMR: New Delhi, 1988.

40. B. Sethi, S.C. Gupta, R. Rajkumar, and P. Kumari. A psychiatric study of 500 rural families. *Indian Journal of Psychiatry* 14:183–196,1972.

41. Sen, D.N. Nandi, S.P. Mukherjee, D.C. Mishra, G. Banerjee, and S. Sarkar. Psychiatric morbidity in an urban slum-dwelling community. *Indian Journal of Psychiatry* 26:185–193, 1984.

42. A. Jablensky. Epidemiology of schizophrenia: A European perspective. *Schizophrenia Bulletin* 12, 52–73, 1986.

43. C.H. Chen. Incidence and prevalence of schizophrenia in a community mental health service from 1975 to 1981. *Zhonghua Shen Jing Jing Shen Ke Za Zhi* Dec;17(6):321–324,1984.

44. B.Y. Rhi, K.S. Ha, Y.S. Kim, Y. Sasaki, D. Young, Woon, et al. The health care seeking behavior of schizophrenic patients in 6 East Asian areas. *International Journal of Social Psychiatry* Autumn;41(3):190–209, 1985.

45. D. Kebede, A. Alem, T. Shibre, A. Fekadu, D. Fekadu, A. Negash, et al. The Bitaijir-Ethiopia study of the course and outcome of schizophrenia and bipolar disorders. I. Description of study settings, methods and cases. Unpublished manuscript, 1999.

46. S. Rajkumar, R. Padmavati, R. Thara, et al. Incidence of schizophrenia in an urban community in Madras. *Indian Journal of Psychiatry* 35:18–21, 1993.

47. F.W. Hickling. Psychiatric hospital admission rates in Jamaica, 1971 and 1988. *British Journal of Psychiatry* 159, 817–821, 1991.

48. E. Mahy, R. Mallett, J. Leff, and D. Bhugra. First contact incidence rate of schizophrenia on Barbados. *British Journal of Psychiatry.* July 175:28–33, 1999.

49. A. McNaught, S.E. Jeffreys, C.A. Harvey, A.S. Quayle, M.B. King, and A.S. Baird. The Hampstead Schizophrenia Survey 1991. II. Incidence and migration in inner London. *British Journal of Psychiatry* 170, 307–311,1997.

50. J. Brewin, R. Cantwell, T. Dalkin, R. Fox, I. Medley, C. Glazebrook, et al. Incidence of schizophrenia in Nottingham. *British Journal of Psychiatry* 171, 140–144, 1997.

51. Gottesman II. Schizophrenia Genesis: The Origin of Madness. Freeman: New York, 1991.

52. K.S. Kendler and S.R. Diehl. The genetics of schizophrenia: A current, genetic-epidemiologic perspective. *Schizophrenia Bulletin* 19: 261–285, 1993.

53. N. Risch. Genetic linkage and complex diseases, with special reference to psychiatric disorders. *Genetic Epidemiology* 7: 3–16, 1990.

54. S.V. Faraone, M.T. Tsuang, and D.W. Tsuang. *Genetics of Mental Disorders.* Guilford: New York, 1999.

55. A. Jablensky and W.W. Eaton. Schizophrenia. In: *Epidemiological Psychiatry,* Jablensky, A., ed. Baillière Tindall: London, p. 294, 1995.

56. J. Kelly and R.M. Murray. What risk factors tell us about the causes of schizophrenia and related psychoses. *Current Psychiatry Report* Oct;2(5):378–385, 2000.

57. E. Fuller-Torrey, R. Rawlings, and R.H. Yolken. The antecedents of psychoses: A case-control study of selected risk factors. *Schizophrenia Research* Nov 30;46(1):17–23, 2000.

58. M.K.C. Dube and N. Kumar. An epidemiological study of schizophrenia. *Journal of Biosocial Science* 4(2), 187–195, 1972.

59. H. Rin and T.Y. Lin. Mental illness among Formosan aborigines as compared with the Chinese in Taiwan. *Journal of Mental Science* 198, 134–146, 1962.

60. C. Brugger. Versuch einer Geisteskrankenzählung in Thüringen. *Zeitschrift für die gesamte Neurologie und Psychiatrie* 133, 252–390, 1931.

61. E. Strömgren. Beiträge zur psychiatrischen Erblehre, auf Grund von Untersuchungen an einer Inselbevölkerung. *Acta Psychiatrica et Neurologica Scandinavica* 19, 1938.

62. S. Bøjholm and E. Strömgren. Prevalence of schizophrenia on the island of Bornholm in 1935 and in 1983. *Acta Psychiatrica Scandinavica* 79, Supplement 348, 157–166, 1989.

63. P. Lemkau, C. Tietze, and M.Cooper. A survey of statistical studies on the prevalence and incidence of mental disorder in sample populations. *Public Health Reports* 58, 1909–1927, 1943.

64. E. Essen-Möller, H. Larsson, C.E. Uddenberg and G. White. Individual traits and morbidity in a Swedish rural population. *Acta Psychiatrica et Neurologica Scandinavica*, Supplement 100, 1956.

65. O. Hagnell. *A Prospective Study of the Incidence of Mental Disorder*. Svenska Bokforlaget: Lund, 1966.

66. G.J. Crocetti, P.V.Lemkau, Z. Kulcar, and B. Kesic. Selected aspects of the epidemiology of psychoses in Croatia, Yugoslavia, II. The cluster sample and the results of the pilot survey. *American Journal of Epidemiology* 94, 126–134, 1971.

67. V.G. Rotstein. Material from a psychiatric survey of sample groups from the adult population in several areas of the USSR (in Russian). *Zhurnal nevropatologii I psikhiatrii* Korsakov 77, 569–574, 1977.

68. L.N. Robins, J.E. Helzer, M.M. Weissman, H. Orvaschel, E. Gruenberg, J.D. Burke, D.A. Regier. Lifetime prevalence of specific psychiatric disorders in three sites. *Archives of General Psychiatry* 41, 949–958, 1984.

69. S.E. Jeffreys, C.A. Harvey, A.S. McNaught, A.S. Quayle, M.B. King, and A.S. Bird. The Hampstead Schizophrenia Survey 1991. I: Prevalence and service use comparisons in an inner London health authority, 1986–1991. *British Journal of Psychiatry* 170:301–306, 1997.

70. A. Jablensky, J. McGrath, H. Herrman, D. Castle, O. Gureje, V. Morgan, and A. Korten: *People Living with Psychotic Illness: An Australian Study 1997–98.* National Survey of Mental Health and Wellbeing Report 4. Commonwealth of Australia, 1999.

71. T.Y. Lin, H.M. Chu, H. Rin, C. Hsu, E.K.Yeh, and C. Chen. Effects of social change on mental disorders in Taiwan: Observations based on a 15-year follow-up survey of general populations in three communities. *Acta Psychiatrica Scandinavica* 79, Supplement. 348, 11–34, 1989.

72. K.W. Bash and J. Bash-Liechti. Psychiatrische Epidemiologie in Iran. In: *Perspektiven der heutigen Psychiatrie,* Ehrhard, H.E., ed. Gerhards: Frankfurt, 1969.

73. M.K.C. Dube and N. Kumar. An epidemiological study of schizophrenia. *Journal of Biosocial Science* 4, 187–195, 1972. Indian Council of Medical Research. *Multicentered Collaborative Study of Factors Associated with Course and Outcome of Schizophrenia.* ICMR: New Delhi, 1988.

74. R. Padmavathi, S. Rajkumar, N. Kumar, A. Manoharan, and S. Kamath. Prevalence of schizophrenia in an urban community in Madras. *Indian Journal of Psychiatry* 31, 233–239, 1987.

75. R. Salan. Epidemiology of schizophrenia in Indonesia (the Tambora I study). *ASEAN Journal of Psychiatry* 2: 52–57, 1992.

76. C.K. Lee, Y.S. Kwak, J. Yamamoto, H. Rhee, Y.S. Kim, J.H. Han, et al. Psychiatric epidemiology in Korea. Part I. Gender and age differences in Seoul. Part II. Urban and rural differences. *Journal of Nervous Mental Disorders* 178: 242–252, 1990.

77. C.N. Chen, J. Wong, N. Lee, M.W. Chan-Ho, J. Tak-Fai Lau, and M. Fung. The Shatin community mental health survey in Hong Kong. II. Major findings. *Archives of General Psychiatry* 50, 125–133, 1993.

78. M.C. Waldo. Schizophrenia in Kosrae, Micronesia: Prevalence, gender ratios, and clinical symptomatology. *Schizophrenia Research* 35: 175–181, 1999.

79. D. Kebede and A. Alem Major. mental disorders in Addis Ababa, Ethiopia. I. Schizophrenia, schizoaffective and cognitive disorders. *Acta Psychiatrica Scandinavica*, Supplement 397: 11–17, 1999.

80. O. Ødegaard. A statistical investigation of the incidence of mental disorder in Norway. *Psychiatric Quarterly* 20, 381–401, 1946.

81. H. Häfner and H. Reimann. Spatial distribution of mental disorders in Mannheim, 1965. In: *Psychiatric Epidemiology*, Hare, E.H. and Wing, J.K., eds. Oxford University Press: London, 341–354, 1970.

82. Y.I. Lieberman. The problem of incidence of schizophrenia: Material from a clinical and epidemiological study (in Russian). *Zhurnal nevropatologii i psikhiatrii Korsakov* 74, 1224–1232, 1974.

83. T. Helgason. Epidemiology of mental disorders in Iceland. *Acta Psychiatrica Scandavica* Supplement 173, 1964.

84. D. Castle, S. Wessely, G. Der, and R.M. Murray. The incidence of operationally defined schizophrenia in Camberwell, 1965–84. *British Journal of Psychiatry* 159, 790–794, 1991.

85. L. Nicole, A. Lesage and P. Lalonde. Lower incidence and increased male:female ratio in schizophrenia. *British Journal of Psychiatry* 161, 556–557, 1992.

86. A. McNaught, S.E. Jeffreys, C.A. Harvey, A.S. Quayle, M.B. King, and A.S. Baird. The Hampstead Schizophrenia Survey 1991. II. Incidence and migration in inner London. *British Journal of Psychiatry* 170, 307–311, 1997.

87. J. Brewin, R. Cantwell, T. Dalkin, R. Fox, I. Medley, C. Glazebrook, et al. Incidence of schizophrenia in Nottingham. *British Journal of Psychiatry* 171, 140–144, 1997.

88. A.C. Raman and H.B.M. Murphy. Failure of traditional prognostic indicators in Afro-Asian psychotics: results from a long-term follow-up study. *Journal of Nervous and Mental Disease* 154:238–247, 1972.

89. D. Bhugra, J. Leff, R. Mallett, G. Der, B. Corridan, and S. Rudge. Incidence and outcome of schizophrenia in Whites, African-Caribbeans and Asians in London. *Psychological Medicine* 27:791–798, 1997.

90. G. Hutchinson, N. Takei, T.A. Fahy, D. Bhugra, C. Gilvarry, P. Morgan et al. Morbid risk of schizophrenia in first-degree relatives in White and African-Caribbean patients with psychosis. *British Journal of Psychiatry* 169:776–780, 1996.

91. M. Marcelis, F. Navarro-Mateu, R. Murray, J.P. Selten, and J. Van Os. Urbanization and psychosis: A study of 1942–1978 birth cohorts in the Netherlands. *Psychological Medicine* Jul;28(4):871–879, 1998.

92. W.W. Eaton, P.B. Mortensen, and M. Frydenberg. Obstetric factors, urbanization, and psychosis. *Schizophrenia Research* Jun 16;43(2–3):117–123, 2000.

93. P.J. Harrison. The neuropathology of schizophrenia. A critical review of the data and their interpretation. *Brain* 122: 593–624, 1999.

94. F. Owen and M.D.C. Simpson. The neurochemistry of schizophrenia. In *Schizophrenia*, Hirsch, S.R and Weinberger, D.R., eds. Blackwell Science: Oxford, pp. 358–378, 1995.

95. S.S. Kindermann, A. Karimi, L. Symonds, G.G. Brown, and D.V. Jeste. Review of functional magnetic resonance imaging in schizophrenia. *Schizophrenia Research* 27: 143–156, 1997.

96. C.D. Frith. *The Cognitive Neuropsychology of Schizophrenia*. Lawrence Erlbaum: Hove, United Kingdom, 1992.

97. K.H. Nuechterlein, M.E. Dawson, and M.F. Green. Information-processing abnormalities as neuropsychological vulnerability indicators for schizophrenia. *Acta Psychatrica Scandinavica* 90(384):71–79, 1994.

98. J.R.J. Finkelstein, T.D. Cannon, R.E. Gur, R.C. Gur, and P. Moberg. Attentional dysfunctions in neuroleptic-naïve and neuroleptic-withdrawn schizophrenic patients and their siblings. *Journal of Abnormal Psychology* 106: 203–212, 1997.

99. R. Toomey, S.V. Faraone, L.J. Seidman, W.S. Kremen, J.R. Pepple, and M.T. Tsuang. Association of neuropsychological vulnerability markers in relatives of schizophrenic patients. *Schizophrenia Research* 31: 89–98, 1998.

100. D.R. Weinberger. *Schizophrenia as a neurodevelopmental disorder*. In: *Schizophrenia*, Hirsch, S.R. and Weinberger, D.R., eds. Blackwell Scientific: Oxford, pp. 293–323, 1995.

101. R.M. Murray. Neurodevelopmental schizophrenia: The rediscovery of dementia praecox. *British Journal of Psychiatry* 165(25):6–12, 1994.

102. D.R. Weinberger and B.K. Lipska. Cortical maldevelopment, anti-psychotic drugs, and schizophrenia: A search for common ground. *Schizophrenia Research* 16:87–110, 1995.

103. H. Häfner, K. Maurer, W. Löffler, and A. Riecher-Rössler. The influence of age and sex on the onset and early course of schizophrenia. *British Journal of Psychiatry* 162, 80–86, 1993.

104. J.M. Sutter, M. Porot, and Y. Pelicier. Algerian aspects of mental pathology. *Algerie Medicale* 63, 891–896, 1959.

105. T. Weaver, A. Renton, G. Stimson, and P. Tyrer. Severe mental illness and substance misuse. *British Medical Journal* 318: 137–138, 1999.

106. J. Smith and S. Hucker. Schizophrenia and substance abuse. *British Journal of Psychiatry* 165: 13–21, 1995.

107. D.H. Linszen, P.M. Dingemans, and M.E. Lenior. Cannabis abuse and the course of recent-onset schizophrenic disorders. *Archives of General Psychiatry* 51: 273–279, 1994.

108. D.C. Mathers and A.H. Ghodse. Cannabis and psychotic illness. *British Journal of Psychiatry* 161: 648–653, 1992.

109. N.E. Waxler. Is outcome for schizophrenia better in nonindustrial societies? The case of Sri Lanka. *Journal of Nervous and Mental Disease* 167, 144–158, 1979.

110. R. Thara, M. Henrietta, A. Joseph, S. Rajkumar, and W.W. Eaton. Ten-year course of schizophrenia—The Madras longitudinal study. *Acta Psychiatrica Scandinavica* 90, 329–336, 1994.

111. P. Kulhara and K. Chandiramani. Outcome of schizophrenia in India using various diagnostic systems. *Schizophrenia Research* 1, 339–349, 1998.

112. A.Verghese, J.K. John, S. Rajkumar, J. Richard, B.B. Sethi, and J.K. Trivedi. Factors associated with the course and outcome of schizophrenia in India. *British Journal of Psychiatry* 154, 499–503, 1989.

113. J.U. Ohaeri. Long-term outcome of treated schizophrenia in a Nigerian cohort. Retrospective analysis of 7-year follow-ups. *Journal Nervous Mental Disorders* 181, 514–516, 1993.

114. A. Kleinman. *Rethinking Psychiatry. From Cultural Category to Personal Experience.* The Free Press: New York, 1988.

115. R. Warner. Recovery from schizophrenia in the Third World. *Psychiatry* 46, 197–212, 1983.

116. C.J.L. Murray and A.D. Lopez. *Global Health Statistics.* Harvard University Press: Cambridge, 1996.

117. J. van Os, N. Takei, H. Verdoux, and P. Delespaul. Early detection of schizophrenia (Letter to Editor), *British Journal of Psychiatry* 170, 579, 1997.

118. M. Birchwood, P. McGorry, and H. Jackson. Early intervention in schizophrenia. *British Journal of Psychiatry* 170: 2–5, 1997.

119. H. Häfner. Disability, stigma and discrimination: A view from outside the USA. In: *Schizophrenia*, Maj, M. and Sartorius, N., eds. Vol. 2, WPA Series Evidence and Experience in Psychiatry. Wiley: Chichester, pp. 288–291, 1999.

120. R.J. Wyatt. Neuroleptics and the natural course of schizophrenia. *Schizophrenia Bulletin* 17, 325–351, 1991.

121. American Psychiatric Association. Practice guidelines for the treatment of patients with schizophrenia. *American Journal of Psychiatry* 154, April 1997 Supplement, 1–49, 1997.

122. K. Wahlbeck, M. Cheine, and M.A. Essali. Clozapine versus typical neuroleptic medication for schizophrenia (Cochrane Review) In: *The Cochrane Library*, Issue 3. Oxford, Update Software, 2000.

123. A. Davies, P.C. Langley, N.A. Keks, S.V. Catts, T. Lambert, and I. Schweitzer. Risperdone versus haloperidol: II. Cost-effectiveness. *Clinical Therapy* 20,196–213, 1998.

124. K.C. Coley, C.S.Carter, S.V. DaPos, R. Maxwell, J.W. Wilson and R.A. Branch. Effectiveness of antipsychotic therapy in a naturalistic setting: A comparison between risperidone, perphenazine, and haloperidol. *Journal of Clinical Psychiatry* 60,850–856, 1999.

125. R. Rosenheck, J. Cramer, E. Allan, J. Erdos, L.K. Fisman, W. Xu et al. Cost-effectiveness of clozapine in patients with high and low levels of hospital use. Department of Veterans Affairs Cooperative Study Group on Clozapine in Refractory Schizophrenia. *Archives of General Psychiatry* 56,565–572, 1999.

126. K.M Lin and M.W. Smith. Psychopharmacology in the context of culture and ethnicity. In: *Ethnicity and Psychopharmacology.* Ruiz, P., ed. *Review of Psychiatry* 19; 1–36, American Psychiatric Press: Washington, D.C., 2000.

127. E.H. Pi and G.E. Gray. Ethnopsychopharmacology for Asians. In: *Ethnicity and Psychopharmacology*, Ruiz, P., ed. *Review of Psychiatry*, 19,91–113, American Psychiatric Press: Washington, D.C., 2000.

128. N.N. Wig, S. Murthy, and T.W. Harding. A model for rural psychiatric services—Raipur Rani experience. *Indian Journal of Psychiatry* 23, 275–290, 1981.

129. S. Murthy. Integration of mental health with primary health care—Indian experience. In *Community Mental Health*. Proceedings of the Indo-U.S. Symposium, Murty, S. and Burns, B.J., eds., *National Institute of Mental Health and Neuro-Sciences*: Bangalore, 1992.

130. N.E. Sokhela and L.R.Uys. The integration of comprehensive psychiatric/mental health care into the primary health system: Diagnosis and treatment. *Journal of Advanced Nursing* 30, 229–237, 1999.

131. F. Schulsinger and A. Jablensky. The national mental health programme in the United Republic of Tanzania: A report from WHO and DANIDA. *Acta Psychiatrica Scandinavica* 83, Suppl 364, 1–132, 1991.

132. W. Xiong, M.R. Phillips, X. Hu, R.Wang, Q. Dai, J. Kleinman, and A. Kleinman. Family-based intervention for schizophrenic patients in China. A randomised controlled trial. *British Journal of Psychiatry* 165, 239–247, 1994.

133. T. Caldera, G. Kullgren, U. Penayo, and L. Jacobsson. Is treatment in groups a useful alternative for psychiatry in low-income countries? An evaluation of a psychiatric outpatient unit in Nicaragua. *Acta Psychiatrica Scandinavica* 92, 386–391, 1995.

134. C. Vaughn, K. Snyder, S. Jones, W.B. Freeman, and I.R. Falloon. Family factors in schizophrenic relapse. *Archives of General Psychiatry* 41, 1169–1177, 1984.

135. S. King and M.J. Dixon. Expressed emotion and relapse in young schizophrenia outpatients. *Schizophrenia Bulletin* 25(2),377–386, 1999.

136. J. Leff, N.N.Wig, H. Bedi, D.K. Menon, L. Kuipers, A. Korten et al. Relatives' expressed emotion and the course of schizophrenia in Chandigarh: A two-year follow-up of a first-contact sample. *British Journal of Psychiatry* 156, 351–356,1990.

137. M.R. Chaudhry. Prevention of disability and stigma: Experience from a developing country. In *Schizophrenia*, Maj, M. and Sartorius, N., eds., vol. 2, WPA Series Evidence and Experience in Psychiatry, Wiley: Chichester, pp. 308–310, 1999.

138. R.P. Liberman. Social skills training. In: *Psychiatric Rehabilitation for Chronic Patients*, Liberman, R.P., ed., American Psychiatric Press: Washington, D.C., pp. 147–198, 1988

139. G. Hogarty, C. Anderson, D. Reiss, S.J. Kornblith, D.P. Greenwald, R.E. Ulrich, et al. Family psychoeducation, social skills training, and maintenance chemotherapy in aftercare of schizophrenia. II. Two year effects of a controlled study of relapse and adjustment. *Archives of General Psychiatry* 48, 340–347, 1991.

140. T.A. Lambo. The importance of cultural factors in psychiatric treatment. In: *Cross-Cultural Studies of Behaviour*, Al-Issa, I. and Dennis,W., eds. Holt, Rinehart & Winston: Austin, TX, 1970.

141. M.R. Phillips. Are Western models of psychiatric rehabilitation feasible and appropriate for developing countries? In: *Schizophrenia, Maj* M. and Sartorius, N., eds. WPA Series Evidence and Experience in Psychiatry, Wiley: Chichester, (2),304–306, 1999.

142. R.M. Chen Rong-Min. An investigation of family environmental alteration affecting short-term recovery from schizophrenia in China. *British Journal of Psychiatry* Feb;166(2),258–261, 1995.

143. K. Lou and D. Yu. Enterprise-based sheltered workshops in Nanjing. A new model for the community rehabilitation of mentally ill workers. *British Journal of Psychiatry* Supplement Aug;(24),89–95, 1994.

144. X. Wang. An integrated system of community services for the rehabilitation of chronic psychiatric patients in Shenyang, China. *British Journal of Psychiatry* Supplement Aug;(24),80–88, 1994.

145. M. Zhang, H. Yan, and M.R. Phillips. Community-based psychiatric rehabilitation in Shanghai. Facilities, services, outcome, and culture specific characteristics. *British Journal of Psychiatry* Supplement Aug;(24),70–79, 1994.

146. M.R. Phillips and V. Pearson. Rehabilitation interventions in urban communities. *British Journal of Psychiatry* Supplement Aug;(24),66–69, 1994.

147. F. Li and M. Wang. A behavioral training programme for chronic schizophrenic patients. A three-month randomized controlled trial in Beijing. *British Journal of Psychiatry* Supplement Aug;(24),32–37, 1994.

148. F. Qiu and S. Lu. Guardianship networks for rural psychiatric patients. A non-professional support system in Jinshan County, Shanghai. *British Journal of Psychiatry* Supplement Aug;(24),114–120, 1994.

149. M.R. Phillips and V. Pearson. Rehabilitation interventions in rural communities. *British Journal of Psychiatry* Supplement Aug;(24),103–106, 1994.

150. Q. Wang, Y. Gong, and K. Niu. The Yantai model of community care for rural psychiatric patients. *British Journal of Psychiatry* Supplement Aug;(24),107–113, 1994.

151. M.R. Phillips and V. Pearson. Future opportunities and challenges for the development of psychiatric rehabilitation in China. *British Journal of Psychiatry* Supplement Aug;(24),128–142, 1994.

152. M.R. Phillips, S.H. Lu, and R.W. Wang. Economic reforms and the acute inpatient care of patients with schizophrenia: the Chinese experience. *American Journal of Psychiatry* Sep;154(9),1228–1234, 1997.

Summary of Findings:
Bipolar Disorder in Developing Countries

- Bipolar disorders account for about 11 percent of the neuropsychiatric disease burden and about 1 percent of the total disease burden in developing countries.

- Between 25 and 50 percent of patients in developed countries with bipolar disorder are estimated to attempt suicide, and as many as 15 percent complete the act.

- Predisposition to bipolar disorder may be inherited; other apparent risk or precipitating factors include substance abuse, living in an urban setting, and lack of education. The significant impact of social and environmental factors on the presentation, course, and incidence of bipolar disorder argues for increased research in developing countries.

- There is no known course of primary prevention for bipolar disorder. Risk factors and the physical and psychological symptoms of the disorder can be reduced and controlled but not eliminated following diagnosis.

- Treatment for bipolar disorder often requires a combination of medications, few of which have been tested in developing countries. Acute episodes of mania are best treated with antipsychotic medications or high doses of mood stabilizers; acute episodes of depression can be treated with antidepressant medication and electroconvulsive treatment.

- Once acute symptoms are under control, active treatment with mood stabilizers, possibly including psychosocial interventions, must be undertaken to prevent the illness from becoming increasingly severe.

8

Bipolar Disorder

DEFINITION

One of the first descriptions of mania dates from 30AD,[1] but it was not until the conceptual separation of schizophrenia from other psychoses and the description of mania by Kraepelin in 1921 [2] that focused research and attempts to define mania accurately began. The discovery of lithium therapy as an effective treatment for mania argued for the origins of this disorder as being biological. The subsequent research precipitated by these findings revealed bipolar disorder (also known as manic-depressive illness) as a distinct diagnosable condition.

Despite the strong neurobiological indicators that have been discovered for bipolar disorder,[3–6] diagnosis is made on the basis of characteristic symptoms of mood disorder, which include alternating episodes of extreme elevation of mood (mania) and severe depression.[7] Elevated mood can be accompanied by delusions, hallucinations, insomnia, and extreme excitement, and depressive states by persistent low mood or sadness that is accompanied by both physical and psychological symptoms of at least 2 weeks duration and an associated impact on social functioning.

Kraepelin characterized manic psychosis by its periodic course, good prognosis, and mood symptoms in the acute phase.[2] It is important to note that bipolar disorder remains a clinical syndrome and that the neurobiology underlying its causes is not yet fully known. There is at present no biological test or marker that can identify the disease (or a predisposition to it) independently of clinical assessment (e.g., recognizing a family history of the disorder). Both standardized diagnostic mechanisms for disease, the *Tenth Revision of the International Classification of Diseases (ICD-10)*,[8] and the (APA) *Diagnostic and*

Statistical Manual, fourth edition (*DSM-IV*) still rely on the course of the illness (see tables 8-1 and 8-2) [9]:

- **Bipolar I = at least one manic (elevated mood) episode (hypomania = less severe presentation without the need for hospitalization or impediment to occupational or social functioning).**
- **Bipolar II = at least one episode of mania or hypomania and a full major depressive episode.**

In contrast with other psychoses, the psychotic symptoms of bipolar disorder must be congruent with the prevailing elated or depressed mood state. For these purposes, irritability is presumed to be congruent with an elated or elevated mood state.

SCOPE OF THE PROBLEM

Mortality

The evidence clearly reveals the exceedingly high mortality rate from suicide exacted by bipolar disorder. Evidence from developed countries has shown varying rates for attempted suicide of between 25 and 50 percent among patients with the disorder.[10, 11] Follow-up studies have found that as many as 15 percent were completed suicides. This rate is approximately 30 times greater than the rate for general populations.[11, 12]

In developing countries, similar rates of suicide have been observed.[13,14] High rates of attempted suicide (24 percent) were found in a study conducted in a psychiatric hospital in Taiwan.[15] An earlier age of onset, interpersonal problems with partners and close family members, and occupational maladjustment rather than demographic characteristics are suggested as collectively identifying those with bipolar disorder at high risk of suicide attempt.

Social and Economic Costs

In light of the findings of the 1996 Global Burden of Disease study and more recent estimates of the same measurements of disability-adjusted life years (DALYs), neuropsychiatric conditions have been recognized as a significant social and economic burden (see Chapter 2).[16,17] Bipolar disorder is considered to represent 11 percent of the disease burden from neuropsychiatric conditions in low- and-middle income countries. Moreover, within these estimates for low- and middle-income countries, bipolar disorder is estimated to account for a full 1.1 percent of all categories of disease burden. When estimating the disability weight measurements for the Global Burden of Disease study, the burden of bipolar disorder was weighted somewhere between that of paraplegic and quadriplegic physical disability.[16]

TABLE 8-1 Overview of the DSM-IV Criteria for Diagnosis of Bipolar Disorder

Bipolar Disorder I	Bipolar Disorder II
(A) Presence of only one manic episode (see Table C) and no past major depressive disorders	(A) Presence of one or more major depressive episodes (see Table D).
(B) The manic episode is not better accounted for by schizoaffective disorder and is not superimposed on schizophrenia, schizophreniform disorder, delusional disorder, or psychotic disorder not otherwise specified.	(B) Presence of at least one hypomanic episode (see Table E).
	(C) There has never been a manic episode (see Table C) or a mixed episode (see Table F).
	(D) The mood symptoms in Criteria A and B are not better accounted for by schizoaffective disorder and are not superimposed in schizophrenia, schizophreniform disorder, delusional disorder, or psychotic disorder not otherwise specified.
	(E) or impairment in social, occupational, or other important areas of functioning.
Specify if: Mixed: if symptoms meet criteria for a mixed episode.	
Specify (current or most recent episode): (a) Severity/Psychotic/Remission specifiers (b) With catatonic features (c) With postpartum onset.	*Specify (current or most recent episode):* (a) Hypomanic: if currently in a hypomanic episode (b) Depressed: if currently (or most recently) in a major depressive episode.
	Specify (for current or most recent major depressive episode only if it is the most recent type of mood episode): (a) Severity/Psychotic/Remission specifiers (b) Chronic (c) With catatonic features (d) With melancholic features (e) With atypical features (f) With postpartum onset.
	Specify: (a) Longitudinal course specifiers (with and without interepisode recovery) (b) With season pattern (c) With rapid cycling.

Source: [9]

TABLE 8-2 Overview of the ICD-10 Criteria for Diagnosis of Bipolar Disorder

---

F.30 Manic Episode

Three degrees of severity are specified here, sharing the common underlying characteristics of elevated mood, and an increase in the quantity and speed of physical and mental activity. All the subdivisions of this category should be used only for a single manic episode. If previous or subsequent affective episodes (depressive, manic, or hypomanic), the disorder should be coded under bipolar affective disorder.

F.32 Depressive Episode

In typical depressive episodes of all three varieties described below (mild, moderate, and severe), the individual usually suffers from depressed mood, loss of interest and enjoyment, and reduced energy leading to increased fatiguability and diminished activity. Marked tiredness after only slight effort is common. Other common symptoms are:

    (a) reduced concentration and attention;
    (b) reduced self-esteem and self-confidence;
    (c) ideas of guilt and unworthiness (even in a mild type of episode);
    (d) bleak and pessimistic views of the future;
    (e) ideas or acts of self-harm or suicide;
    (f) disturbed sleep;
    (g) diminished appetite.

The lowered mood varies little from day to day, and is often unresponsive to circumstances, yet may show a characteristic diurnal variation as the day goes on. As with manic episodes, the clinical presentation shows marked individual variations, and atypical presentations are particularly common in adolescence. In some cases, anxiety, distress, and motor agitation may be more prominent at times than the depression, and the mood change may also be masked by added features such as irritability, excessive consumption of alcohol, histrionic behaviour, and exacerbation of pre-existing phobic or obsessional symptoms, or by hypochondriacal preoccupations. For depressive episodes of all three grades of severity, a duration of at least 2 weeks is usually required for diagnosis, but shorter periods may be reasonable if symptoms are unusually severe and of rapid onset.

Source: [8]

Bipolar disorder is a chronic disease with high frequencies of relapsing symptoms that often worsen over time, even when appropriate pharmacotherapy is administered.[18] During both manic and depressive states, sufferers are often limited in their social, familial, and employment roles.[19,20] Several recent studies in developed countries found that patients with bipolar disorder had substantial impairment in health-related quality of life in comparison with the general population.[21,22] Bipolar patients were less compromised in areas of physical functioning than chronic back pain patients, but had similar impairment in overall mental health and social functioning.[23]

Despite the identification of bipolar disorder early in the 20th century and prevalence rates in developed countries that are higher than those for nonaffective psychoses, less research has been conducted in these countries on this disorder in comparison to other psychiatric conditions (including those discussed elsewhere in this report). In developing countries, an even smaller and similarly inconclusive body of research exists. For the purposes of this report, we include, where applicable, data from one or both settings and where possible make comparisons between them. After reviewing the literature, the committee concluded that more investigation into the etiology of and interventions for bipolar disorder are needed to reduce its long-term debilitating effects. Recent advances in genetic research have greatly increased the potential for unraveling the complex neurobiology of bipolar disorder and meeting the challenges involved in its treatment.

PREVALENCE AND INCIDENCE

According to the U.S. National Comorbidity Survey,[24] bipolar affective disorder is nearly three times more prevalent than nonaffective psychoses. However, bipolar disorder has not been investigated on the same scale, for example, in a large-scale international comparative study on schizophrenia (such as the study described in chapter 7), to validate the cross-cultural reliability of diagnosis between developed- and developing-country settings. Nevertheless, in a cross-cultural study that included two developing countries and used a single, standardized diagnostic method, lifetime rates of bipolar disorder were found to be similar across populations (0.3/100 in Taiwan and 1.5/100 in New Zealand).[25] Another study in India using standard DSM-III-R criteria found rates of diagnosis and course of illness in children and adolescents to be similar to the findings in developed countries.[26]

However, when comparisons are made both within and between countries the evidence points to some variation in both the incidence and prevalence of the symptoms of bipolar affective disorder.[27–33] In the United States, the Epidemiologic Catchment Area Study used DSM-III criteria.[27] It reported a lifetime prevalence of 2.7 percent for a manic episode. Manic symptoms were more common in the 18–29 age group and more common in men than women. Yet there was no significant sex difference in actual bipolar disorder. The lifetime prevalence of Bipolar I was 0.8 (0.7 male, 0.9 female), and that of Bipolar II was 0.5 (0.4 male, 0.5 female). There was also no ethnic difference in the rate of these disorders. However, there was a difference in the rates of illness among study sites.

Population-based studies in Italy showed a higher 1-year prevalence in women (1.86 percent) than in men (0.65 percent), with an overall Bipolar II rate of 0.2 percent.[28] In Taiwan, the prevalence for a manic episode was found to be between 0.7 and 1.6 percent, depending on whether a city or small town was studied.[29] In Puerto Rico, the prevalence of a manic episode was 0.7 for males and 0.4 for females,[30] and similar rates were found in Alberta, Canada.[31] A study in the Netherlands found much lower rates of 0.1 percent for a manic episode in both genders.[32]

Prevalence is dependent not only on the rate of new illness, but also on the availability of medical interventions and social buffers to the development of symptoms. Incidence studies are a better index of illness rates, but there are few such studies. Incidence studies in Scandinavia have reported rates of 9.2–15.2

cases per 100,000 for men and 7.4–32.5 cases per 100,000 for females.[33] A retrospective study of hospital admission rates in Denmark and the United Kingdom has been used as a proxy measure for incidence—virtually identical rates of 2.6 per 100,000 were found in both centers.[34]

A recent WHO study found comparable rates of mood disorders in Mexico and Brazil as compared with the United States, Canada, Germany, and the Netherlands.[35] However, the results included no indication of the proportion of mood disorders that were unipolar and bipolar. Research has shown significant variations among countries in the ratio of unipolar to bipolar illness, but even the most conservative estimate would identify bipolar illness as a significant health problem in the developing countries.

Few studies of bipolar disorder have been conducted in developing countries and many of these have offered inconclusive and variable evidence, as illustrated by the examples described below.

In India, Brown et al. looked at affective psychosis in Chandigarh and found that all 24 patients with mania experienced full recovery within a 1-year period. At 1-year follow-up, 75 percent of manic patients demonstrated no symptoms or social impairment. The mean episode duration was 10.2 weeks, and the rate of relapse was 21 percent. Overall, these outcomes are considerably more favorable than those found in comparable studies of affective disorders in developed-country settings.[36]

Higher rates of bipolar disorder were found among some Indonesian groups and the Hutterites in North America [37] as compared with their overall population rates. Among Jewish people of European background in the United States, the rates are higher than among those of North African background.[38] Bazzoui found that 44 percent of patients admitted with affective disorder in Iraq suffered from bipolar disorder.[39] Though only a fifth of people suffering from affective disorders in Sweden suffer from bipolar disorder, one in three such patients in Jerusalem suffers from the disorder.[40]

Khanna et al. investigated the course of bipolar disorder in India. In their consecutive admission sample, they found that recurrent mania was common, and there was a significantly greater frequency of manic compared with depressive relapses.[41] They also found a marked preponderance of male subjects. This finding may have been due in part to their methodology, but this is unlikely to be a complete explanation. It may be that the low female admission rates reflect sociocultural determinants of admission. The greater tendency for men to display aggressive behavior may mean that their symptoms are less well tolerated socially than in females. Moreover, the greater economic impact of men's incapacity to work may influence their admission rate, and the stigma of mental illness in a culture in which marriages are arranged may decrease the rate of female admission.

RISK FACTORS
Genetic

Evidence for high aggregates of familial risk and results of recent research conducted in developed countries to elicit genetic linkage in families with bipolar disorder supports the argument for a significant genetic contribution to the etiology of bipolar disorder.[42–48] However, the findings reported to date are inconsistent and larger-scale replication of many of these studies will be required before the evidence is conclusive.[3] Data from a recent French study suggest that early- and late-onset bipolar disorders differ in clinical expression and familial risk, and may therefore foreshadow findings of different subforms of the disorders within genetic research.[49]

It is known that there is a 1.5 percent lifetime risk for the children of an affected person, 6 percent for brothers, 4.1 percent for mothers, and 6.4 percent for fathers.[24] In a recent U.S. study, the offspring of parents with early-onset bipolar disorder were found to experience high levels of psychopathology.[50] Studies in both developed and developing countries showing high familial risk for bipolar disorder indicate that establishing the diagnosis of a family member with the disorder can be an important factor in attempting to diagnose children who may present with symptoms common to other disorders, such as attention-deficit hyperactivity disorder as well as adults who may present only with symptoms of unipolar depression.[26,51–53] Correct diagnosis is, of course, essential to ensure the appropriate course of treatment, which differs significantly among these disorders.

Substance Abuse

Data from both developed and developing countries countries reveal high levels of comorbidity in bipolar illness. Data collected on bipolar disorder show rates of substance abuse that are 5–6 times greater than those among general populations.[13,54] Three studies found the rate of substance misuse in those with Bipolar I disorder to be over 60 percent, and at least 35 percent of total bipolar disorder cases were complicated by alcohol abuse.[24,55] A diagnosis of an underlying bipolar illness may be missed because of the high rate of comorbidity and the more conspicuous signs and symptoms of substance abuse.[56]

Strakowski and DelBello's recent review of the existing literature on the co-occurrence of bipolar disorder and substance abuse found evidence to support four distinct hypotheses to explain this association: 1) substance abuse occurs as a symptom of bipolar disorder; 2) substance abuse is an attempt by bipolar patients to self-medicate symptoms; 3) substance abuse causes bipolar disorder; and 4) substance use and bipolar disorders share a common risk factor. The variability in findings from the existing evidence suggests that additional studies to examine the relationship between substance abuse and bipolar disorder are needed. Future studies that increase the understanding of this frequent co-occurrence may eventually provide guidance toward improved prevention and treatment strategies for both conditions.[57]

Environmental

Several studies have indicated that social conditions and experiences contribute to both the onset and recurrence of relapse in bipolar disorder. Striking urban–rural differences have been found, with the illness being three times more common in urban than in rural populations.[58] It is still unclear whether variations in the rates of mania among different populations are due to genetic loading or societal factors.

Associations with Age and Gender

Findings of recent studies in developed as well as developing countries estimate the peak age of onset for bipolar disorder between 18 and 24.[26,58,59] Though the age of onset and number of affective episodes of each polarity have not been shown to differ between men and women,[24] some studies have shown that women experience depressive episodes of the disorder more frequently and men have been shown to be at greater risk for manic episodes.[60–63]

Several studies have yielded similar findings for childhood-onset bipolar disorder. Irritability was the predominant affective disturbance in younger manic children, but prepubertal bipolar children began their illness with cycles of dysphoria, hypomania, and agitation intermixed, and increasingly extreme cycles of manic and depressive states became more common with the onset of puberty.[64,65] Adolescents who are early into their illness are often prone to highly elevated mood states and grandiose delusions resulting in poor adherence to treatment.[11,53] Similar findings on the course of bipolar disorder in children have been reported in India.[25,51]

Factors Affecting Course and Outcome

Bipolar disorder is quite disabling because of its recurrent course, frequency of suicidal ideation, and significant impact on social functioning during acute episodes of both polarities.[66] Data on the frequency of variable levels of recurrence are inconsistent, yet telling. An older study found that patients averaged as many as 12 episodes during a 25-year period.[67] Winokur et al. (1994) estimated that over a 10-year period, patients averaged three episodes and five hospitalizations.[68] Even with pharmacological intervention, those suffering one manic episode almost always go on to have another.[69,70] Ongoing and significant symptoms between major episodes occur even in individuals who suffer infrequent acute episodes.[71]

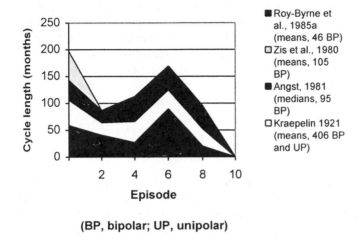

(BP, bipolar; UP, unipolar)

Figure 8-1 Increasing probability of relapse with each episode of manic-depressive illness.
Source: [11]

Despite the likely significant mortality, morbidity, and burden on families developing countries is very limited. If the epidemiology in the developed world is applicable, the burden in developing countries would be significant. The impact of social and environmental factors on the presentation, course, and incidence of the illness argues for the need for much more work to delineate the treatment needs in developing countries. This work could also lead to vital etiological data that could inform primary prevention interventions in both developed and developing countries.

Recommendation 8-1. Research to determine the applicability of current diagnostic methods in the local settings of developing countries should be conducted to better understand the epidemiology of bipolar disorder in developing countries and to ensure the effectiveness of efforts to identify and treat the disease within various health care settings. Research to determine the local risk factors and patterns of heredity for bipolar disorder should also be undertaken to further inform effective courses of intervention.

Recommendation 8-2. Large-scale population-based studies in developing countries should be carried out to expand and validate the findings of previous studies relative to bipolar disorder, particularly in the area of genetic research. The existence of isolated populations and extended family environments in parts of the developing world may provide uniquely appropriate settings for such research. Collaborative efforts between researchers in developing countries and well-equipped research institutions in developed countries should be emphasized, in part to build the research capacity of developing-country centers.

INTERVENTIONS

Prevention

Currently, there is no known method or strategy of primary prevention for bipolar disorder. Even for those at risk because of familial history, no method to eliminate or preempt the origins of the disease exists. Once the disorder has been diagnosed, risk factors and the physical and psychological symptoms can be reduced and controlled, but not eliminated. Nevertheless, research into presymptomatic detection of bipolar disorder is important,[72] and the prospect of prevention is likely to become increasingly realistic with advances in knowledge of the genetic basis for the disorder and its neurodevelopmental pathophysiology.

Treatment

Though no current data are available, the conspicuous lack of research on bipolar disorder in developing countries would support the argument that effective treatments currently available in developed countries are not reaching those suffering from the disorder elsewhere. Even in developed countries, the treatment of bipolar disorder is underinvestigated. The complexity of the disorder and the variability of its symptoms make clinical treatment a complicated endeavor.[72] Treatment often requires a combination of medications, and caution must be exercised because of the high rate of significant side effects. Because of the lack of available data from developing countries, the following discussion on treatments for bipolar disorder is based on the research literature of developed countries. Where very limited information from developing countries is available, it is noted.

The difficulty of clinical diagnosis for bipolar disorder is twofold. First, those who are experiencing the manic phase of the disorder do not usually seek treatment because this period is characterized by highly elevated mood states. Often it is only when patients present with high levels of agitation or aggression that treatment will be pursued. Second, those who seek treatment when experiencing the depressed state of the disorder are frequently diagnosed with unipolar depression. Though bipolar and unipolar disorders are clinically recognized as distinct, the lack of research on distinguishing the pathophysiology of the conditions provides little support for more accurate diagnosis.[41,61] Moreover, the stigma associated with mental illness in developing countries (see Chapter 2) is often a major deterrent in individuals seeking treatment for psychological problems or feelings of emotional distress.

For the majority of patients in developed countries, treatment and care need to be provided on a lifelong basis, with periodic reviews of outcome and adjustment of the mix of interventions according to need and the phase of the illness. It is of overriding importance to recognize that the symptoms and behavioral impairments associated with bipolar disorder are shaped by interactions between intrinsic vulnerabilities caused by the disease and the psychosocial environment. Good practice in the management and treatment of bipolar disorder requires addressing both sides of this interaction.

TABLE 8-3 Critical Challenges in the Stages of Pharmacological and Psychosocial Treatment

Stage	Goals of Treatment	Issues for Patient/Family
Acute	Gain control over severe symptoms	Trauma and shock, dealing with police and/or hospitalization (in some cases), making sense of what has happened
Stabilization	Hasten recovery from the acute episode, address residual symptoms/impairment, encourage medication compliance	Adapting to post-episode symptoms and social–occupational deficits, financial stress, accepting a regular medication regime, uncomfortable discussions about medication and illness, denial about the realities of the disorder
Maintenance	Prevent recurrences, alleviate residual affective symptoms, continue to encourage medication compliance	Fears about the future, accepting the illness and the vulnerability to future episodes, coping with ongoing deficits in social–occupational functioning, issues surrounding long-term medication adherence

SOURCE: [66]

Pharmacotherapy

Recurrent affective disorders often require treatment to prevent relapse, as well as to alleviate acute episodes. Acute episodes of mania are best treated with antipsychotic (typical and atypical) medication (see Chapter 7 on considerations for the use of antipsychotics in developing countries), though they can be treated with high doses of mood stabilizers. Because the significant side effects from typical antipsychotics, particularly tardive dyskinesia, tend to occur with greater frequency in bipolar patients as compared with those suffering from schizophrenia and other psychoses,[73–75] their use should be minimized, and preference may be given to high doses of mood stabilizers.[76] Acute episodes of depression can be treated with antidepressant medication and electroconvulsive treatment (ECT) (see Chapter 9 on considerations for the use of antidepressants and ECT in developing countries). However, particular caution must be exercised in the use of tricyclic antidepressants because the data suggest that they can trigger episodes of mania, hypomania, and rapid cycling in bipolar patients.[77] Once acute symptoms are under control, decisions about prophylaxis need to be made. It is important to treat bipolar disorder actively because each episode of mania increases the risk of progression of the illness, with increasingly severe episodes occurring with greater frequency.[78]

Mood Stabilizers

The following commonly used mood stabilizers have some antidepressant effect, but are prescribed mainly for the prophylaxis of bipolar disorder.

Lithium is the best-investigated mood stabilizer. It is used for the treatment of mania and for the prophylaxis of bipolar and unipolar affective disorders.[79–81] Retrospective studies ranging from 4 months to 3 years indicate that the relapse rate for bipolar patients treated with placebo is 80 percent, while the relapse rate for those treated with lithium is as low as 35 percent.[78,82] Lithium has been shown to decrease the severity as well as the frequency of episodes.[11,83,84] Those with a family history of bipolar affective disorder and complete recovery between relapses are likely to respond to lithium. Patients whose first episode is manic rather than depressive and those who have a good response to lithium during the acute episode tend to respond to prophylaxis. Lithium has been noted as the most influential medication for preventing suicidal behavior.[85] Patients with neurological signs or mania secondary to cerebral injury respond less well, as do patients who are rapid cycling and those with histories of drug abuse.[79,80]

The side effects of lithium reflect its effects on numerous bodily systems. Most patients experience at least one side effect.[84] Thyroid function may be reduced; patients with existing thyroid illness or family histories of the illness are at increased risk for this side effect.[84] In one-third of patients, changes in the architecture of the kidneys are apparent within the glomerulus and tubules. However, these changes rarely lead to deterioration in renal function, except when toxicity has occurred.[84] A fine tremor is reported by 25 percent of patients. A few patients develop Parkinsonian features, which are not amenable to treatment with anticholinergic drugs.[80] A number of other side effects have been described,[86] including reversible t-wave flattening and abdominal discomfort. In the first trimester of pregnancy, 4–12 percent of exposed babies will develop congenital malformations.[87] Lithium toxicity can be life-threatening, and patients who have survived it may be left with permanent cerebellar signs.[88]

Lithium is currently considered the first-line, most appropriate medication for acute bipolar depression and the first-line monotherapy for the treatment and prophylaxis of bipolar disorder.[89,90] Data from a recent study in Iran show a lower ratio of lithium to side effects in patients treated only with lithium than in those treated with combinations of lithium and neuroleptics.[91]

Carbamazepine has been tested for efficacy in only a few small placebo-controlled trials.[92] The mood-stabilizing action of carbamazepine was first reported in 1973.[93] Carbamazepine has shown possible antimanic and antidepressant effects as a monotherapy or in combination with lithium.[94,95] Patients with dysphoric mania, mixed states, no family history of bipolar disorder, mania following brain injury, or a history of rapid cycling may be more likely to respond initially to carbamazepine than to lithium. However, there is some evidence that the effects of carbamazepine decrease 3 years or so into treatment.[96] A combination of lithium and carbamazepine is more effective than either monotherapy in the treatment of rapid cycling.[97]

The most common side effects are nausea, dizziness, diplopia, and ataxia. Among 15 percent of patients, an itchy rash develops within 2 weeks of starting treatment. A number of idiosyncratic side effects have been described as well, such as a small percentage of patients who develop agranulocytosis.[98–100]

Sodium valproate has been shown to be effective for mania and for mixed affective states. It is useful in patients who are resistant to lithium and carbamazepine, and may be especially valuable in preventing relapse of depression, rapid cycling, or mixed states in bipolar patients,[101] as well as in treating elderly patients.[78] There are a number of dose-dependent side effects, including nausea and stomach cramps, hair thinning, lethargy, and elevated liver function, which can be managed by decreasing the dose. Agranulocytosis, liver failure, and pancreatitis are idiosyncratic reactions that contraindicate further treatment. A fetal valproate syndrome has been described that includes congenital malformations, jitteriness, and seizures in the fetus.[102]

Other Mood Stabilizers

A number of other drugs have been used as mood stabilizers, either by themselves or as adjunctive therapy. Clonazepam is used as adjunctive therapy with lithium, and verapamil and lamotrigine are used acutely and also as pro-phylaxis in cases of treatment failure with lithium or carbamazepine. There are also a number of new drugs currently undergoing trials, but to date none of these equals current treatments in risk-benefit analysis and their effects on unipolar disorder have not been adequately reported. Most of these mood stabilizers are relatively expensive as compared with lithium, carbamazepine, and valproate. Additionally, despite concerns about the described side effects of lithium, a recent review of existing research regarding the use of lithium for the treatment of acute mania in bipolar disorder concluded that it should remain the first-line treatment.[103]

In developed countries, the drugs discussed previously have been shown to be effective and because they are available in generic form they are relatively low cost. Only limited analysis has been done to determine actual cost-effectiveness, but given the highly disabling effects of this disorder it is likely that cost-effectiveness will bear out in future studies.[22,104] No evidence exists for developing countries, but the need for blood monitoring poses unique challenges even when low-cost medications may be available. Problems encountered with the development of therapeutic drug monitoring in India have been high-lighted by Gogtay et al.[105] They found that the service was available only in large teaching hospitals or in the private sector. Lack of funding and problems with the quality of medicines and the availability of generic products made quality control difficult and increased the risks associated with drug toxicity.

The limitations imposed by the cost of long-term prophylaxis drug treatment in India affect the current practice regarding the use of prophylaxis treatment beyond five years. Upon review of the first five years of treatment, the occurrence of relapse is examined and if no relapse has occurred then drug treatment is stopped. Decisions regarding the continuation of drug treatment for patients still experiencing relapse are based on the frequency of relapse and periodic review of the course of illness thereafter.[106]

Better epidemiological and treatment outcome data is needed in developing countries to determine the need for and course of treatment for bipolar disorder in local health care settings.

Psychosocial Treatment

Bipolar disorder is characterized by high rates of relapse of the acute states of polarity even when patients are maintained on proper pharmacotherapy. It has been argued that stressful life events and disturbances in social-familial support systems affect the cycling of the disorder in the context of other genetic, biological, and cognitive vulnerabilities.[107,108] Some current models of psychosocial treatment focus on modifying the effects of social or familial risk factors and may help improve the course of the disorder.[109–112]

Adjunctive psychotherapy may assist patients in understanding the implications of having bipolar disorder and assist with more positive attitudes about compliance with drug therapy to avoid more frequent relapses involving manic or depressive episodes. Individual, family, or group psychotherapy may help both patients and families address feelings of denial, difficulties with interpersonal functioning, and concerns about worsening of the disorder.[11,113] Therapeutic and nonjudgmental environments allow for open discussion of symptoms, treatments, and their side effects. Such discussion can create long-term stability, optimize compliance, and allow for early identification and intervention when relapsing episodes occur.[114]

Preliminary research has been conducted on three models of psychotherapy that are beneficial for bipolar disorder and may be applicable in developing countries: **problem-solving therapy**, **interpersonal therapy**, and **family-focused treatments** for psychoeducation and communication enhancement.[66,115–117] Where resources are limited, it may be difficult to implement psychotherapy treatments that require specialized knowledge of mental illness and lengthy periods of training.

> **Recommendation 8-3. Lithium, carbamazepine, and valproate, considered by WHO to be "essential medications" for bipolar disorder, should be made readily available to developing-country medical facilities for the treatment of the disorder. Additionally, treatment programs that make mobile facilities for blood monitoring more readily available to more remote populations should be developed to enable appropriate courses of treatment that avoid the toxic and sometimes lethal side effects of mood stabilizers.**

> **Recommendation 8-4. Side effects of treatment can be intolerable for some patients, and lack of adherence to drug treatment is a frequent obstacle to effective treatment of bipolar disorder with mood stabilizers. Stressful life events and other social factors are suspected to contribute to the onset and frequency of relapse as well. Programs that promote adherence to drug treatment in conjunction with psychosocial therapy should therefore be implemented within community-based management programs for health care. Training for family-based therapy should be provided to those in the households of bipolar patients.**

> **Recommendation 8-5. Current knowledge of bipolar disorder suggests that biological vulnerability affecting brain development and function and environmental influences, including psychosocial factors, interact and potentiate each other at every stage of the disorder—preclinical, acute, and residual. Programs aiming at early treatment, stabilization, and rehabilitation of those afflicted must**

consider this essential feature of bipolar disorder and engage the system as a whole—the patient, the family, and the community. Programs to limit the chronicity of bipolar disorder should also address substance abuse and suicidal behavior frequently associated with patients suffering from this disorder.

Recommendation 8-6. Randomized controlled trials (in the form of large-scale demonstration projects) of pharmacotherapeutic and psychosocial treatments should be conducted to identify locally cost-effective methods of treatment.

CAPACITY

The generic primary health care model (see Chapter 3) is probably the single most important vehicle for providing essential care within the community to the majority of patients with bipolar disorder in the developing world. The model is well adapted to the acute shortage of medical staff in rural areas and redefines the role of psychiatrists and other mental health professionals as being focused primarily on providing training; designing methodological tools, such as problem detection and treatment guidelines; and offering tertiary consultation.[27–30]

The primary health care model has been implemented in a number of developing countries. The lack of systematic data collection and exchange of information across the developing world, however, makes it impossible to determine if bipolar disorder is being properly diagnosed or treated within these settings. The findings of large-scale epidemiological studies would inform the process of priority setting and health planning for developing countries. Currently, the high prevalence and significantly disabling effects of bipolar disorder, found in developed countries and a limited number of developing countries along with the disproportionately high rates of suicide associated with the disease, argue for placing effective interventions on the public health agenda of national and local planners.

Recommendation 8-7. Randomized controlled trials of the efficacy and feasibility of affordable community-based management programs for those with bipolar disorder (within the context of the extended health care system) should be conducted to determine the most appropriate programs for treatment. Using the evidence from developed countries as a guide, initial trial programs should have three specific aims:

- **Reduce the frequency of manic and depressive relapses;**
- **Reduce the risk of premature mortality due to suicide; and**
- **Reduce stigma, and protect the patient's human rights.**

Such a program should involve at least three operational components:

- Adaptation of existing screening and diagnostic tools for bipolar disorder, with a view to accounting for differences in the local presentation of the disorder and making them suitable for use by personnel in the primary care setting.
- Pharmacological treatment, with specific guidelines for symptom control in acute episodes, maintenance of stabilization and prevention of relapse, and means of ensuring adherence to the treatment protocol.
- Mobilization of family and community support, including providing education on the nature of the disorder and its treatment, involving the family in simple problem-solving training, and involving the local community in providing a supportive and nonstigmatizing environment.

REFERENCES

1. F. Adams. The extant works of Aretaeus, the Cappadocian. London, The Syndenham Society 1856. Reprinted in the Classics of Medicine Library Series. Gryphon Editions Inc.: Birmingham, AL, 1990.
2. E. Kraepelin. Manic-depressive insanity and paranoia. E&S Livingstone: Edinburgh, 1921.
3. C. Friddle, R. Koskela, K. Ranade, J. Hebert, M. Cargill, C.D. Clark, M. McInnis, S. Simpson, F. McMahon, O.C. Stine, D. Meyers, J. Xu, D. MacKinnon, T. Swift-Scanlan, K. Jamison, S. Folstein, M. Daly, L. Kruglyak, T. Marr, J.R. DePaulo, and D. Botstein. Full-genome scan for linkage in 50 families segregating the bipolar affective disease phenotype. *American Journal of Human Genetics* 66:205–215, 2000.
4. D.H.R. Blackwood, L. He, S.W. Morris, A. McLean, C. Whitton, M. Thomson, et al. A locus for bipolar affective disorder on chromosome 4p. *Nature Genetics* 12:427–430, 1996.
5. E.I. Ginns. A genome-wide search for chromosomal loci linked to bipolar affective disorder in the Old Order Amish. *Nature Genetics* 12:431–435, 1996.
6. N.B. Freimer, et al. Genetic mapping using haplotype, association and linkage methods suggests a locus for severe bipolar disorder (BPI) at 18q22–q23. *Nature Genetics* 12: 436–441, 1996.
7. A.L. Stoll, M. Tohen, Baldessarini, D.C. Goodwin, S. Stein, S. Katz, et al. Shifts in the diagnostic frequencies of schizophrenia and affective disorders from 1972 through 1998; A combined analysis from four North American psychiatric hospitals. *American Journal of Psychiatry* 151:130–132, 1994.
8. World Health Organization. The ICD-10 Classification of Mental and Behavioural Disorders. Clinical descriptions and diagnostic guidelines. World Health Organization: Geneva, 1992.
9. American Psychiatric Association. *Diagnostic and Statistical Manual of Mental Disorders, Fourth Edition.* American Psychiatric Association: Washington D.C., 1994.

10. M.A. Oquendo, C. Waternaux, B. Brodsky, B. Parsons, G.L. Haas, K.M. Malone, and J.J. Mann. Suicidal behavior in bipolar mood disorder: Clinical characteristics of attempters and nonattempters. *Journal of Affective Disorders* 59(2):107–117, 2000.

11. F.K. Goodwin and K.R. Jamison. *Manic-Depressive Illness*. Oxford University Press: New York, 1990.

12. G.K. Brown, A.T. Beck, R.A. Steer, and J.R. Grisham. Risk factors for suicide in psychiatric outpatients: A 20-year prospective study. *Journal of Consulting and Clinical Psychology* 68(3):371–377, 2000.

13. S.Y. Tsai, J.C. Lee, and C.C. Chen. Characteristics and psychosocial problems of patients with bipolar disorder at high risk for suicide attempt. *Journal of Affective Disorders* 52(1–3):145–152, 1999.

14. A. Ucok, D. Karaveli, T. Kundakei, and O. Yazici. Comorbidity of personality disorders with bipolar mood disorders. *Comprehensive Psychiatry* 39(2):72–74, 1998.

15. C.Y. Liu, Y.M. Bai, Y.Y Yang, C.C. Lin, C.C. Sim, and C.H. Lee. Suicide and parasuicide in psychiatric inpatients: Ten years experience at a general hospital in Taiwan. *Psychological Reports* 79(2):683–690, 1996.

16. C. Murray and A. Lopez, eds. *The Global Burden of Disease*. Boston: The Harvard Press, 1996.

17. WHO (World Health Organization). *The World Heath Report*. Geneva: 1999.

18. T.C. Monschreck and A.H. Leighton. Reducing disability in mood disorders and schizophrenia. *Hospital and Community Psychiatry* 43:262–265, 1992.

19. J.M. Murphy, D.C. Oliver, A.M. Sobol, R. R. Monson, and A.H. Leighton. Diagnosis and outcome: Depression and anxiety in a general population. *Psychological Medicine* 16:117–126, 1986.

20. P. Martin. Impacts économiques des troubles bipolaires de l'humeur. *Encephale* 23(Spec No 1):49–54, 1997.

21. G.M. MacQueen, L.T. Young, J.C. Robb, M. Marriott, R.G. Cooke, and R.T. Joffe. Effect of number of episodes on wellbeing and functioning of patients with bipolar disorder. *Acta Psychiatrica Scandinavica* 101(5):374–381, 2000.

22. K.B. Wells and C.D. Sherbourne. Functioning and utility for current health of patients with depression or chronic medical conditions in managed, primary care practices. *Archives of General Psychiatry* 56(10):897–904, 1999.

23. L.M. Arnold, K.A. Witzeman, M.L. Swank, S.L. McElroy, and P.E. Keck Jr. Health-related quality of life using the SF-36 in patients with bipolar disorder compared with patients with chronic back pain and the general population. *Journal of Affective Disorders*. 57(1-3):235–239, 2000.

24. R.C. Kessler, K.A. McGonagle, S. Zhao, C.B. Nelson, M.Hughes, S. Eshleman, et al. Lifetime and 12 month prevalence of DSM-III-R, psychiatric disorders in the United States. *Archives of General Psychiatry* 51:8–19, 1994.

25. M.M. Weissman, R.C. Bland, G.J. Canino, C. Faravelli, S. Greenwald, H.G. Hwu, et al. Cross-National Epidemiology of Major Depression and Bipolar Disorder. *Journal of the American Medical Association* Jul 24/31; 276(4), 1996.

26. Y.C. Reddy, S. Girimaji, and S. Srinath. Clinical profile of mania in children and adolescents form the Indian subcontinent. *Canadian Journal of Psychiatry* 42(8):841–846, 1997.

27. L. N. Robins, J. E. Helzer, M. M. Weissman, H. Orvaschel, E. Gruenberg, J. D. Burke, et al. Lifetime prevalence of specific psychiatric disorders in three sites. *Archives of General Psychiatry.* 41:949–958, 1984.

28. C. Faravelli, B.C. Deg'lInnocenti, L. Azzi, G. Incerpi, and S. Pallanti. Epidemiology of mood disorders: A community survey in Florence. *Journal of Affective Disorders* 20:135–141, 1990.

29. H. G. Hwu, E. K Yeh, and L.Y. Chang. Prevalence of psychiatric disorders in Taiwan defined by the Chinese Diagnostic Interview Schedule. *Acta Psychiatrica Scandinavica* 79:136–147, 1989.

30. G.J. Canino, H.R. Bird, P.E. Shrout, M. Rubio-Stipee, M. Bravo, M. Sesman, et al. Prevalence of specific psychiatric disorders in Puerto Rico. *Archives of General Psychiatry* 44:727–735, 1987.

31. R.C. Bland, S.C. Newman, H. Orm, eds. Epidemiology of psychiatric disorders in Edmonton. *Acta Psychiatrica Scandinavica* 77 (Suppl 338), 1988.

32. P. Hodiamont, N. Peer, and N. Syben. Epidemiology aspects of psychiatric disorder in a Dutch health area. *Psychological Medicine* 17:495–505, 1987.

33. J.H. Boyd and M.M. Weissman. Epidemiology of affective disorders: A re-examination and future directions. *Archives General Psychiatry* 38:1039–1046, 1981.

34. J.O. Leff, M. Fisher, and A. Bertelsen. A cross national epidemiological study of mania. *British Journal of Psychiatry* 129:428–442, 1976.

35. WHO (World Health Organization). International consortium in psychiatric epidemiology. Cross national comparisions of the prevalences and correlates of mental disorders. *Bulletin of the World Health Organization* 78(4):413–426, 2000.

36. A.S. Brown, V.K.Varma, S.Malhotra, R.C. Jiloha, S.A. Conover, and E.S. Susser. Course of acute affective disorders in a developing country setting. *Journal of Nervous & Mental Disease* 186(4);207–213, 1998.

37. J.W. Eaton and R.J. Weil. Culture and mental disorders: A comparative study of the Hutterites and other populations. New York: New York Free Press, 1955.

38. E. S. Gershon and J.H. Liebowitz. Socio-cultural and demographic correlates of affective disorders in Jerusalem. *Journal of Psychiatric Research* 12:37–50, 1975.

39. W. Bazzoui. Affective disorders in Iraq. *British Journal of Psychiatry* 117:195–203, 1970.

40. R.H. Belmaker and H.M. Van Praag. Mania and evolving concept. New York: Spectrum, 1980.

41. R. Khanna, N. Gupta, and S. Shanker. Course of bipolar disorder in eastern India. *Journal of Affective Disorders* 24:35–41, 1992.

42. D.F. MacKinnon, K.R. Jamison, and J.R. DePaulo. Genetics of manic depressive illness. *Annual Review of Neuroscience* 20:355–373, 1997.

43. W.H. Berrettini, T.N. Ferraro, L.R. Goldin, D.E. Weeks, S. Detera-Wadleigh, J.I. Nurnberger Jr, et al. Chromosome 18 DNA markers and manic-depressive illness: Evidence for a susceptibility gene. *Proceedings of the National Academy of Science USA* 91:5918–5921, 1994.

44. O.C. Stine, J. Xu, R. Koskela, F.J. McMahon, M. Gschwend, C. Friddle, et al. Evidence for linkage of bipolar disorder to chromosome 18 with a parent-of-origin effect. *American Journal of Human Genetics* 57:1384–1394, 1995.

45. F.J. McMahon, P.J. Hopkins, J. Xu, M.G. McInnis, S. Shaw, L. Cardon, et al. Linkage of bipolar affective disorder to chromosome 18 markers in a new pedigree series. *American Journal of Human Genetics* 61:1397–1404, 1997.

46. L.A. McInnes, M.A. Escamilla, S.K. Service, V.I. Reus, P. Leon, S. Silva, et al. A complete genome screen for genes predisposing to severe bipolar disorder in two Costa Rican pedigrees. *Proceedings of the National Academy of Science USA* 93:13060–13065, 1996.

47. D. Curtis. Chromosome 21 workshop. *American Journal of Medical Genetics* 88:272–275, 1999.

48. C. Van Broeckhoven and G. Verheyen. Report of the chromosome 18 workshop. *American Journal of Medical Genetics* 88:263–270, 1999.

49. F. Schuhoff, F. Bellivier, R. Jouvent, M.C. Mouren-Simeoni, M. Bouvard, J.F. Alli-laire, et al. Early and late onset bipolar disorders: Two different forms of manic-depressive illness? *Journal of Affective Disorders* 58(3):215–221, 2000.

50. K. D. Chang, H. Steiner, and T. A. Ketter. Psychiatric phenomenlogy of child and adolescent bipolar offspring. *Journal of American Academy of Child Adolescent Psychiatry* Apr 39(4):453-460, 2000.

51. P.J. Alexander and R. Raghavan. Childhood mania in India. *Journal of the American Academy of Child and Adolescent Psychiatry* 36(12):1650–1651, 1997.

52. G.S. Sachs, C.F. Baldassano, C.J. Truman, and C. Guille. Comorbidity of attention deficit hyperactivity disorder with early- and late-onset bipolar disorder. *American Journal of Psychiatry* 157(3):466–468, 2000.

53. J. Biederman, R. Russell, J. Soriano, J. Wozniak, and S.V. Faraone. Clinical features of children with both ADHD and mania: Does ascertainment of source make a difference? *Journal of Affective Disorders* 51(2):101–112, 1998.

54. D.A. Regier, M.E. Farmer, D.S. Rae, B.Z. Locke, S. J. Keith, L.L. Judd, et al.. Comorbidity of mental disorders with drug and alcohol abuse: Results from the Epidemiologic Catchment Area (ECA) study. *Journal of the American Medical Association* 264:2511–2518, 1990.

55. M. Tohen and F. Goodwin. Epidemiology of Bipolar Disorder. In: M.T. Tsuang, M. Tohen, and G. E.P. Zahner, eds., *Textbook in Psychiatric Epidemiology*. Wiley-Liss: New York, pp.301–317, 1995.

56. J.E. Helzer, A Burnam, and L.T. McEvoy. Alcohol abuse and dependence. In: L.N. Robins and D.A. Regier, eds. *Psychiatric Disorders in America*. Free Press: New York. pp. 81–129, 1991.

57. S.M. Strakowski and M.P. DelBello. The co-occurrence of bipolar and substance use disorders. *Clinical Psychology Review* Mar;20(2):191–206, 2000.

58. M.M. Weissman, M.L.Bruce, P.J. Leaf et al. In: L.N. Robins and D.A. Reiger, eds. *Psychiatric Disorders in America*. Free Press: New York, pp. 53–81,1991.

59. S. Sethi and R Khanna. Phenomenology of mania in Eastern India. *Psychopathology* 26:274–278, 1993.

60. J.C. Robb, L.T. Young, R.G. Cooke, R.T. Joffe. Gender differences in patients with bipolar disorder influence outcome in the medical outcomes survey (SF-20) subscale scores. *Journal of Affective Disorders* 49(3):189–193, 1998.

61. J. Angst. The course of affective disorders, II: Typology of bipolar manic-depressive illness. *Archiv fur Psychiatrie und Nervenkrankheiten* 226:65–73, 1978.

62. L. Tondo and R.J. Baldessarini. Rapid cycling in women and men with bipolar manic-depressive disorders. *American Journal of Psychiatry* 155:1434–1436, 1998.

63. P. Roy-Byrne, R.M. Post, T.W. Uhde, T. Porcu, and D. Davis. The longitudinal course of recurrent affective illness: Life chart data from research patients at the National Institute of Mental Health. *Acta Psychiatrica Scandinavica Supplement* 317:5–34, 1985.

64. J. Wozniac, J. Biederman, K. Kiely, J.S. Ablon, S.V. Faraone, E. Mundy, et al. Mania-like symptoms suggestive of childhood onset bipolar disorder in clinically referred children. *Journal of the American Academy of Child and Adolescent Psychiatry* 34:867–876, 1995.

65. T. Shiratsuchi, N. Takahashi, T. Suzuki, and K. Abe. Depressive episodes of bipolar disorder in early teenage years: Changes with increasing age and the significance of IQ. *Journal of Affective Disorders* 58(2):161–166, 2000.

66. D.J. Miklowitz and M.J. Goldstein. Bipolar disorder: A family-focused treatment approach. The Guilford Press: New York, 1997, p. 36.

67. J. Angst, W. Felder and R. Frey. The course of unipolar and bipolar affective disorders In: M Schou and E. Stromgren, eds. *Origin, prevention and treatment of affective disorders.* New York: Academic Press. p. 20, 1979.

68. G. Winokur, W. Coryell, J.S. Akiskal, J. Endicaott, M. Keller, and T. Mueller. Manic-depressive (bipolar) disorder: The course in light of prospective ten-year follow-up of 131 patients. *Acta Psychiatrica Scandinavica* 89:102–110, 1994.

69. F.K. Goodwin and K.R. Jamison. The natural course of manic-depressive illness. In: R.M. Post and J.C. Ballenger, eds. *Neurobiology of mood disorders.* Williams & Wilkins: Baltimore, pp. 20–37, 1984.

70. T. Silverstone and S. Romans-Clarkson. Bipolar affective disorder: Causes and prevention of relapse. *British Journal of Psychiatry* 154:321–335, 1989.

71. M.J. Gitlin, J. Swendsen, T.L. Heller, and C. Hammen. Relapse and impairment in bipolar disorder. *American Journal of Psychiatry* 152:1635–1640, 1995.

72. M.T. Compton and C.B. Nemeroff. The treatment of bipolar depression. *Journal of Clinical Psychiatry* 61(9):57–67, 2000.

73. P.E. Keck Jr, S.L. McElroy, S.M. Strakowski, C.A. Soutullo. Antipsychotics in the treatment of mood disorders and risk of tardive dyskinesia. *Journal of Clinical Psychiatry* 61(Suppl 4):33–38, 2000.

74. S. Mukherjee, A.M. Rosen, G. Caracci, and S. Shukla. Persistent tardive dyskinesia in bipolar patients. *Archives of General Psychiatry* 43:342–346, 1986.

75. M.A. Frye, T.A. Ketter, L.L. Altshuler, K. Denicoff, R.T. Dunn, T. A. Kimbrell, et al. Clozapine in bipolar disorder: Treatment implications for other atypical antipsychotics. *Journal of Affective Disorders* 48:91–104, 1998.

76. M.A. Brotman, E.L. Fergus, R.M. Post, G.S. Leverich. High exposure to neuroleptics in bipolar patients: A retrospective review. *Journal of Clinical Psychiatry* 61(1):68–72, 2000.

77. M. Srisurapanont, L.N. Yathan, and A.P. Zis. Treatment of acute bipolar depression: A review of the literature. *Canadian Journal of Psychiatry* 40(9):533–544, 1995.

78. J.C. Masters. When lithium does not help: The use of anticonvulsants and calcium channel blockers in the treatment of bipolar disorder in the older person. *Geriatric Nursing* 17(2):75–78, 1996.

79. J. Cookson. Lithium and other drug treatments for recurrent affective disorder. In: S. Checkley, ed. *The Management of Depression*. Blackwell, U.K., 1998.
80. A.Coppen and M.T. Abou-Saleh. Lithium in prophylaxis of unipolar depression. *Journal of the Royal Society of Medicine* 76:297–301, 1983.
81. P. Vestergaard. Clinically important side effects of long term lithium treatment: A review. *Acta Psychiatrica Scandinavica* 305:1–36, 1983.
82. P.E. Keck Jr. and S.L. McElroy. Outcome in the pharmacologic treatment of bipolar disorder. *Journal of Clinical Psychopharmacology* 16(2 Suppl):15S–23S, 1996.
83. L. Tondo, K.R. Jamison, and R.J. Baldessarini. Effect of lithium maintenance on suicidal behavior in major mood disorders. *Annals of the New York Academy of Science* 836:339–351, 1997.
84. P. Vestergaard, A. Adisen, and M. Schou. Clinically significant side effects of lithium treatment: A survey of 237 patients in long term treatment. *Acta Psychiatrica Scandanavica* 62:193–200, 1980.
85. L. Tondo and R.J. Baldessarini. Reduced suicide risk during lithium maintenance treatment. *Journal of Clinical Psychiatry* 61(9):97–104, 2000.
86. G. Johnson. Lithium. *Medical Journal of Australia* 141:595–601, 1984.
87. L.S. Cohen, J.M. Friedman, J.W. Jefferson, E.M. Johnson, and M.L. Weiner. A re-evaluation of risk of in utero exposure to lithium. *Journal of the American Medical Association*. 271:146–150, 1994.
88. S. M Long. Lasting neurological sequelae after lithium intoxication. *Acta Psychiatrica Scandanavica* 70:594–602, 1984.
89. A.J. Frances, D.A. Kahn, D. Carpenter, J.P. Docherty, and S.L. Donovan. The Expert Consensus Guidelines for treating depression in bipolar disorder. *Journal of Clinical Psychiatry* 59(Suppl 4):73–79, 1998.
90. G.L. Zornberg, H.G. Pope. Treatment of depression in bipolar disorder: New directions for research. *Journal of Clinical Psychopharmacology* 13:397–408, 1993.
91. A.R. Dehpour, E.S. Emamian, S.A. Ahmadi-Abhari and M Azizabadi-Farahant. The lithium ratio and the incidence of side effects. *Progress in Neuro-Psychopharmacological & Biological Psychiatry* 22:959–970, 1998.
92. R. M. Post, G. S. Leverich , A. S. Rosoff, and L. L. Altshuler. Carbamazepine prophylaxis refractory affective disorders: A focus on long-term follow-up. *Journal of Clinical Psychopharmacology* Oct;10(5):318–327, 1990.
93. Okuma, A. Kishimoto, K Inoue et al. Anti-manic and prophylactic effects of carbamazepine on manic depressive psychosis: A preliminary report. *Folia Psychiatric Neurology*, Japan 283–297, 1973.
94. D.G. Folks, L.D. King, S.B. Dowdy, W.M. Petrie, R.A. Jack, J.C. Koomen, B.R. Swenson, and P. Edwards. Carbamazepine treatment of selected affectively disordered inpatients. *American Journal of Psychiatry* 139:115–117, 1982.
95. Y. Kwamie, E. Persad, and H. Stancer. The use of carbamazepine as an adjunctive medication in the treatment of affective disorders: A clinical report. *Canadian Journal of Psychiatry* 29:605–608, 1984.
96. R.M. Post, T.W. Uhde, P.P. Roy-Byrne, and R.T. Joffe. Correlates of antimanic responses to carbamazepine. *Psychiatric Research* 21:71–84, 1987.
97. K.D. Denicoff, E.E. Smith-Jackson, E.R. Disney, S.O. Ali, G. S. Leverich, and R.M Post. Comparative prophylactic efficacy of lithium, carbamazepine, and the combination in bipolar disorder. *Journal of Clinical Psychiatry* 58:470–478, 1997.

98. L. Banfi, M. Ceppi, M. Colzani, F. Guzzini, R. Morena, and P. Novati. [Carbamaz-epine-induced agranulocytosis. Apropos of 2 cases]. *Recenti Progressi in Medicina* [Article in Italian] Oct;89(10):510–513, 1998.

99. D.W. Kaufman, J.P. Kelly, J.M. Jurgelon, T. Anderson, S. Issaragrisil, B. E. Wi-holm, et al. Drugs in the aetiology of agranulocytosis and aplastic anaemia. *European Journal of Haematology* supplement 60:23–30, 1996.

100. H. Askmark and B.E. Wilholm. Epidemiology of adverse reactions to carbamezepine as seen in a spontaneous reporting system. *Acta Neurologica Scandinavica* Feb;81(2):131–140, 1990.

101. J. R. Calabrese and M. J. Woyshville. A medication algorithm for treatment of bi-polar rapid cycling? *Journal of Clinical Psychiatry* 56(3):11–18, 1995.

102. E. Thisted and F. Ebbeson. Malformations, withdrawal manifestations and hypogly-caemia after exposure to valproate in utero. *Archives of Diseases of Childhood* 69:288–291, 1993.

103. N. Poolsup, A. Li Wan Po, and H.R. de Oliveira. Systematic overview of lithium treatment in acute mania. *Journal of Clinical Pharmacy and Therapeutics* 25(2):139–156, 2000.

104. J. Novacek and R. Raskin. Recognition of warning signs: A consideration for cost-effective treatment of severe mental illness. *Psychiatric Services* 49(3):376–378, 1998.

105. N.J. Gogtay, N.S. Kshirsagar, and S.S. Dalvi. Therapeutic drug monitoring in a de-veloping country: An overview. *British Journal of Clinical Pharmacology.* 48(5):649–654, 1999.

106. R.S. Murthy, personal communication, 2000.

107. B.O. Rothbaum and M.C. Astin. Integration of pharmacotherapy and psychotherapy for bipolar disorder. *Journal of Clinical Psychiatry* 61(Suppl 9):68–75, 2000.

108. D.J. Miklowitz and L.B. Alloy. Psychosocial factors in the course and treatment of bipolar disorder: Introduction to the special section. *Journal of Abnormal Psychology* 108(4):555–557, 1999.

109. K.C. Wilson, M. Scott, M Abou-Saleh, R. Burns, and J.R. Copeland. Long-term effects of cognitive-behavioural therapy and lithium therapy on depression in the elderly. *British Journal of Psychiatry* 167(5):653–658, 1995.

110. N.A. Huxley, S.V. Parikh, and R.J. Baldessarini. Effectiveness of psychosocial treatments in bipolar disorder: State of the evidence. *Harvard Review of Psychiatry* 8(3):126–140, 2000.

111. E.M. Van Gent. Follow-up study of 3 years group therapy with lithium treatment. [Article in French] *Encephale* 26(2):76–79, 2000.

112. D. Dudek and A. Zieba. Development and application of cognitive therapy in affec-tive disorders. [Article in Polish] *Psychiatria Polska* 34(1):81–88, 2000.

113. S.A. Hlastala, E. Frank, A.G. Mallinger, M.E. Thase, A.M. Ritenour, and D.J. Kup-fer. Bipolar depression: An underestimated treatment challenge. *Depression and Anxiety* 5(2):73–83, 1997.

114. American Psychiatric Association. Practice guideline for the treatment of patients with bipolar disorder. *American Journal of Psychiatry* 151(Suppl 12):1–36, 1994.

115. N.A Reilly-Harrington, L. B. Alloy, D.M. Fresco, and W.G. Whitehouse. Cognitive styles and life events interact to predict bipolar and unipolar symptomatology. *Journal of Abnormal Psychology* 108:567–578, 1999.

116. T.L. Simoneau, D.J. Miklowitz, J.A. Richards, R. Saleem, and E.L. George. Bipolar disorder and family communication: Effects of a psychoeducational treatment program. *Journal of Abnormal Psychology* 108:588–597, 1999.
117. E. Frank, Swartz H.A., A.G. Mallinger, M.E. Thase, E.V. Weaver, and D.J. Kupfer. Adjunctive psychotherapy for bipolar disorder: Effects of changing treatment modality. *Journal of Abnormal Psychology* 108(4):579–587, 1999.

Summary of Findings:
Depression in Developing Countries

- Depression, estimated to be the leading cause of disability worldwide, accounts for more than 1 in 10 years of life lived with disability, as well as for significant premature mortality due to suicide and physical illness. By 2020, unipolar major depression will rank second only to ischemic heart disease as the leading source of disease burden worldwide.

- Major risk factors for depression appear similar in developed and developing countries and include family history of the disease, life events, chronic social adversity, poverty, and gender.

- The course of depression is influenced by several factors, including the type, causes, severity, duration prior to treatment, and underlying presence of chronic minor depression. Depression in children and adolescents is often chronic and continues into adulthood with higher rates of overall impairment and significant rates of attempted suicide.

- Because depression typically results from a combination of causes, effective prevention and treatment demands a multifaceted approach. In developing countries, this may translate into a combination of health care, health education, community care, and socioeconomic development.

- Effective pharmacotherapies and psychosocial treatments exist for depression. Though no treatment has been shown to cure all forms of the illness, a large number of efficacious and low-cost treatments are available.

9

Depression

DEFINITION

The term "depression" can apply to a transient mood, a sustained change in mood, a symptom, or a disorder. In this chapter, the term is used to refer to unipolar/major depression that is characterized by persistent low mood or sadness and accompanied by both physical and psychological symptoms of at least 2 weeks duration and with associated impact on social functioning. Both genetic and environmental factors are implicated in the etiology of depression.[1–3]

Depression can present as acute episodes with depressive psychosis that are severely disabling yet often treatable, and when recurrent are controllable with maintenance pharmacotherapy. More often depression presents as an overlapping syndrome of depression, anxiety, and somatization forms such as bodily aches and pain, persistent backache, or genitourinary complaints.

The diagnosis of a depressive illness is based on symptomatology, the severity and duration of the symptoms, and their impact on social functioning. Cases may be identified by means of self-rating on a questionnaire or observer assessment. In the latter case, the patient is interviewed by a health professional with training in assessment and diagnosis (the level of training being consistent with the local resources available for mental health services). The use of operational criteria strengthens the reliability of a conventional clinical interview. Operational diagnosis of psychiatric disorders, which seeks to identify patterns of symptoms that characterize a given illness most reliably, has been one of the major advances in psychiatry within the last 40 years. This diagnostic method allows clinicians to classify illnesses even when etiology is unknown, and hence to communicate about and conduct research on patients with similar characteristics.[4–6]

While criteria for diagnosis have been standardized by the American Psychiatric Association [7] and the *International Classification of Disease*, 10th revision,[8] their criteria are often of limited applicability in non-psychiatric settings, especially by primary care physicians, who often see patients with significant physical comorbidity. The accurate and timely diagnosis of depression is also complicated by the reluctance of patients to seek help because of the stigma associated with mental illness and by the nature of the complaints, which may often be thought to have a physical origin.[9]

There have been continuing studies on the reliability and validity of various methods of assessing depression, and in parallel there has been continuing work on evolving the classification systems and criteria used for these disorders. Current standardized classification systems used for depression appear in Tables 9-1 and 9-2.

TABLE 9-1 DSM-IV Criteria for Major Depressive Episode

A. *Five (or more) of the following symptoms have been present during the same 2-week period and represent a change from previous functioning: at least one of the symptoms is either (1) depressed mood or (2) loss of interest or pleasure.*

(1) Depressed mood most of the day, nearly every day, as indicated by either subjective report or observation made by others;
(2) Markedly diminished interest or pleasure in all, or almost all, activities most of the day, nearly every day;
(3) Significant weight loss when not dieting or weight gain, or decrease or increase in appetite nearly every day;
(4) Insomnia or hypersomnia nearly every day;
(5) Psychomotor agitation or retardation nearly every day;
(6) Fatigue or loss of energy nearly every day;
(7) Feelings of worthlessness or excessive or inappropriate guilt nearly every day;
(8) Diminished ability to think or concentrate, or indecisiveness, nearly every day;
(9) Recurrent thoughts of death, recurrent suicidal ideation without a specific plan, or a suicide attempt or a specific plan for committing suicide.

B. The symptoms do not meet criteria for a Mixed Episode (see Table F).

C. The symptoms cause clinically significant distress or impairment in social, occupational, or other important areas of functioning.

D. The symptoms are not due to the direct physiological effects of a substance or a general medical condition.

E. The symptoms are not better accounted for by bereavement, i.e., after the loss of a loved one, the symptoms persist for longer than 2 months or are characterized by marked functional impairment, morbid preoccupation with worthlessness, suicidal ideation, psychotic symptoms, or psychomotor retardation.

Source: [7]

TABLE 9-2 ICD–10 Criteria for depressive episode

General	Episode must have lasted at least two weeks with symptoms nearly every day
	Change from normal functioning
Key symptoms (n = 3)	Depressed mood Anhedonia Fatigue/loss of energy
Ancillary symptoms	Weight and appetite change Sleep disturbance Subjective or objective agitation/retardation Low self esteem/confidence Self reproach/guilt Impaired thinking/concentration Suicidal thoughts
Criteria	Mild episode: 2 key , 4 symptoms in total Moderate episode: 2 key , 6 symptoms in total Severe episode: 3 key , 8 symptoms in total
Exclusions	No history ever of manic symptoms Not substance related Not organic

Source: [8]

The vast majority of research on the clinical features of depression has been conducted in the United States and Europe. Although far fewer in number, comparable studies from the developing world deserve careful attention, for they reveal significant differences in the presentation of depression among cultures, as well as core features common to all societies. Where possible in this chapter, we examine and compare findings from research in both developed and developing countries. For the purposes of comprehensive reporting, developed-country data are noted and used alone when findings from developing countries are not available.

Although symptoms of depression are found everywhere, the Western biomedical definition of depressive illness does not fit local concepts of illness in many developing communities.[10,11] Diagnoses of some mental disorders, including depression, have no conceptual equivalent in many languages. In non-European cultures, for example, use of the term "depression" often leads to the mistaken belief that sadness is an essential presenting feature of the disorder. While the experience of dysphoric mood may be universal, the concept of depressive disorder that focuses on mood must be recognized as having evolved within Western cultures, and therefore may not be universally applicable.[12]

Several authors also imply that Cartesian mind–body dichotomies are absent from certain cultural worldviews. Nichter (1982), for example, noted that South Havik Brahmin women express distressed emotions and other social problems in terms of dietary preference for certain foods, religious metaphors, or humoral imbalance in the body.[13] Chinese popular explanations of mental illness ascribe problems to an imbalance in the psychosocial, physiological, or supernatural environment.[14,15] In African societies, health is viewed as more social than biological, and a unitary concept of psychosomatic interrelationship exists, with an apparent reciprocity between mind and matter.[16] Because these conceptualizations strongly influence how people express the experience of psychological distress and dysphoric mood, standardized instruments may not be applied accurately without regard to cultural differences among populations. Nevertheless, studies show that depression is found in countries around the world with significantly different cultural traditions and levels of economic development.[17–19]

The majority of people with depression eventually consult primary care doctors or nurses. While the overall symptoms of depression are ubiquitous in population surveys, research has shown somatic symptoms to be the most common presenting features of depression in developed as well as developing societies.[20–22] Most commonly, patients present with physical symptoms such as lack of energy or vitality, fatigue, and aches and pains.[20,23–25] Several studies in developing countries indicate that when people with depression present with somatic symptoms, they will upon questioning also report that they have experienced classic psychological symptoms of depression.[20,26,27]

SCOPE OF THE PROBLEM

Depressive disorders are common around the world and are associated with significant disability.[18,28–31] Depression is a long-term illness that produces significant psychological, physical, and functional disability.[28,32–34]. In a study conducted in Malaysia, over half the patients with chronic depression had dysfunctional behavior and experienced significant disabilities.[35] Indeed, depression is estimated to be the leading cause of disability worldwide, accounting for more than 1 in 10 years of life lived with disability. Those suffering from depressive disorders also have high premature mortality, both from suicide and from physical illness.[17,18,35,36] Prevalence rates for depression vary among and between countries, but age of onset, social and environmental risk factors, and the preponderance of depressive disorders within families are similar across many cultures.

Once recognized, depression can often be treated effectively. Though treatments are often not entirely curative, they offer significant relief from many of the debilitating symptoms of depression and can significantly improve the level of social functioning. Yet depressive disorders still remain largely underdiagnosed and untreated around the world. Even in developed nations, depressed patients consistently receive either no medication or dosages that are ineffective in treating their symptoms.[19,37,38]

Mortality

Suicide

Suicide is estimated to be the 10th leading cause of death worldwide.[31] These estimates are based on nationally collected official data on suicide, which are thought to be significantly underestimated because of the stigma often associated with suicide. Reported rates of suicide vary widely throughout the world, with some of the highest rates being found in developing countries. For example, Sri Lanka [39] has the highest suicide rate in the world, followed closely by China.[40] Factors affecting the suicide rate among a given population include the rate of depression; the prevalence of alcohol abuse; the presence of high-risk occupational and demographic groups, including people with severe mental illness; the availability of easy means of suicide; the degree of social integration; and cultural attitudes toward suicide.

Psychological autopsy studies (which gather detailed information about the deceased from multiple key informants) indicate that more than 90 percent of people who commit suicide suffer from depression, substance abuse, psychosis, or some other form of mental illness.[41–43] In a major review of all studies of suicide reported in the English literature, Harris and Barraclough (1998) found that people with affective disorders combined (major depression, bipolar disorder, and affective disorder not otherwise specified) were 20 times more likely to kill themselves than the general population.[44] In non-Western countries, however, completed suicides may be less likely to have received a psychiatric diagnosis because of the paucity of mental health services.

Suicides often appear to be precipitated by a "last-straw phenomenon": a recent social stress or life event in the context of multiple preexisting social stresses and an underlying mental illness. Official statistics tend to highlight the existence of social stresses rather than any underlying depression or other mental disorder. In settings where police officers, coroners, or physicians without mental health training are recording data about the principal causes of suicide, they are likely to focus on social and situational problems, rather than on preexisting depression. However, community surveys reveal that social problems are correlated with high rates of depression and anxiety.[45–47]

Individuals with limited or dysfunctional social networks have been shown to be predisposed to depression, suicidal thoughts, and suicide.[48] Similarly, at the broader societal level, social disruption in contemporary industrialized society is believed to contribute to anomie, depression, and suicide.[49] The suicide rate in Sri Lanka rose from 6.5 per 100,000 in 1950 to 47 per 100,000 in 1991 following a period of profound social upheaval and violence.[39] War and social disruption have been associated with dramatically different suicide rates in various settings.

Access to means of suicide has a major influence on the suicide rate.[50] Where rapid and effective means of self-destruction are readily available, people making impulsive gestures may commit suicide inadvertently. This may explain at least in part the extremely high rates of self-poisoning with insecticides among young women in China, Sri Lanka, and Western Samoa.[39,40,51,52] Medicines that can be obtained without prescription and are lethal in overdose may also be used for self-poisoning. Barbiturates are frequently used in this way in Nigeria, as are chloroquine in East Africa [53] and paracetamol in Europe.[54] In addition, potentially lethal features of urban or rural landscapes appeal to those at risk by virtue of their symbolic association as an effective means of suicide. For example, tall buildings in Singapore and Hong Kong are popular sites for suicidal jumpers.[55]

Physical Illness

A growing body of evidence links untreated depression to severe and life-threatening physical illness.[56] Depression is associated with high premature mortality from physical causes, irrespective of premature mortality from suicide and trauma.[57–59]

In a 40-year study, Ford and colleagues (1998) found that increased risk of coronary heart disease among people with major depression persisted for years after their first depressive episode. The increased risk was present even for myocardial infarctions occurring 10 years after the first depressive episode.[59] Examining data from the Baltimore, Maryland, site of the Epidemiological Catchment Area Study, Pratt and co-workers (1996) found a fivefold increase in the risk of myocardial infarction following major depression and a twofold increase in those who suffered from less severe (subsyndromal) depression. The increased risk of cardiovascular disease with depression appears to apply equally to men and women.[60–62]

Conversely, high rates of depression have been found in older patients suffering from cerebrovascular disease.[63,64] The significant disability often associated with recovering stroke patients may account for episodes of depression.[63,65] A recent study has suggested that cerebrovascular disease may have an etiopathological role in late-life depression. The increased damage to frontal and subcortical brain circuitry following stroke, transient ischemia, and hypertension may explain the high prevalence of depression in older individuals with vascular risk factors.[66]

Hormonal changes may go a long way toward explaining how depression results in physiological harm. For example, major depression leads to increased activation of the hypothalamic-pituitary-adrenal axis, which has in turn been associated with decreases in bone mineral density and increases in intraabdominal fat, a known risk factor for coronary artery disease.[67–69] Researchers have examined the link between depression and osteoporosis.[70,71] One such study reported that depression-associated loss of bone density could be expected to increase hip fractures by more than 40 percent in 10 years.[68]

Social and Economic Costs

The most comprehensive analysis to date of the worldwide impact of depression was performed in 1990 as part of the *Global Burden of Disease* (GBD) study. A major finding of this study, released in 1996, was that conditions such as mental disorders that disable, may cause less mortality than a number of physical conditions, but exact a high cost in disability throughout the world. Previous public health assessments, derived only from mortality data, did not rank mental disorders among the most burdensome diseases. Once disability was entered into the equation, mental disorders joined the ranks of cardiovascular and respiratory diseases, revealing a burden that surpassed both AIDS and all combined malignancies.[31]

The disability-adjusted life years (DALYs) methodology employed in the GBD (see Appendix B) provides a way of linking information on disease occurrence to information on short- and long-term outcomes, including disabilities and restrictions on participation in usual life situations. The disability component is weighted according to the severity of the disability. For example, in the original GBD study, disability caused by major depression was weighted as being equivalent to blindness or paraplegia. Thus calculated, the GBD study ranked depressive disorders (considered as a single diagnostic category) as the leading cause of disability worldwide.

The GBD study also resulted in the prediction that in 2020, as the result of a combination of several demographic and epidemiological trends, unipolar major depression will rank second only to ischemic heart disease as the leading cause of disease and injury worldwide. These trends include the breakdown of extended family networks; increasing urbanization, migration, and mobility; and alcohol and drug abuse. In addition, the expected growth of the world's population, overall increases in life expectancy, and relative decreases in other communicable disorders are likely to result in depressive disorders becoming the leading cause of disability and overall disease burden worldwide.

Continuing debate and further scientific studies will be required to confirm and refine the findings of the GBD study. However, it is important to note several limitations of the study:

- The figures used to calculate the burden due to depressive disorders are very low compared with the recent findings from large-scale epidemiological studies, such as the (U.S.) National Comorbidity Survey [72] and the British national psychiatric morbidity survey.[73]

• The GBD study considered unipolar depression to be an episodic illness, while current concepts of the disorder describe it as a chronic relapsing medical illness.

• Likewise, the study considered depression only as an adult disease, yet overwhelming evidence suggests that depression also occurs with considerable frequency in childhood and adolescence.[74]

• Only two disability weights were used to calculate the global burden of depressive disorders—one for treated cases, the other for untreated cases.[31]

• The impact of comorbidity of depression with other mental and substance abuse disorders was not addressed.[75]

• The burden on families, which is particularly significant for depression, was also not addressed.

Given all of the above limitations, it is clear that the GBD estimates of the global burden of disability caused by depression are conservative at best, and more likely significantly underreport the worldwide burden exacted by depressive illness. Thus there is a pressing need for more precise information on the prevalence of and disability associated with these disorders in low-income countries.

As noted above, the burden on family members of patients was not included in the GBD. However, the findings of several studies in both developed and developing countries reveal the significant toll exacted by depressive illness on family members and family stability.[76–78] Family members of depressed individuals may have increased rates of physical illness and frequent symptoms of fatigue.[79,80]

As described in Chapter 2, the stigma associated with mental illness is often great in both developed and developing countries. The burden of stigma is experienced not only by those who suffer from the illness, but also by their family members. This burden can lead to lost social and employment opportunities, social isolation, and unwillingness to assist the ill family member in seeking treatment.[81]

A few studies in developed countries have begun to examine the cost to the workforce caused by depression. Findings indicate that depressive illness has resulted in more days of disability and lost work time than chronic physical conditions such as heart disease, hypertension, and lower back pain.[82,83] The governments and employers of developing countries would be likely to see similar results. Studies to determine this economic burden may reinforce the argument for robust, proactive efforts on the part of governments and communities to prevent and treat depression.

Recommendation 9-1. Depressive disorders exhibit high incidence and prevalence in the developing world, lead to disability and mortality, and exact high social costs. Therefore, they should be given high national priority as a public health problem of relevance to all government ministries, and be accorded high local priority by district planning committees.

PREVALENCE AND INCIDENCE

Over the last four decades, community surveys of mental disorders have provided diagnostic information, based on standardized methods of assessment, that permits comparison of research from different locations. Here we summarize selected epidemiological studies on depression conducted at the community level (Table 9-3) and on common mental disorders (which include depression) conducted at both the community (Table 9-4) and primary care (Table 9-5) levels.

The accumulated evidence from these studies reveals the widespread prevalence of depression within both the developing and developed worlds, ranging from 8–43 percent. The variation in rates reported by these studies also appears to be due in part to cultural and environmental differences among the populations studied. Overall rates are higher in surveys of primary care attenders than in surveys of community populations. Precise case rates vary among locations and populations, and depend partly on the methodology used.[17,83] Differing rates of depression among population groups are discussed in greater detail in the subsequent discussion of risk factors.

The most common psychiatric syndrome seen in community studies is a combination of depression and anxiety. For example, about one-half of those with a primary diagnosis of DSM-IV major depression also have an anxiety disorder.[84,85] This condition is sometimes referred to as comorbidity, but such a definition appears to be an artifact of classification systems designed primarily for hospital patients, rather than for the general population. When examined at the more universal level of primary care, anxiety and depression appear to coexist in the majority of depressed patients in both developing and developed countries.[86–89] Indeed, many mental health professionals now support the grouping of depression, anxiety, and other conditions often found to coexist in a single category—referred to as common mental disorders (CMD).[90–93] This chapter at times includes research that has examined CMD because it not only provides data that would eitherwise be absent, but also offers an accurate reflection of the high frequency with which these coexisting mental disorders occur.

In addition to anxiety, several other conditions frequently coexist with depression; these include panic and dissociative disorders, neurasthenia, and sleep problems.[94] Recent studies rank CMD among the most important causes of morbidity in primary care settings.[95] For example, a review of the recent literature on CMD from South Asia [11] indicated that these disorders can be detected in more than a third of people who seek primary health care.

A World Health Organization (WHO) collaborative study provided important information on the form, frequency, and outcome of psychological disorders seen in general health care settings. This study was carried out in 14 countries in different parts of the world: Brazil, Chile, the Federal Republic of Germany, France, Greece, India, Italy, Japan, the Netherlands, Nigeria, the People's Republic of China, Turkey, the United Kingdom, and the United States.[96] In the study, 25,916 people aged 18 to 65 who consulted health care services were screened. Well-defined psychological problems were found in 24 percent of these subjects; most common were depressive disorders, anxiety disorders, alcohol use disorders, somatoform disorders, and neurasthenia.

The results of the WHO study indicate a strong association between CMD and disability, defined as impairment of physical and social functioning. Disability levels were found to be greater on average among primary care patients with a psychological disorder than among those with common chronic diseases such as hypertension, diabetes, arthritis, and back pain. This finding of enhanced disability for psychological disorders was consistent across centers, across time, and across individual diagnoses.[33,34,97,98] The conditions categorized as CMD were also found frequently to be chronic. Approximately half of those with CMD when they first sought primary care continued to be afflicted a year later.[19]

People with CMD frequently seek primary care for physical symptoms. The latter may either serve as a risk factor for mental illness or result from somatization of psychological symptoms. As a result, CMD contributes significantly to the workload in both primary health care clinics and specialty medical clinics (Table 9-5).[94,97,98]

TABLE 9-3 Selected Prevalence Studies of Depression

Country	Population	Method	Prevalence per 1,000 Population at Risk
Lesotho [99]	Rural village (n = 356); age 19–93	Sample survey Modules of DIS	88.5
South Africa [100]	Rural village (n = 481); age > 18	Two-stage sample survey SRQ and PSE	180
Uganda [101]	Two rural villages (n = 206); age > 18	Homestead survey PSE/SPI	143 males 226 females
Taiwan [102]	Rural		6
Taiwan [102]	Urban, small town		11
Taiwan [102]	Taipei (urban)		8
Taiwan [18]	Urban and rural (n = 11,004); age 18–65	DIS	8
South Korea [18]	National sample (n = 5,100); adults 18–65	DIS	23
India [103]	Rural (n = 4,481)	Interviews by trained field worker	430
India [104]	Urban (n = 4,481)	Interviews by field worker	10
China [105]	(n = 388,136)		Neurotic depression, 0.37 affective psychosis, 13 neurasthenia
Brazil [106]	3 urban localities	Household survey	13–67 across different localities
Dubai [107]	Females (n = 300)		137
Australia [108]	Canberra (n = 756)	Household survey PSE	26 male 67 female 48 total
United Kingdom [109]	Camberwell (n = 800)	Household survey PSE	48 male 90 female 70 total
Holland [110]	Nijmegen (n = 3,232)	Household survey PSE	55
Finland [111]	(n = 742)	Household survey PSE	46
United Kingdom [112]	Camberwell Cypriot community in inner London (n = 307)	Household survey PSE	42 male 71 female 56 total
Italy [113]	Sardinia (n = 374)	Household survey PSE	52 male 110 female 83 total
United States of America [114]	48 contiguous states (n = 8098); age 15–54	Household survey	77 male 129 female annual prevalence
United Kingdom [73]	Sample of total population excluding Northern Ireland and the highlands and islands of Scotland (n = 10,1108); age 18–64	Household survey CIS-R and SCAN	18 male 27 female one week prevalence

RISK FACTORS

A variety of social, psychological, and biological factors may predispose an individual to depressive illness. Studies of risk factors for depression in developed and developing countries have yielded similar findings with regard to social and economic variables, such as life events, chronic social adversity, poverty, and gender. The vast majority of research concerning biological risk factors for depression, such as neuroendocrinological and genetic factors, derives from the developed world. This section briefly reviews the evidence for a variety of risk factors for depression and points, where possible, to data from developing countries.

TABLE 9-4 Prevalence of Common Mental Disorders in Community Studies

Country	Population	Method	Prevalence
Ethiopia [115]	Rural (n = 337); all ages	Lujik's method	190
South Africa [116]	Urban	Structured questio nnaire	118–230
Lesotho [99]	Rural (n = 356); age 19–93	DIS	228
Ethiopia [117]	Urban (n = 40); age > 18	SRQ	120
Uganda [101]	Rural (n = 206); age > 18	PSE	204
Sudan [118]	Urban (n = 204); age 22–35	SRQ	166
South Africa [100]	Rural (n = 481); age > 18	SRQ/PSE	270
Ethiopia [119]	Rural (n = 2000); age 15–55	SRQ	172
South Africa [120]	Urban and rural (n = 139); age > 65	PSE/MMSE	237
South Africa [121]	Urban and rural (n = 400); age > 65	SRQ	390
South Africa [122]	Urban (n = 365); age > 60	Short Care	252
West Bengal, India [123]	Urban and rural (n = 1424)	Trained field investiga tors	23–40
Pakistan [45]	Rural Punjab (n = 664)		660 female 250 male
Pakistan [124]	Rural Chitral		460 female 150 male
India [125]	Rural (n = 2,183 in 1972 and 3,488 in 1992); ages-all	Bengali case detection schedule	117 in 1972 105 in 1992
Brazil [126]	Urban	SRQ-20	350
Brazil [127]	Urban	CIS-R	
United Kingdom [128]	Urban and rural (n = 1,277)	Household survey	160

TABLE 9-5 Prevalence of Common Mental Disorders in Studies of Primary Care Attenders

Country	Population	Method	Prevalence
Nigeria [129]	Urban (n = 277); Pregnant women	GHQ 28/PAS	157
Guinea-Bissau [130]	Rural (n = 251); age > 16	SRQ/PSE	120–180
Kenya [131]	Urban (n = 200); age 18–55	SRQ/SPI	258
Kenya [132]	Rural/semi-urban (n = 388); age > 16	SRQ	290
Senegal [133]	Rural (n = 933); adults	SRQ	162
South Africa [134]	Urban/rural (n = 363); age > 16	SRQ/PSE	83
Ethiopia [115]	Rural (n = 337); all ages	Lujik's	190
Zimbabwe [135]	Urban (n = 448); age > 16	SRQ	105
4 developing countries [136]	Rural (n = 360); age > 18	SRQ/PSE	106
Ethiopia [117]	Urban (n = 30); age > 18	SRQ	270
South Africa [137]	Rural (n = 159); age > 15	GHQ 28	45
South Africa [138]	Urban (n = 301); age 16–60	SRQ/PSE	103–143
Sri Lanka [139]	Urban (n = 3,000); age	Clinical Interview	210
India			
Karnataka [140]	Urban (n = 300); age	GHQ/IPSS	360
Maharashtra [141]	Urban (n = 500); age	GHQ/Clinical Interview	570
Karnataka [142]	Urban (n = 882); age	GHQ/IPSS	360
West Bengal [88]	Urban (n = 202); age	SRQ/CIS	250
Bangalore [143]	Urban (n =1366); age	GHQ/CIDI	240
Haryan [144]	Rural (n = 218); age	SRQ/Clinical Interview	420
Goa [26]	Rural (n = 303); age	GHQ/CIS-R	465
Gujarat [145]	(n = 200); age	BDI/Clinical Inter view	210

Environmental

Life events that lead to the threat of loss or to actual loss, such as the death of a family member, marital separation, maternal deprivation, or loss of employment, have been shown to cluster before the onset of depressive episodes and to influence the course of depression in both developed and developing countries.[1,2,146–148] Beck has described a cognitive triad that may contribute to the onset or reoccurrence of depressive episodes by increasing the risk for exposure to stressful life events: (1) negative self-view, (2) negative interpretation of experience, and (3) negative view of the future.[149] Personality traits found to be associated with depression include avoidance, dependence, reactivity, and impulsiveness.[150] People with such personality traits may cope less effectively with stress and may also tend to encounter continuing adversity. These traits that often contribute or predispose individuals to experience depressive episodes are both genetically and socially influenced.[151,152] Most people with depression do not have personality disorders. It is important to remember that efforts to assess personality during times of acute illness are misleading, and personality assessments frequently change when patients recover.

Rates of depression are increased in a variety of vulnerable groups, including refugees, neglected ethnic minority groups, and those exposed to war trauma. As discussed in Chapter 2, a large body of evidence demonstrates the association between poverty and CMD. For example, five cross-sectional surveys of people who sought treatment in primary care and community samples from Brazil, Zimbabwe, India, and Chile were collated to examine the economic risk factors for CMD.[153] In all five studies, a consistent and significant relationship was found between low income and risk of CMD. Similarly, a population-based study from Indonesia revealed that people with less education and material possessions were more likely to suffer from depression.[154] It appears that both absolute and relative poverty are important in the genesis of depression.

Further investigation to disentangle the complex relationship among stressful life events, social behavior, the interpretation of life events, and genetic influence (see below) would contribute to more effective methods for identifying individuals at high risk and appropriate methods of intervention.

Genetic

Understanding of the biological basis for depression has been one of the more recent and important findings regarding the etiology and risk factors for this disorder. Family, twin, and adoption studies have provided evidence of the genetic contribution to the etiology of depressive disorders and clearly shown the transmission of increased risk through heredity.[3,155–158] Twin studies, in particular, also point to a strong role of the nonshared (i.e., individually experienced) environment in the causation of depression.[2] However, understanding of the genetics of behavioral variation and of mental illness has proven enormously complex and has been constrained by small sample populations with sometimes unclear or limited ranges of environmental variation.[159] Future genetic studies would benefit from the collection and analysis of one or more of the following types of data sets [160]:

- Large numbers of pedigrees from outbred populations containing multiple individuals affected with a given mental disorder;
- Pedigrees from genetically isolated populations; and
- Large numbers of affected individuals and control samples.

Examination of gene-environment interactions is essential to future research and could benefit from a much wider range of variation in the psychosocial environments studied, making it possible to better delineate the etiological contribution of each, including such environmental factors as socioeconomic adversity, pervasive stress, and the breakdown of social support networks. The populations and environments of many developing countries provide such conditions for research and may prove particularly useful in elucidating the complex nature of depressive disorders.

It is currently understood that multiple genes act in conjunction with other, nongenetic factors to produce a risk for mental disorder. Future discoveries in genetics and neuroscience can be expected to lead to better models for understanding the complexity of the interactions between the brain and behavior and the development of both. These discoveries are likely to have significant impacts on clinical practice in both developed and developing countries.[161,162]

Gender and Reproductive Health

Both community-based and primary care studies indicate that women are often affected disproportionately by depression in both developing and developed countries (see also Chapter 2).[153,163,164] Women often develop the disorder in response to life events, social adversity, and other environmental factors.[164–166] The multiple roles assumed by women—including the bearing and rearing of children; responsibility for the home; caring for both healthy and ill relatives; and, increasingly, earning income—can lead to considerable stress. Women in both developed and developing countries also encounter difficulties related to their social position, aspirations, social support networks, and domestic problems, which may include physical or sexual abuse.[153,167–169] Additionally, because mental illness in women may engender a greater amount of shame and dishonor and have a greater impact on family life because of the woman's role in running the household, the condition is often hidden and treatment not pursued (see also Chapter 2).[9,170,171]

Initial scientific evidence has suggested that hormonal changes in and imbalances of such hormones as oxytocin, estrogen, and vasopressin may contribute to the onset of depressive disorders.[172,173] Periods after childbirth and during menopause for women involve significant hormonal changes whose examination may provide further evidence regarding the higher rates of depression in women.[174–177]

Postpartum depression has been identified in both developed and developing countries.[178–183] The greatest risk for postpartum depression is within the first 30 days of childbirth and the condition can persist for up to 2 years.[184] Certain practices in developing countries such as isolation of recent mothers from family and the new infant, are disruptive to the initial mother–infant relationship and eliminate the benefits of positive social supports. These practices have been identified as possible contributing factors to the onset of postpartum depression.[179–181,183] In a recent study conducted in Zimbabwe, a brief screening questionnaire proved effective in identifying women (in the eighth month of pregnancy) as being at higher risk of postpartum depression. Such a tool may be useful in devising preventive measures aimed at identifing high-risk individuals and implementing appropriate interventions shortly after childbirth.[178]

Neuroendocrine

Defective neurotransmission [185,186] and defective neuroendocrine receptor responses [187–189] are associated with depression. Three monoamines have been implicated: 5-hydroxytryptamine (serotonin), noradrenaline, and dopamine. Conclusive evidence on the impact of these defects on the course of depressive disorders remains to be found. It is still unclear whether associations with neurological function represent cause or effect in the pathogenesis of depression.

Comorbidity

Comorbidity (the coexistence of two or more current disorders) has been found to be common among patients suffering from depression, and typically to involve a combination of physical and mental disorders.[36,59,63,89] In one study of patients attending primary care, of nearly 21 percent of patients with clinically significant depressive symptoms, only 1.2 percent cited depression as the reason for their visit to the physician.[190]

Comorbidity of physical and mental illness has been found to increase with age, as described earlier with regard to stroke and ischemic heart disease.[24,191,192] Substance abuse is a frequent comorbid condition with depressive illness. Studies in both developed and developing countries point to substance abuse as both a cause and effect of depression linked to both genetic and environmental factors.[193–195] Depression has been shown to be a major factor in contributing to relapse in women abusing alcohol and drugs.[196,197] Identifying substance abuse in patients presenting with depressive illness is an important component of determining an effective course of treatment. Depression is also a common concomitant of HIV/AIDS.[198]

Associations with Age

Several studies conducted in developing countries have indicated a greater risk for depression among the aged.[199–201] Other large studies have found the highest rates of the disorder among those aged 25 to 34.[114,202,203] Additionally, the rates of suicide are increasing rapidly among adolescents and young adults in developed countries and more recently in developing countries.[204,205] This inconsistency in findings arises from age bias (instruments do not have equivalent validity across the age span) and covarying risk factors, including sociodemographic factors and rates of physical illness.[206] A cross-national study of both developed and developing countries using the standardized DSM-III diagnostic criteria found the mean age of onset to be 24.8–34.8

years[18] Studies that use standardized measurements are still needed in developing countries to determine more conclusively the role of age as a risk factor for depression.

Factors Affecting Course and Outcome

The course of depression is influenced by the type of depression, its causes, its severity, its prior duration, and the underlying presence of chronic minor depression. Patients who are genetically predisposed to develop depression have a less favorable long-term prognosis than those who become depressed following a specific life event.[207] The prognosis for depression also appears to worsen for cases that are either severe or long-standing at the outset of treatment.[208,209] Early-onset depression (in both children and adolescents) is often chronic and continues into adulthood with higher rates of overall impairment and significant rates of attempted suicide.[74,210,211]

On the basis of data from 11,242 outpatients in New Zealand, Wells and colleagues concluded that depressive symptoms produce impairment comparable to that associated with chronic medical conditions such as diabetes, lung disease, hypertension, and heart disease.[202] Approximately 40 percent of patients with major depression remained functionally impaired 2 years after treatment, while 54 percent of those previously treated for dysthymia had a major depressive episode during this period. Similarly, a WHO cross-national study of more than 5,000 outpatients in developing as well as developed countries has shown that psychiatric disorder produces significant functional disability over and above any associated physical health problems.[96]

Recovery rates for depression depend on how recovery is measured: by complete remission of symptoms or by remission to below case-threshold levels. Data from the U.S. National Institute of Mental Health's collaborative study on the psychobiology of depression indicate that the rate of recovery from a first depressive episode declines over time. Although 70 percent of patients in this study were found to recover during the first year, only an additional 18 percent had recovered by the fifth year.[212] A review of 51 follow-up studies of depressed adults treated by inpatient or outpatient psychiatric services in developed countries assessed outcome in terms of recovery, recurrence, and persistent depression. The authors estimated that 50 to 60 percent of patients with major depression recovered at least briefly over 1 year, while up to 90 percent experienced short-term recovery or better over 5 years.[213] However, only 43 percent of these patients reported that they experienced sustained recovery after 1 year, a figure that declined to 24 percent after 10 years. Significant numbers of people with depression suffer from chronic versions of the disease. A variety of studies indicate that between 10 and 25 percent of patients with depression suffer non-remitting episodes lasting 2 years or more.[212–217]

Recommendation 9-2. Trained health care providers (health care workers, nurses, and general physicians), particularly those in primary care settings, should be prepared to identify patients at risk for depression, who include those with a family history of the disorder, postpartum women and those of childbearing age, and those who experienced early-onset depressive episodes in childhood or adolescence. These providers should be adequately trained and informed to recommend additional sources of information, and counseling in available support systems, and to provide treatment. Severe cases should be referred to specialist mental health personnel that maintain oversight of primary care facilities.

INTERVENTIONS

Because depression typically results from a combination of causes, effective prevention and treatment of the disorder and its consequences demands a multifaceted approach. In developing countries, this may translate into a combination of health care, public health awareness, community care, and socioeconomic development, as has been the case, for example, in India and Iran (see Boxes 9-1 and 9-2). Many prevention and treatment interventions have not been proven conclusively to be cost-effective in developing countries. However, where developing-country data exist for the following interventions, this is noted. In other instances, comparable evaluations have been included from developed countries, and implementation of their findings in developing countries is addressed.

Prevention

Evidence on the effectiveness of depression prevention strategies remains inconclusive, and it is likely that no single strategy could ameliorate the occurrence of the disorder, but only serve to reduce its cumulative effects. The multiple issues to be considered in preventing depression include precipitating life events, efforts to enhance the use of coping strategies, the provision of social and community support, and the need for general educational support for mental health.

BOX 9-1 Primary Mental Health Care in India

Like other developing countries, India has limited resources for mental health care. In 1999, 3,000 psychiatrists served its 1 billion people. To cope with this disparity, India has taken a community approach to promoting mental health through a variety of initiatives. Most important, mental health care has become an integral part of the country's program of primary care, which provides mechanisms for mental health planning at both the state and national levels.

Several studies have shown not only that mental disorders are common in India, but also that few physicians diagnose and treat them appropriately. In response to this situation, simple, rapid training programs on mental health have been developed for primary health care personnel. Manuals of mental health for different categories of health personnel, recording systems, training videos, assessment forms, and public education materials have also been developed. A demonstration project on primary mental health care, conducted between 1985 and 1990, showed that it is possible to provide basic mental health care with limited reliance on mental health specialists.

Psychiatry in India is showing strong signs of growth as culturally sensitive interventions are developed. At this time, research efforts are limited, and longitudinal studies remain to be done. However, existing findings on mental disorders, their antecedents, and patterns of care are sufficient to prompt a reexamination of long-held concepts regarding mental health care. Increasing efforts toward this goal promise to benefit the practice of mental health care throughout the world.

Source: [218–227]

BOX 9-2 Primary Mental Health Care in Iran

Prior to 1985, mental health care in Iran was based on institutional care by medical specialists and was based primarily in cities. With the debut of a national program of universal coverage, mental health care became integrated into Iran's existing primary health care system. The village-based primary care system in Iran was implemented in the 1970s and has spread to over 60 regions. Highlighting the importance of comprehensive, well-supported primary care, the program has continued to link village-based care centers to surrounding hospitals and medical schools. Iran's national health program supports training in mental health for all personnel, development of a district-level mental health support system, and an annual mental health week.

One male and one female village health worker serve every 2,000 people in the rural regions of Iran. Workers are trained in assessment, diagnosis, and management of priority conditions, which include depression, anxiety, psychosis, epilepsy, infectious diseases, childbirth, and, as of 1999, substance abuse. They use good-practice guidelines for assessment, diagnosis, and management, and they are able to prescribe a limited list of essential medicines, including antidepressants and lithium for depression and bipolar disorder. Village health workers practice prevention and mental health promotion, regularly visiting each person in their area to screen for illness. They also see patients in the clinic, and are expected to collect routine data on diagnosis, consultations, and health outcomes, which are collated annually.

Quality control is achieved by health psychologists who make monthly visits to each village health center to provide support to the village health workers and ensure quality of treatment. Village health workers refer complex or severely ill patients to a primary care doctor who is responsible for 10,000 people. He or she is also trained in the use of good-practice guidelines in the priority conditions. Because Iran's Ministry of Health and Medical Education is responsible for education as well as for the administration of care, the medical curriculum taught in universities is consistent with and supportive of the role of primary care for mental health. At present the program is active in almost half of the nation's rural areas, with 9,200 of the total 15,500 "houses of health" of the country being engaged in mental health programs. To date, 18,200 behvarzes (multipurpose health workers) and 5,500 general practitioners have received the appropriate training. Within the 14 years since the program was introduced, 12.7 million rural residents have been covered by the program. The total population covered by the program at this point is 16.4 million, which constitutes one-fourth of the country's total population.

Additional innovative programs in Iran include the following:

• An urban mental health program, which was introduced into the primary health care system during the past 3 years and at present time covers 10 percent of the urban population (3.7 million). It is hoped that this percentage will increase to 20 percent by the end of 2000.

• Primary prevention of mental disorders with emphasis on depression and suicide has been planned and initiated in four districts since 1999.

• Integration of a prevention program on substance abuse into the primary health care system is planned for five districts as pilot studies during 2000.

• Other new mental health programs and activities for the Ministry of Health and Medical Education include:

• A second revision of the National Program of Mental Health, scheduled for late 2000.

• Preparation of a comprehensive mental health act.

• Development of a school mental health program.

• Development of a child abuse prevention program.

• A second independent evaluation of the National Mental Health Program during 2000.

Source: [228–231]

Social and Public Health Models

Public education campaigns to raise awareness about depression have been undertaken in a number of developed countries.[232–234] These campaigns have included messages that identify depression as a treatable and common condition to reduce the stigma surrounding the disease and to encourage afflicted individuals to seek treatment. These campaigns have also included strong anti-suicide messages.[235] Though limited in scope, recent evaluation has shown that some of these campaigns have resulted in improved attitudes toward seeking treatment.[236]

Educational programs aimed at promoting mental health should provide information on prevention and treatment; reduce the stigma associated with mental disorders; and offer ways to improve every person's capacity to cope with predictable life events, as well as with crises. In some cases, programs might be targeted at community leaders who are in key positions to affect the lives of others (e.g., clergy, teachers, employers, and doctors). Similarly, both national and local policy makers must be kept informed about mental health issues through the efforts of mental health professionals and advocates. Mental health programs in schools aim chiefly to improve life skills. Within communities, mental health initiatives that involve a variety of local organizations (e.g., schools, social services, and law enforcement agencies) may also serve to increase community awareness of health issues, such as children's welfare, rape, and domestic violence.[237,238] Such cooperative participation and intersectoral funding from national- and-local level government agencies and other organizations serves to reinforce and expand prevention efforts. One such program instituted in Pakistan is described in Box 9-3.

An important role for primary health care personnel is to recognize and address mental disorders in children, as well as to provide support for school programs on mental health. In Zanzibar, primary care teams include health education workers who link with schools on a local basis. In some countries, moreover, such as India and Pakistan, school children play a vital role by recognizing adults with epilepsy, schizophrenia, and other disorders and bringing them to medical attention.[239]

BOX 9-3 School Mental Health Program of Pakistan

Pakistan has an estimated population of 136 million. The fertility rate is 5.8 per 100, and the literacy rate has been estimated between 27 percent and 30 percent. In rural areas, school-going children are often the only members of the community who are able to read and write. They are thus in a unique position to be the agents of change for their communities. In rural areas, school, along with the family, is the strongest social institution. Therefore, schools are a possible point of access to the community.

A school mental health program was initiated as part of the Community Mental Health Program in the Rawalpindi District by the Institute of Psychiatry in 1987, with the objective of raising awareness about health in general and mental health in particular among school children, teachers, and the community. The program was carried out in a phased manner. In the familiarization phase, education administrators were sensitized to the application of mental health principles in the field of education. In addition, baseline data regarding knowledge and attitudes about mental health among the schoolteachers and students were collected. This was followed by training. Male and female teachers were trained with the aim of providing knowledge and counseling skills. This training was reinforced by regular visits to the schools by the community support team, who assisted with the organization of parent–teacher associations; speech and essay contests on mental health; and the development of slogans carrying primary, secondary, and tertiary prevention health messages such as the following:

- Smoking is the gateway to substance use;
- Mental illnesses are treatable like physical illness and not due to jinns and possessions; and
- The mentally ill may be different, and it is a sin to laugh at somebody's disability.

Evaluation of the program is currently in progress.

The impact of the school mental health program on raising awareness about and reducing the stigma attached to mental illness among school children, their parents, friends not attending school, and neighbors was assessed. Significant improvement in awareness and attitudes was seen among school children and those at increasing social distance (i.e., parents, friends not attending school, and neighbors.)

It would be safe to conclude that the establishment of school mental health programs is a cost-effective means of raising mental health awareness and reducing the stigma attached to mental illness.

Source: [240]

To date, evidence for the effectiveness of these school-level interventions has included a reduced requirement for special education classes and fewer occurrences of bullying behavior.[241] Such programs aimed at empowerment and enhanced coping capacity may be expected to have long-term effects on conditions such as depression that often result from an inability to cope with life stresses. Longitudinal research is needed to provide evidence for these effects.

Recommendation 9-3. Intersectoral funding should be provided for population-based strategies aimed at preventing depression and their evaluation. This support should be directed at interventions as the following:

- **School mental health programs;**
- **Public education programs designed to reduce the stigma associated with mental disorders;**
- **Workplace mental health programs; and**
- **Mental health care in prisons.**

Preventing Suicide

As with efforts to prevent depression, interventions to reduce suicide should take place on multiple levels. General approaches must be complemented by specific strategies directed toward high-risk groups (based on such factors as demography, occupation, and health status). A 1996 survey of suicide prevention programs in nine countries [242] revealed several common themes for intervention, including:

- Improving the detection and treatment of depression through better basic training and continuing education of health professionals [243] and through access to crisis intervention.
- Promoting responsible media reporting so that suicide is not glamorized, and the method of suicide is not reported.[244]

Additional key interventions should include:

- Training health care personnel to assess and counsel individuals who have attempted suicide.[245]
- Identifying alcohol abuse as a pathway to suicide.[39,246]
- Reducing access to the means of suicide. For example, restricting packet sizes, retail outlets, and advertising to prevent overdoses of over-the-counter medicines, such as paracetamol; restricting access to guns; and, restricting access to and labeling of pesticides.[54]
- Recognizing that self-destructive and risk-taking behaviors, particularly in young people, often precede formal suicide attempts. The peak incidence of these behaviors occurs between ages 15 and 24, a group for which, in males,

suicide rates have been rising for three decades in developed countries; indeed, there is considerable concern that a similar rise may be under way in developing countries. Suicide rates in young women are already known to be extremely high in Southeast Asia.[39]

• Conducting routine clinical audits of suicides as a way of better understanding their causes and establishing and assimilating the implications for prevention.[247,248]

In addition to the above interventions, effective strategies to prevent suicide must be supported by comprehensive national policy. The United Nations (1996) has identified several key traits of successful national suicide prevention plans. These include government backing, specific aims and goals, measurable objectives, plans for implementation, and mechanisms for monitoring and evaluation. [249]

> **Recommendation 9-4. The consequences of depression have an impact on all levels of society and the economy. Therefore, increased intersectoral funding should be allocated by all relevant ministries (e.g., education, employment, environment, housing, tourism, youth, information, home affairs, criminal justice, and finance, as well as health) for programs aimed at the prevention of depression and suicide, with consideration of the strategies discussed above.**

Treatment

Effective treatment strategies exist for depression in the form of both pharmacotherapies [250] and psychosocial treatments.[251] Though no treatment interventions have proven entirely curative for all forms of depression, a large number of efficacious and low-cost treatments are available.[250–253] Despite the availability of these interventions, however, many individuals in developed countries and an even greater number in developing countries remain underdiagnosed and untreated.[254–259] Particular gaps in treatment remain for children experiencing depression and in the appropriate sequencing of treatment for adults.[260,261]

Medical interventions

Antidepressants. Because of their efficacy and cost-effectiveness, antidepressant medications represent the mainstay of treatment for depression in developed countries. Research indicates that 70 percent of patients prescribed an antidepressant will show a worthwhile clinical improvement in their symptoms.[262,263] Antidepressants have also been found to be effective in prophylaxis; treatment has been shown to reduce the relapse rate for recurrent depression from 80 percent (when untreated) over 3 years to 22 percent.[264] The use of antidepressants in developing countries has not been as widespread, but the limited available evidence shows similar rates of efficacy, through there have been variations in treatment dosage and sequencing.[265,266] Additional research in developing countries will be necessary to determine appropriate treatment guidelines for the use of these medications in different populations.

Two of the three main types of antidepressants—tricyclic antidepressants (TCAs) and monoamine oxidase inhibitors (MAOIs) [267,268]—have been in use for four decades, while selective serotonin re-uptake inhibitors (SSRIs) are more recent. TCAs are broad-spectrum drugs that treat most types of depression effectively.[269,270] Traditional TCAs and the newer SSRIs have similar efficacy for moderate depression.[271] Meta-analysis has shown that traditional TCAs produce clinical improvements more quickly than SSRIs, but the two have similar efficacy at 6 weeks.[272]

Studies to date indicate that SSRIs and TCAs have similar effectiveness. However, the reduced side effects of SSRIs are likely to enhance patient compliance and therefore improve overall treatment outcomes.[266,273,274] Tricyclic anti-depressants are currently the first line of treatment in many developing countries because the higher costs of SSRIs remains prohibitive.[275,276] However, as SSRIs become affordable, they should also be considered first-line treatments in developing countries.

MAOIs are an important option for patients who are refractory to TCA treatment, who have responded to them before, or who have marked anxiety/panic features. They work best in patients with specific symptom combinations, such as anxiety or phobias. Despite the efficacy of MAOIs, their clinical use is limited because of a frequently occurring side effect that induces a rapid rise in blood pressure (associated with certain food intake such as cheese or pickles) and can contribute to long-term hypertensive conditions or acute cardio- and cerbrovascular episodes.[277] The difficulty for many developing countries in monitoring blood pressure [278] would prohibit use of these drugs.

Many low-income countries have insufficient psychotropic medicines available in secondary care, and hardly any such medicines in primary care. It is possible, using basic epidemiological data, to calculate the requirements for essential medicines provided by a primary health care unit (e.g., for a population of 10,000).

Evaluations of cost-effectiveness will depend on the actual costs of specific drugs, which vary among countries and will decrease as newer drugs come off-patent. Requisite long-term follow-up studies (which would include attention not only to recovery from symptoms and disability, but also to reduction of family, social, and economic burden over 5 years) have not been conducted. Such studies are needed before cost-effectiveness can be definitively established.

Future research developments associated with tolerability, drug-to-drug interactions, and levels of efficacy in preventing relapse will continue to increase the desirability of many antidepressants as a first-line treatment for depression.[279,280] Research into these new drug developments may benefit from examining clinical environments in developing countries. Collaborations on such research that will benefit developing country populations should be encouraged by the establishment of national research and training centers in these countries (as recommended in Chapter 4).

> **Recommendation 9-5. An adequate supply of essential medicines (TCAs and low-cost SSRIs), based on epidemiological estimates of need, should be made available to all primary and secondary care facilities. Training of staff will be required to ensure appropriate monitoring for possible side effects of these drugs and to determine when changes in treatment regimens are required.**

Electroconvulsive Therapy. Numerous studies have shown electroconvulsive therapy (ECT) to be an effective treatment for severe depressive illness.[281,282] However, its nature and fears regarding long-term cognitive side effects have significantly curtailed its use, although follow-up studies have failed to show such effects or structural damage to the brain.[281–283]

Patients with severe depression, delusions, agitation, or retardation are particularly likely to improve if treated with ECT. Such symptoms are often found among the elderly, who represent a substantial fraction of the treatment population in developed countries.[284] Modern practice of ECT also poses less risk to pregnant women than the risk associated with some psychotropic drugs used in the treatment of depression. In contrast, ECT is considered a treatment of last resort among children and adolescents.[281,284] The risk of death from ECT is similar to that for general anesthesia for minor surgical procedures—about 2 deaths per 100,000 treatments.[285]

It is important to note that when used appropriately, ECT is an effective treatment for severe and refractory depression. Because ECT works more rapidly than antidepressants (which typically take more than 2 weeks before improvement starts and 6 weeks to achieve full effect), it can be life-saving for those who are suicidal and not responding quickly enough to antidepressants, or those who are mute and refusing to eat and drink.[286] However, caution must be exercised to ensure that the treatment is not misused or overused because of its inexpensive cost relative to antidepressant medication.[287]

Psychosocial interventions

Four main factors support the psychosocial treatment of depression: recognition that the effects of pharmacological treatments can be enhanced when administered with adjunctive psychotherapy; evidence of the effectiveness of psychosocial treatments; increased understanding of the psychosocial causes of depression (e.g., life events and lack of social support); and the increasing role of nonmedical professionals (e.g., psychologists and social workers) in caring for people with depression.

Psychosocial therapy can be an important means of reinforcing the social support networks involved in overall mental health for patients suffering from depression. The use of psychosocial interventions in combination with antidepressant medications targets both the biological and social causes of the disease and provides a comprehensive approach to treatment.[288–290] Patients involved in such therapy can benefit from both the more immediate effects of medication and the longer-term successes that are achieved in psychotherapeutic environments.[290] Furthermore, psychosocial treatments are frequently used with patients who have become depressed as a result of suffering a physical illness, such as coronary artery disease, AIDS, or cancer.[291,292] Psychosocial treatments have been suggested as particularly useful in the case of postpartum depression.[293,294]

Though limited evidence of effectiveness is available on the many varieties of psychosocial interventions used in developed countries, *cognitive behavior therapy*,[295,296] *problem-solving therapy*,[297–299] and *family-focused therapy* [300] have met with proven success in the treatment of depression. A small number of published reports address the use of psychosocial interventions to treat depression in developing countries.

Problem-solving therapy has been suggested as an effective psychosocial treatment, particularly because it seeks to provide the patient with a technique for coping with future problems, thereby potentially preventing a recurrence of depressive symptoms or enabling the patient to dealt with them more effectively when they recur.[298,301] Problem-solving therapy has been conducted effectively by trained community nurses in primary care settings,[297] making the approach particularly attractive for resource-poor settings where psychiatrists and specially trained general physicians are often not regularly available. Additional research should be conducted in developing countries to determine the cost-effectiveness of this strategy in primary health care settings.

Results of an open trial of *cognitive behavior therapy* with 25 depressed patients from Bangalore indicate the feasibility and effectiveness of the treatment.[302] Similarly, a recent randomized controlled trial of cognitive behavior therapy for medically unexplained symptoms in patients attending general medical clinics in Sri Lanka revealed significant improvements in psychiatric morbidity and number of medical consultations.[303] Yet cognitive behavior therapy requires levels of training most likely to appear in secondary levels of care in developing countries (such as district hospitals or more urban centers) and is therefore recommended for use in such settings.[304]

Family-focused therapy for psychoeducation and communication enhancement has proven effective in facilitating greater support for family members with depression. Therapeutic and nonjudgmental environments allow for open discussion about symptoms, treatment, and their side effects, which can create long-term stability, optimize compliance, and allow for early identification and intervention when relapsing episodes occur.[300] Definitive research on family burden exploring attitudes and beliefs about depressive illness would provide valuable guidance for the design of locally appropriate educational interventions designed to decrease the impact of family and other relationship stresses on the patient and to enhance the family's support for the patient.

Current models of psychosocial treatment focus on modifying the effects of social or familial risk factors and may help improve the course of the disorder. Indeed, the psychosocial treatments described above may prove especially advantageous in developing countries because most can be administered by trained, nonspecialist health care personnel and can help empower patients to attain and maintain recovery.

Traditional healers

Traditional healers are common in most low-income countries and, despite the presence of practitioners of modern Western medicine, are routinely consulted in the first instance. In developing countries, consultation of traditional healers is common even among the well educated, and a high proportion of people consult both traditional and modern systems.[305–307]

Traditional and religious healers frequently play a major role in treating mental disorders.[304,308–310] Many healers are familiar with concepts of psychosis, depression, epilepsy, and alcohol abuse; some recognize the value of hospital tests and encourage their clients to use orthodox care.[311] As a result, some health care services in developing countries are attempting to forge collaborations with these kinds of traditional healers to foster more efficacious and culturally sensitive treatments for depression.[312,313]

Cost Analysis

Despite the acknowledged need for economic analysis of mental health care strategies, few such studies have been conducted in either the developed or developing world.[314–320] Where cost-effective models of care exist, it may not always be possible to transfer them directly from developed to developing countries, or from one developing country to another. Nevertheless, strategies for cost-effective mental health care have been adapted by several developing nations, including Brazil, India, Guinea-Bissau, China, Pakistan, and South Africa (See Boxes 3.1–3.3 in Chapter 3).[104,130,321–325]

The refinement of mental health economics and policy analysis in industrialized countries have paved the way for the creation of appropriate frameworks for evaluating health care costs in developing countries.[326–329] In addition, a recently completed demonstration project conducted in India and Pakistan illustrates the feasibility of applying economic analysis to community mental health programs in low-income countries (see Chapter 3 for a description of this analysis).[330]

Encouraging evidence has also emerged to support the cost-effectiveness of depression management through primary care in developed countries.[19,331–333] However, more extensive prospective studies are required to provide definitive evaluation of alternative interventions for depression.[334–336] Cost-effective treatments for depression appear likely to produce measurable benefits, such as reducing disability in the workplace [337] and averting indirect human, social, and family costs.[338,339]

CAPACITY

Because depression is common throughout populations, the existing capacity and location of psychiatric specialists in both developed and developing countries cannot meet the needs of those suffering from mental disorders.[19,34,37] As a result, the integration of mental health with primary care services has become a significant policy objective in both wealthy and low-income areas of the world (see Chapter 3).[340–345] Countries differ in the extent to which they have achieved this objective. Some of the most proactive examples are to be found in low-income countries, where programs have often been assisted by WHO and have followed a public health model modified for the needs of mental health.[301,341–345]

Each country has its own unique health care delivery system, and what makes sense in one country may not in another country. In formulating health care policy, it is important to examine the existing primary and secondary care systems, staffing, basic training and continuing education for each of the professional groups involved, and the system for data collection. The composition of primary care teams will vary from country to country. In low-income countries, the team may contain no doctors and perhaps a few medical assistants, and be staffed largely by nurses and trained health workers. In some countries, health workers with months rather than years of training are on the front line, dealing with screening and case finding, assessment, and maintenance treatments (see Box 9-3).

In Zanzibar, the first tier is the primary health care unit, which usually contains several male and female nurses responsible for a population of 10,000. In Tanzania, the front line is the first-aid volunteer, who attends to the simple health needs of approximately 50 people; the second tier is the dispensary, which is responsible for a population of 2,000; and the third tier is the primary health care unit, which is run by nurses and medical assistants who care for a population of 10,000. In Pakistan, the first tier comprises health workers, usually married women with adult children, who receive brief training; the second tier is the primary care doctor, often responsible for a population of approximately 2,000.

Training

Currently, the limited number of psychiatrists and other mental health professionals dictates in developing countries that their roles be defined as being focused primarily on providing training; designing methodological tools, such as problem detection and treatment guidelines; and confirming initial diagnosis and course of treatment through secondary and tertiary consultation.[96] For these purposes, the curriculum and training of both psychiatrists and general physicians should be adapted to consider not only the clinical presentation of these disorders in tertiary centers, but also the frequently somatized conditions that present in both primary and secondary settings. Diagnostic training should be problem-solving based and rooted in national and community health priorities.[346] Acquiring training skills that are effective in reaching multiple levels of health care personnel will be important for transferring the necessary knowledge base. Specialists and general physicians must be prepared for their critical responsibility in the establishment and continuing oversight of programs in both urban and rural areas and in promoting sound health policy for efforts to address depression and other mental illnesses.[347,348] Where there are few physicians in primary care, nurses can play an effective role in the management of those with mental disorders if given appropriate training.[128,349,350] It is also important to provide mental health education to midwives and traditional birth attendants in low-income countries so they can identify cases of postpartum depression and other psychoses.

When establishing mental health care programs, it is important to assess the basic training needs of each level of personnel for all levels of care in the health care system and the extent to which mental health training is already included. In Iran, health workers receive several months of training in a few priority topics that include depression, and medical students are given extensive training in psychiatric disorders, including depression. In Zanzibar, the College of Health Sciences runs a 4-year basic nurse training course, of which the fourth year for men is psychiatry and the fourth year for women is midwifery. A similar situation exists in Tanzania, so that these countries now have a substantial population of nurses in primary and specialist care who have received at least a year of basic training in psychiatry.

In Asia, there have been evaluative studies of methods of training multipurpose health care workers in the delivery of basic mental health care.[351] In Zanzibar, education coordinators organize and deliver continuing education for primary health care staff. This continuing education takes place during several weekends per year, and the primary care workers receive transport allowances and incentive payments to attend. Unfortunately, continuing education programs in most countries focus largely on physical illness; mental health topics tend to be considered optional or extra, and thus are not an integral component of general training.

Research in the United States has demonstrated the success of primary care programs that train general physicians to diagnose depression at night, more valid rates.[258,352,353] However, this research has also shown that even after proper diagnosis, appropriate drug treatment and referral to psychosocial therapy remain inadequate.[260] Recognizing and addressing similar limitations in developing country primary care settings will be important for both treatment and training models.

Maintaining standards is crucial to providing cost-effective primary health care. In Iran, for example, health psychologists monitor the performance of health workers, visiting every month to provide support and to supervise and check on the quality of the work.[228] In many countries, especially in rural areas with little or no public transport, outreach from primary care to the community and from secondary care to primary care and to the community cannot occur without access to transportation. Program planning must account for the provision of these services to ensure that efforts to provide care reach those in need.

Recommendation 9-6. A feasible and affordable community-based management program to diagnose and treat depressive illness should have five specific aims:

- **Reduce the frequency of depressive episodes.**
- **Reduce the social withdrawal and isolation commonly associated with the disease that leads to high levels of disability and impairment of social functioning.**
- **Reduce the risk of premature mortality due to suicide or physical disease.**
- **Identify those at risk because of familial history or negative life events.**
- **Reduce stigma and protect the patient's human rights.**

Such a program should involve at least three operational components:

- **Pharmacological treatment, with specific guidelines for symptom control in acute episodes, maintenance for stabilization and prevention of relapse, and means of ensuring adherence to the treatment protocol.**
- **Problem-solving psychosocial therapy programs to encourage recovery and assist patients in developing techniques for coping with future events to potentially prevent the severity or occurrence of relapse.**
- **Mobilization of family and community support, including providing education about the nature of the disorder and its treatment, involving the family in simple problem-solving skills training,**

and involving the local community in providing a supportive and nonstigmatizing environment.

Recommendation 9-7. Implementation of comprehensive primary care programs for depression should include the following elements:

- **Basic training (undergraduate and graduate) and continuing education of primary care personnel at all levels (from village-level health workers to primary care physicians);**
- **Organized periodic support and supervision from mental health specialists;**
- **Good-practice guidelines on the distribution of antidepressant medications and psychosocial treatments for depression;**
- **Concise and meaningful materials for increasing awareness and self-management and for monitoring and evaluating outcomes; and**
- **Public education efforts to enhance the impact of these programs.**

Research

Adequate planning is not possible without good systems for routine data collection within the health care system. Prevalence and outcome data may be gathered, as is routinely done in Iran (see Box 9-2). However, existing standard forms for recording consultations in primary care pay inadequate attention to mental disorders. For example, committee members have noted that the primary care diagnostic form in use in several East African countries includes 34 categories for separate physical illnesses, but only a single category for "mental disorder." Diagnostic recording forms that are appropriately modified to identify separately each of the main mental disorders, including depression, would greatly improve local capacity to determine and evaluate mental health needs.

Research capacity for mental health services and training is essential to appropriate evaluation and implementation strategies. Local health researchers should be empowered to conduct and lead research programs, including the development of methods for screening and outcome measurement. The establishment of national centers for research and training and of standard protocols would facilitate these developments (see Chapter 4 for a description of these centers).

Recommendation 9-8. To better inform ongoing and future programs in developing countries aimed at reducing the burden of depression, research is needed on the following topics, with responsibility at the indicated levels:

Local

- Locally appropriate practice guidelines for prevention and treatment in primary care;
- Aspects of disability and burden of depression in different population groups to determine priority strategies for local and national programs;
- Development and evaluation of communication strategies for education at the national and local levels, including public awareness programs to reduce stigma; and
- Cost-effectiveness evaluations of local prevention and treatment programs.

National

- Aspects of disability and burden of depression in different population groups to determine priority strategies for local and national programs;
- Impact of the social determinants for depression (e.g., poverty, illiteracy, violence at home, unemployment);
- Evaluation of preventive interventions based on knowledge of risk factors (including the establishment of long-term cohorts);
- Evaluation of programs for chronic disease management (including depression) in primary care;
- Evaluation of programs for continuing education for primary health care personnel;
- Development and evaluation of communication strategies for mental health education at the national and local levels, including public awareness programs to reduce stigma; and
- Methods for disseminating model programs to create successful intervention policies at the national level.

Collaborative

- Genetic etiology of depression, to include gene–environment interactions; and
- Treatment outcome and dosage studies for TCAs and SSRIs to determine population-specific needs.

Recommendation 9-9. To assist in the widespread implementation of improved prevention and care for people with depression, a series of demonstration projects should be undertaken in low-income countries. These projects should incorporate the following:

- Practice guidelines for prevention and treatment in primary care;
- Scientific evaluation of outcomes and cost-effectiveness; and

- **Capacity to support dissemination and generalization within countries.**

Support for these projects should be provided by a wide range of international and local organizations, including the World Health Organization Nations for Mental Health Initiative; the World Bank; the U.S. National Institute of Mental Health; government development agencies; national ministries of health, education, welfare, and finance; and international and local professional and patient advocacy organizations.

REFERENCES

1. N. Husain, F. Creed, and B. Tomenson. Depression and social stress in Pakistan. *Psychological Medicine* Mar;30(2):395–402, 2000.
2. K.S. Kendler, M.D. Karkowski, and C.A. Prescott. Causal Relationship Between Stressful Life Events and the Onset of Major Depression. *American Journal of Psychiatry* Jun;156:6:837–841, 1999.
3. A. Bertelsen, B. Harvald, and M. Gauge. A Danish Twin Study of manic depressive disorders. *British Journal of Psychiatry* 130:330–351, 1997
4. J. Heinik, P. Werner, A. Mendel, B. Raikher, and A. Bleich. The Cambridge Cognitive Examination (CAMCOG): Validation of the Hebrew version in elderly demented patients. *International Journal of Geriatrics Psychiatry* Dec;14(120:1006–1013, 1999.
5. A.K. Lehman, B. Ellis, J. Becker, I. Rosenfarb, R. Devine, A. Khan, et al. Personality and depression: A validation study of the depressive experiences questionnaire. *Journal of Personality Assessment* Feb;68(1):197–210, 1997.
6. V. Patel, J. Pereira, L. Coutinho, and R. Fernandes. Is labeling of common mental disorders as psychiatric illness useful in primary care? *Indian Journal of Psychology* 39:239–246, 1997.
7. American Psychiatric Association. *Diagnostic and statistical manual of mental disorders* (DSM-IV), APA, Washington, D.C.,1994.
8. World Health Organization. *The ICD-10 Classification of mental and behavioural disorders: diagnostic criteria for research.* Geneva: WHO, 1993.
9. A. Sarin. Depression. *The National Medical Journal of India* 10(2):77–79, 1997.
10. T. Sivik, N. Delimar, and R. Schoenfeld. Construct validity of the Sivik Psychosomaticism Test and test of operational style: Correlations with four Minnesota Multiphasic Personality Inventory (MMPI) subscales. *Intergration of Physiology and Behaviorial Science* Apr–Jun;34(2):79–84, 1999.
11. V. Patel and C. H. Todd. The validity of the Shona version of the Self Report Questionnaire (SRQ) and the development of the SRQ8. *International Journal Methods of Psychiatric Research* 6:153–160, 1996.
12. V. Patel. The epidemiology of mental disorders in South Asia. *National Institute of Mental Health and Neurological Sciences Journal* (in press), 2000.
13. M. Nichter. Idioms of distress: Alternatives in the expresion of psychosocial distress: A case study from South India. *Culture, Medicine and Psychiatry* Dec;5(4):379–408, 1981.

14. C.W. Aakster. Concepts in alternative medicine. *Social Science and Medicine* 22(2):265–273, 1986.

15. L. Keh-Ming. Traditional Chinese Medical Beliefs and Their Relevance for Mental Illness and Psychiatry. In: *Normal and abnormal behavior in Chinese Culture,* Kleinman, A. and Lin, T.Y., eds. Reidal: Dordrecht, pp.95–111, 1981.

16. T.A. Lambo. The village of Aro. *Lancet* 2:513–514, 1964.

17. J.D.A. Makanjuola and E.A. Olaifa. Masked depression in Nigerians treated at Neuro-Psychiatric Hospital Aro, Abeokuta. *Acta Psychiatrica Scandinavica* 76:480–485, 1987.

18. M. M. Weissman, R.C. Bland, G.J. Canino, C. Faravelli, S. Greenwald, H.G. Hwu, et al. Cross-National Epidemiology of Major Depression and Bipolar Disorder. *Journal of the American Medical Association* Jul;24–31:276(4):293–299, 1996.

19. D. Goldberg and R. Gater. Implications of the World Health Organization study of mental illness in general health care for training primary care staff. *British Journal of General Psychiatry* Aug;46(409):483–485, 1996.

20. G.E. Simon, M. VonKorff, M. Piccinelli, C. Fullerton, and J. Ormel. An international study of the relation between somatic symptoms and depression. *New England Journal of Medicine* 341(18):1329–1334, 1999.

21. A. Bhatt, B. Tomenson, and S. Benjamin. Transcultural patterns of somatization I primary care: A preliminary report. *Journal of Psychosomatic Research* 33:671–680, 1989.

22. W. Katon and E. Walker. Medically Unexplained Symptoms in Primary Care. *Journal of Clinical Psychology* 59 (supplement 20)15–21, 1998.

23. V. Patel, F. Gwanzura, E. Simunyu, K. Lloyd, and A. Mann. The phenomenology and explanatory models of common mental disorder: A study in primary care in Harare, Zimbabwe. *Psychological Medicine* Nov 25(6):1191–1199, 1995.

24. O. Gureje, G. E. Simon, T. B. Ustun, and D. P. Goldberg. Somatization in cross-cultural perspective: A World Health Organization study in primary care. *American Journal of Psychiatry* Jul;154(7):989–995, 1997.

25. J.M. Simon. Chronic pain syndrome: Nursing assessment and intervention. *Rehabilitative Nursing* Jan–Feb;21(1):13–9, 1996.

26. V. Patel, J. Perieira, L. Coutinho, R. Fernandez, J. Fernandez, and A. Mann. Psychological disorder and disability in primary care attenders in Goa, India. *British Journal of Psychiatry* 171:533–536, 1998.

27. R. Araya, W. Robert, L.Richard, and G. Lewis. Psychiatric morbidity in primary health care in Santiago, Chile. Preliminary findings. *British Journal of Psychiatry* 165:530–532. 1994.

28. L.L. Judd, H.S. Akiskal, P.J. Zeller, M. Paulas, A.C. Leon, J.D. Masar, et al. Psychosocial disability during the long-term course of unipolar major depressive disorder. *Archives of General Psychiatry* Apr;57(4):375–380, 2000.

29. C.D. Mathers, E.T. Vos, C. E. Stevenson, and S. J. Begg. The Australian Burden of Disease Study: Measuring the loss of health from diseases, injuries, and risk factors. *Medical Journal of Australia* Jun 19;172(12):592–596, 2000.

30. P.L. Reddy, S. Khanna, M. N. Subhash, S.M. Channabasavanna, and B.S. Rao. CSF amine metabolites in depression. *Biology and Psychiatry* Jan 15;31(2):112–118, 1992.

31. C. Murray and A. Lopez, eds. *The Global Burden of Disease.* The Harvard Press: Boston, 1996.

32. T.B. Ustun and N. Sartorius. *Mental illness in general health care—An international study*. John Wiley & Sons: Chichester, 1995.
33. J. Ormel, M. Von Korff, A.J. Oldenhinkel, G. Simon, B.G. Tiemens, and T.B. Usten. Onset of disability in depressed and non-depressed primary care patients. *Psychological Medicine* July 29(4):847–853, 1999.
34. M. Von Korff, T.B. Usten, J. Ormel, I. Kaplan, G.E. Simon. Self-report disability in an international primary care study of psychological illness. *Journal of Clinical Epidemiology* Mar;49(3):297–303, 1996.
35. M.B. Rahman and S.K. Indran. Disability in schizophrenia and mood disorders in a developing country. *Social Psychiatry and Psychiatric Epidemiology* Oct;32(7):387–390, 1997.
36. J.L. Coulehan, H.C. Schulberg, M.R. Block, J.E. Janosky, and V.C. Arena. Medical comorbidity of major depressive disorder in a primary medical practice. *Archives of Internal Medicine* Nov;150(11):2363–2367, 1990.
37. M. Linden. Theory and practice in the management of depressive disorders. *International. Clinic of Psychopharmacology* Jun 14(3):S15–S25, 1999.
38. A.S. Brown, B.K. Varma, S. Malhotra, R.C. Jiloha, S.A. Conover, and E.S. Susser. Course of acute affective disorders in a developing country setting. *Journal of Nervous and Mental Disease* 186(4);207–213, 1998.
39. R.N. Kearney and B.D. Miller. The spiral of suicide and social change in Sri Lanka. *Journal of Asian Studies* 45:81–101, 1985.
40. J. Jianlin. Suicide rates and mental health services in modern China. *Crisis* 21(3):118–121, 2000.
41. G.E. Murphy and R.D. Wetzel. The lifetime risk of suicide in alcoholism. *Archives of General Psychiatry* Apr 47:383–392, 1990.
42. M.M. Henriksson, H.M. Aro, M.J. Marttunen, M.E. Heikkinen, Isometsä, K.I. Kuoppasalmi, et al. Mental disorders and comorbidity in suicide. *American Journal of Psychiatry* 150:935–940, 1993.
43. P.M. Marzuk, K. Tardiff, A.C. Leon, M. Stajic, E.B. Morgan, and J.J. Mann. Prevalence of cocaine use among residents of New York City who committed suicide during a one-year period. *American Journal of Psychiatry* 149(3):371–375, 1992.
44. E. C. Harris and B. Barraclough. Excess mortality of mental disorder. *British Journal of Psychiatry* Jul;173:11–53, 1998.
45. D.B. Mumford, K. Saeed, I. Ahmad, S. Satif, and M.H. Mubbashar. Stress and psychiatric disorder - in rural Punjab. *British Journal of Psychiatry* 170:473–478, 1997.
46. R.C. Kessler. The effects of stressful life events on depression. *Annual Review of Psychology* 48;191–214, 1997.
47. D.B. Mumford, M. Nazir, F.U.M. Jilani, and I.Y. Bang. Stress and Psychiatric Disorder in the Hindu Kush: A Community Survey of Mountain Villages in Chitral, Pakistan. *British Journal of Psychiatry* 168:299–307, 1996.
48. H. Meltzer, B. Gill, M. Petticrew, and K. Hinds. Economic activity and social functioning of adults with psychiatric disorders, *OPCS Surveys of Psychiatric Morbidity in Great Britain* Report 3. HMSO: London, 1995.
49. E. Durkheim. *Suicide*. Routledge and Kegan Paul: London, 1952.
50. C.H. Cantor and P.J.M. Baume. Access to methods of suicide—What impact? *Australian and New Zealand Journal of Psychiatry* 32:8–14, 1998.

51. W. Van der Hoek, F. Konradsen, K. Athukorala, and T. Wanigadewa. Pesticide poisioning: A major health problem in Sri Lanka. *Social Science and Medicine* Feb-Mar;46(4–5):495–504, 1998.

52. J.R. Bowles. Suicide and attempted suicide in contemporary Western Samoa. In: *Culture, Youth and Suicide in the Pacific: Papers from an East-West Centre Conference,* Hezel, F.X., Rubinstein, D.H., and White, G.H., eds. East -West Centre: Honolulu, pp. 15–35, 1985.

53. G.P. Kilonzo. *Development of mental health services in Tanzania. Working Paper,* International Mental Health Project. Centre for the Study of Culture and Medicine, Harvard Medical School: Boston, 1993.

54. D. Gunnell, K. Hawton, V. Murray, R. Garner, C. Bismuth, J. Fagg, et al. Use of paracetamol for suicide and nonfatal poisoning in the U.K. and France: Are restrictions on availability justified? *Journal of Epidemiology and Community Health 51(2),* 175–179, 1997.

55. P.S. Yip and R.C. Tan. Suicides in Hong-Kong and Singapore: A tale of two cities. *International Journal of Social Psychiatry* Winter;44(4):267–279, 1998.

56. K.B. Wells, A. Stewart, R.D. Hays, M.A. Burnam, W. Rogers, M. Daniels, et al. The functioning and well-being of depressed patients. Results from the Medical Outcomes Study. *Journal of the American Medical Association* Aug 18;262(7):914–919, 1989.

57. G.E. Vaillant, J. Orav, S.E. Meyer, L. McCullough Vaillant, and D. Roston. 1995 IPA/Bayer Research Awards in Psychogeriatrics. Late-life consequences of affective spectrum disorder. *International Psychogeriatrics* Spring;8(1):13–32, 1996.

58. S. A. Everson, D E. Goldburg, G. A. Kaplan, R. D. Cohen, E. Pukkala, J. Tuomeilehto, et al. Hopelessness and risk of mortality and incidence of myocardial infarction and cancer. *Psychosomatic Medicine* Mar–Apr. 58(2):113–121, 1996.

59. D.E. Ford, L.A. Mead, P.P. Chang, L. Cooper-Patrick, N.Y. Wang, and M.J. Klag. Depression is a risk factor for coronary artery disease in men: The precursors study. *Archives of Internal Medicine* Jul 13;158(13):1422–1426, 1998.

60. R.Schulz, R. Scott, D. Ives, L. Martire, A. Abraham, and W. Kop. Association Between Depression and Mortality in Older Adults: The Cardiovascular Health Study. *Archives of Internal Medicine* Jun 26; 160:1761–1768, 2000.

61. B.S. Jonas and M.E. Mussolino. Symptoms of depression as a prospective risk factor for stroke. *Psychosomatic Medicine* Jul–Aug;62(4):463–471, 2000.

62. J.C. Barefoot and M. Schroll. Symptoms of depression, acute myocardial infarction and total mortality in a community sample. *Circulation* June1;93(11);1976–1980, 1996.

63. P. Langhorne, D.J. Stott, L. Robertson, J. MacDonald, L Jones, C. McAlpine et al. Medical complications after stroke: A multicenter study. *Stroke* Jun;31(6):1223–1229, 2000.

64. R. Ramasubbu. Relationship between depression and cerebrovascular disease: Conceptual issues. *Journal of Affective Disorders* Jan–Mar;57(1–3):1–11, 2000.

65. R.M. Post. Stroke depression impedes recovery. *Health News* Sep;6(9):7, 2000.

66. R. Rao. Cerebrovascular disease and late life depression: An age old association revisited. *International Journal of Geriatrics Psychiatry* May;15(5):419–433, 2000.

67. J.H. Thakore, P.J. Richards, R.H. Reznek, A. Martin, and T.G. Dinan. Increased intraabdominal fat deposition in patients with major depressive illness as measured by computed tomography. *Biology and Psychiatry* June 1;41(11):1140–1142, 1997.

68. R.B. Majess, H. Barden, M. Ettinger, and F. Schultz. Bone density of the radius, spine and proximal femur in osteoporosis. *Journal of Bone and Mineral Research* 3: 13–18,1988.
69. W. Mayo-Smith, C.W. Hayes, B.M. Biller, A. Klibanski, H. Rosenthal, and D.I. Rosenthal. Body fat distribution measured with CT: Correlations in healthy subjects, patients with anorexia nervosa, and patients with Cushing's syndrome. *Radiology* Feb;170(2):515–518, 1989.
70. D. Michelson, C. Stratakis, L. Hill, J. Reynolds, E. Galliven, G. Chrousos, and P. Gold. Bone mineral density in women with depression. *New England Journal of Medicine* Oct 17;335(16): 1176–1181, 1996.
71. M.J. Schweiger, R.P. McMahon, M.L. Terrin, N.A. Ruocco, M.N. Porway, A.H. Wiseman et al. Comparison of patients with <60% to > or = 60% diameter narrowing of the myocardial infarct-related artery after thrombolysis. The TIMI Investigators. *American Journal of Cardiology* July 15;74(2) 105–110, 1994
72. R.C. Kessler, C.B. Nelson, K.A. McGonagle, J.Liu, M. Swartz, and D.G. Blazer. Comorbidity of DSM-III-R major depressive disorder in the general population: Results from the U.S. National Comorbidity Survey. *British Journal Psychiatry* 30:17–30, 1996.
73. R. Jenkins, G. Lewis, P. Bebbington, T. Brugha, M. Farrell, B. Gill, et al. The National Psychiatric Morbidity surveys of Great Britian—Initial findings from the household survey. *Psychological Medicine* Jul;27(4):775–789, 1997.
74. G. Masi, L. Favilla, and M. Mucci. Depressive disorder in children and adolescents. *European Journal of Paediatrics and Neurology* 2(6):287–295,1998.
75. E.J. Costello, A. Erkanli, E. Federman, and A. Angold. Development of psychiatric comorbidity with substance abuse in adolescents: Effects of timing and sex. *Journal of Clinical Child Psychology* 28:298–311, 1999.
76. M. Jacob, E. Frank, D.J. Kupfer, and L.L. Carpenter. Recurrent depression: An assessment of family burden and family attitudes. *Journal of Clinical Psychiatry* Oct;48(10):395–400, 1987.
77. S. Chakrabarti, P. Kulhara, and S.K. Verma. The pattern of burden in families of neurotic patients. *Social Psychiatry and Psychiatric Epidemiology* Aug;28(4):172–177, 1993.
78. J.A. Cook, H.P. Lefley, S.A. Pickett, and B.J. Cohler. Age and family burden among parents of offspring with severe mental illness. *American Journal of Orthopsychiatry* Jul;64(3):435–447, 1994.
79. M. Sobieraj, J. Williams, J. Marley, and P. Ryan. The impact of depression on the physical health of family members. *British Journal of General Practice* Oct;48(435):1653–1655, 1998.
80. S. Chakrabarti, P. Kulhara, and S.K. Verma. Extent and determinants of burden among families of patients with affective disorders. *Acta Psychiatrica Scandinavica* Sep;86(3):247–252, 1992.
81. J.C. Phelan, E.J. Bromet, and B.G. Link. Psychiatric illness and family stigma. *Schizophrenia Bulletin* 24(1):115-126, 1998.
82. R.A. Williams and P.B. Strasser. Depression in the workplace. Impact on employees. *American Association of Occupational Health Nurses Journal* Nov;47(11):526-537;quiz 538–539, 1999.

83. B.G. Druss, R.A. Rosenheck, and W.H. Sledge. Health and disability costs of depressive illness in a major U.S. corporation. *American Journal of Psychiatry* Aug;157(8):1274–1278, 2000.

84. J.G. Barbee. Mixed symptoms and syndromes of anxiety and depression: Diagnostic, prognostic and aetiological issues. *Annals of Clinical Psychiatry* 10:15–29, 1998.

85. D.A. Regier, D.S. Rae, W.E. Narrow, C.T. Kaelber, and A.F. Schatzberg. Prevalence of anxiety disorders and their comorbidity with mood addictive disorders. *British Journal of Psychiatry* Supplement34:24–28, 1998.

86. V. Patel. Defeating depression in Zimbabwe. *British Journal of Psychiatry* Aug;165(2):270–271, 1994.

87. D. Goldberg and Y. Lecrubier. Form and Frequency of Mental Disorders across cultures. In: *Mental illness in General Health Care: an international study.* Ustun, T.B. and Sartorius, N., eds. John Wiley & Sons: Chichester, pp.323–334, 1995.

88. B. Sen and P. Williams. The extent and nature of depressive phenomena in primary health care: A study in Calcutta, India. *British Journal of Psychiatry* 151:486–493, 1987.

89. K. Jacob, B. S. Everitt, V. Patel, S. Weich, R. Araya, and G. Lewis. A comparision of latent variable models of nonpsychotic psychiatric morbidity in four culturally different populations. *Psychological Medicine* 28:145–152, 1998.

90. G. Shah and R. Sharma. The validity of clinical differentiation between anxiety and depressive neuroses by factor analysis. *Indian Journal of Psychology* 28:205–210, 1986.

91. M. B. Stein, P. Kirk, V. Prabhu, M. Grott, and M. Terepa. Mixed anxiety-depression in a primary care clinic. *Journal of Affective Disorders* May 17;34(2):79–84, 1995.

92. Z. Stein, M. Durkin, L. Davidson et al. Guidelines for identifying children with mental retardation in community settings. In: *World Health Organization. Assessment of people with mental retardation.* World Health Organization: Geneva, 1992.

93. W. Acuda and H.G. Egdell. Anxiety and depression, and the general doctor. *Tropical Doctor* Apr;14(2):51–55, 1984.

94. T.B. Ustun, D. Goldberg, J. Cooper, G.E. Simon, and N. Sartorius. New classification of mental disorders with management guidelines of use in primary care: ICD-10PHC chapter five. *British Journal of General Practice* (393):211–215, 1995.

95. WHO (World Health Organization). The World Health Report 1995: Bridging the Gaps. World Health Organization: Geneva, 1995.

96. N. Sartorius, T.B. Ustun, J.A. Costa de Silva, D. Goldberg, Y. Lecrubier, J. Ormel, et al. An international study of psychological problems in primary care. Preliminary report from the World Health Organization Collaborative Project on Psychological Problems in General Health Care. *Archives of General Psychiatry* Oct;50(10):819–824, 1993.

97. J. Ormel, M. Von Korff, T.B. Ustun, S. Pini, A. Korten, and T. Oldeninkel. Common mental disorders and disability across cultures. *Journal of the American Medical Association* 272:1741–1748, 1994.

98. M. Von Korff and G. Simon. The relationship between pain and depression. *British Journal of Psychiatry* June (30)101–108, 1996.

99. M. Hollifield, W. Katon, D. Spain, and L. Pule. Anxiety and depression in a village in Lesotho, Africa: A comparison with the United States. *British Journal of Psychiatry* 156:343–350, 1990.

100. R.H. Rumble and K. Morgan. Longitudinal trends in prescribing for elderly patients: two surveys four years apart. *British Journal of General Practice* Dec. 44(389):571–575, 1994.
101. J. Orley and J.K. Wing. Psychiatric disorders in two African villages. *Archives of General Psychiatry* May 36(5):513–520, 1979.
102. H.G. Hwu, E.K. Yeh, and L.Y. Chang. Prevalence of psychiatric disorders in Taiwan defined by the Chinese Diagnostic Interview Schedule. *Acta Psychiatrica Scandinavica* 79:136–147, 1989.
103. D.N. Nandi, S.P. Mukherjee, G.C. Boral, G. Banerjee, A. Ghosh, S. Sarkar, and S. Ajmany. Socio-economic status and mental morbidity in certain tribes and castes in India—A cross cultural study. *British Journal of Psychiatry* Jan 136:73–85, 1980.
104. B.B. Sethi, S.C. Gupta, R.K. Mehendru, and P. Kumari. Mental health and urban life: A study of 850 families. *British Journal of Psychiatry* Mar;124:243–246, 1974.
105. J. Cooper and N. Sartorius, eds. *Mental Disorders in China, Results of the National Epidemiological Survey in 12 Areas* Gaskell Royal College of Psychiatrists: London, 1996.
106. F. Allmeido-Filho, J. de J. Mari, e. Coutinho, J. F. Fanca, J. Fernandes, S.B. Andreoli, and E.D. Busnello. Brazilian multicentric study of psychiatric morbidity. Methodological features and prevalence estimates. *British Journal of Psychiatry* 171:524–529, 1997.
107. M.T. Abou-Saleh and R. Ghubash. The prevalence of early postpartum psychiatric morbidity in Dubai: A transcultural perspective. *Acta Psychiatrica Scandinavica* May;95(5):428–432, 1997.
108. S. Henderson, P. Duncan-Jones, D.G. Byrne, S. Adcock, and R. Scott. Neurosis and social bonds in an urban population. *Australian New Zealand Journal of Psychiatry* Jun 13;(2):121–125, 1979.,
109. P.E. Bebbington, J. Hurry, C. Tennant, E. Sturt, and J. Wing. The epidemiology of mental disorders in Camberwell. *Psychological Medicine* 11:561–580, 1981.
110. P. Hodimont, N. Peer, and N. Syben. Epidemiological aspects of psychiatric disorders in a Dutch health area. *Psychology and Medicine* May 17(2):495–505, 1987.
111. V. Lehtinen M. Joukamaa K. Lahtela, R. Rouitasalo, E. Jyrkinen, J. Maatela, and A. Aromaa. Prevalence of mental disorders among adults in Finland: Basic results from Mini-Finland Health Survey. *Acta Psychiatrica Scandinavica* May 81(5):418–425, 1990.
112. V.G. Mavreas and P.E. Beggington. Psychiatric Morbidity in London's Greek Cypriot community I. Association with sociodemographic variables. *Social Psychiatry* 22, 150–159, 1987.
113. M.G. Carta, B. Carpinello, P.L. Morosini, and N. Rudas. Prevalence of mental disorders in Sardinia: A community study in an inland mining district. *Psychology and Medicine* Nov 21(4):1061–1071, 1991.
114. R.C. Kessler, K.A. McGonagle, S. Zhao, C.B. Nelson, M. Hughes, S. Eshleman, et al. Lifetime and twelve month prevalence of DSM-II-R psychiatric disorders in the US: results from the National Comorbidity Study. *Archives of General Psychiatry* 51:8–19, 1994.
115. R. Giel and J.N. Van Luijk. Psychiatric Morbidity in a Small Ethiopian Town. *British Journal of Psychiatry* 115:149–162, 1969.

116. L.S. Gillis, J.B. Lewis, and M. Slabbert. Psychiatric disorder amongst the Coloured people of the Cape Peninsula. An epidemiologic study. *British Journal of Psychiatry*. Dec;114(517):1575–1587, 1968.

117. F. Kortman. Psychiatric case findings in Ethiopia: Shortcomings of the Self Reporting Questionnaire. *Culture, Medicine, and Psychiatry* 14, 381–391, 1990.

118. S.I. Rahim and M. Cederblad. Epidemiology of mental disorders in young adults of a newly urbanized area in Khartoum, Sudan. *British Journal of Psychiatry* Jul:155;44–47, 1989.

119. S. Tarafi, F.E. Abound, and C.P Larson. Determinants of mental illness in a rural Ethiopian adult population. *Social Science and Medicine* 32(2):197–201, 1991.

120. O. Ben Aire, L. Swartz, A.F. Teggin, and R. Elk. The colored elderly Cape Town— A psycosocial, psychiatric and medical community survey: Part II Prevalence of psychiatric disorders. *South African Medical Journal* Dec 24;64(27):1056–1061, 1983.

121. F.C. Bester, D.J. Weich, H.C. Barnard, and W.J. Vermaak. Biochemical reference Values in elderly black subjects. *South African Medical Journal* Apr 20;79(8):490–495, 1991.

122. L.S. Gillis, M. Welman, A. Koch, and M. Joyi. Psychological distress and depression in urbanizing elderly black persons. *South African Medical Journal* Apr 20;79(8):490–495, 1991.

123. D. Nandi, G. Banerjee, A. Chowdhury, T. Banarjee, G. Boral, and S Biswajit. Urbanization and mental morbidity in certain tribal communities in West Bengal. *Indian Journal of Psychiatry* 34:334–339, 1992.

124. D.B. Mumford, J.T. Bavington, K.S. Bhatnagar, Y. Hussain, S. Mirza, and M.M. Naraghi. The Bradford Somatic Inventory: A multiethnic inventory of somatic symptoms reported by anxious and depressed patients in Britain and the Indo-Pakistan subcontinent. *British Journal of Psychiatry* 158:379–386, 1991.

125. D.N. Nandi, G. Banerjee, S.P. Mukherjee, A. Ghosh, P.S. Nandi, and S. Nandi. Psychiatric morbidity of a rural Indian community. Changes over a 20-year interval. *British Journal of Psychiatry* 176:351–356, 2000.

126. A.B. Ludermir. Socioeconomic status, employment, migration and common mental disorders in Olinda, NE Brazil. Ph.D. dissertation, London School of Hygiene and Tropical Medicine, 1998.

127. M.S. Lima, J.U. Beria, E. Tomasi, A.T. Coneicao, and J.J. Mari. Stressful life events and minor psychiatric disorders: An estimate of the population attributable fraction in a Brazilian community-based study. *International Journal of Psychiatry in Medicine* 26;213–224, 1996.

128. R. Jenkins. Linking epidemiology and disability measurement with mental health service policy and planning. *Epidemiology and Psychiatry and Sociology* 7(2):120–126, May –Aug 1998.

129. A. Aderibigbe and O. Gureje. The validity of the 28-item General Health Questionnaire in a Nigerian antenatal clinic. *Social Psychiatry and Psychiatric Epidemiology.* Nov27(6):280–283, 1992.

130. J.V.T.M. De Jong. A comprehensive public mental health programme in Guinea-Bissau: A useful model for African, Asian and Latin American countries. *Psychological Medicine* 26:97–108,1986.

131. M. Dhadphale, R.H. Ellison, and L. Griffin. Frequency of mental disorders among outpatients at a rural district hospital in Kenya. *Central African Journal of Medicine* Apr. 28(4):85–89, 1982.
132. M. Dhadphale, R.H. Ellison, and L. Griffin. The frequency of psychiatric disorders among patients attending semi-urban and rural general out-patient clinics in Kenya. *British Journal of Psychiatry* 142:379–383, 1983.
133. B. Diop, R. Collingnon, M. Gueye, and T.W. Harding. Diagnosis and symptoms of mental disorder in a rural area of Senegal. *African Journal of Medicine and Science* Sep; 11(3):95–103, 1982.
134. M. Freeman. Psychiatry for a new South Africa. *South African Medical Journal* Aug 3; 80(3):124–126, 1991.
135. A. Hall and H. Williams. Hidden Psychiatric Morbidity: I. A study of prevalence in an out-patient population in Bindura Provincial Hospital. *Central African Journal of Medicine* 33:239–242, 1987.
136. T.W. Harding, M.V. DeArango, J. Baltazar, C.E. Climent, H.H.A. Ibrahim, L. Ladrgolgnacio, et al. Mental disorders in primary health care: A study of their frequency and diagnosis in four developing countries. *Psychological Medicine* 10:231–241, 1980.
137. N.S. Miller and R.M. Swift. Primary Care Medicine and Psychiatry: Addictions treatment. *Psychiatry Annals* 27(6):408–416, 1997.
138. R.G. Thom, R.M. Zwi, and S.G. Reinach. The prevalence of psychiatric disorders at a primary care clinic in Soweto, Johannesburg. *South African Medical Journal* Sep;83(9):653–655, 1993.
139. A. Nikapota, V. Patrick, and L. Fernandes. Aspects of psychiatric morbidity in the out-patient population of a general hospital in Sri Lanka. *Indian Journal of Psychiatry* 23:219–223, 1981.
140. S.K. Murthy, C. Shamasundar, O. Prakash, and N. Prabhakar. Psychiatric morbidity in general practice—A preliminary report. *Indian Journal of Psychiatry* 23:40–43, 1981.
141. V. Bagadia, K. Ayyar, P. Lakdawala, U. Susainathan, and P. Pradhan. Value of the general health questionnaire in detecting psychiatric morbidity in a general hospital out-patient population. *Indian Journal of Psychiatry* 27:293–296, 1985.
142. C. Shamasundar, S.K. Murthy, O. Prakash, N. Prabhakar, and D.K. Subbakrishna. Psychiatric morbidity in general practice in an Indian city. *British Medical Journal* 292:1713–1714, 1986.
143. S.M. Channabasavanna, T. Sriram, and K. Kumar. Results from the Bangalore Centre. In: *Mental Illness in General Health Care: An international study,* Ustun, T.B., Sartorius, N., eds. John Wiley & Sons: Chichester, pp.79–97, 1995.
144. J. Kishore, V. Reddaiah, V. Kapoor, and J. Gill. Characteristics of mental morbidity in a rural primary health centre of Haryana. *Indian Journal of Psychiatry* 38:137–142, 1996.
145. G. Amin, S. Shah, and G.K. Vankar. The prevalence and recognition of depression in primary care. *Indian Journal of Psychiatry* 40:364–369, 1998.
146. E.S. Paykel. Contribution of life events to causation of psychiatric illness. *Psychological Medicine* 8, 245–253, 1978.
147. G.W. Brown, T.O. Harris, and M.J. Eales. Etiology of anxiety and depressive disorders in an inner city population. *Psychological Medicine* 23, 155–165, 1993.

148. T.A. Brown, D.H. Barlow, and M.R. Liebowitz. The empirical basis of generalized anxiety disorder. *American Journal of Psychiatry* 151:1272–1280, 1994.

149. A.T. Beck. Depression: Clinical, experimental, and theoretical aspects. Harper and Row: New York, 1967.

150. R. Hirschfeld and T. Shea. *Personality*. In: *Handbook of affective disorders,* Paykel, E., ed. Guilford Press: New York, 185–194, 1992.

151. J.G. Tubman and M. Windle. Continuity of difficult temperament in adolescence: Relations with depression, life events, family support, and substance use across a one-year period. *Journal of Youth Adolescence* 24:133–153, 1995.

152. D.M. Fergusson and L.J. Horwood. Vulnerability to life event exposure. *Psychology Medicine* 17:739–749, 1987.

153. V. Patel, R. Araya, M. S. Lima, A. Ludermir, and C. Todd. Women, Poverty and Common Mental Disorders in four restructuring societies. *Social Science and Medicine* 49(11) 1461–1471, 1999.

154. E. Behar, A.S. Henderson, and A.J. Mackinnon. An epidemiological study of mental health and socioeconomic conditions in Sumatera, Indonesia. *Acta Psychiatrica Scandinavica* 85:257–263, 1992.

155. P. McGuffin, R. Katz, and S. Watkins. A hospital based twin register of the heritability of DSM-IV unipolar depression. *Archives of General Psychiatry* 53: 129–136, 1996.

156. K.S. Kendler, A.M. Gruenberg, and D.K. Kinney. Independent diagnosis of adoptees and relatives as defined by DSM-III in the provincial and national samples of the Danish Adoption Study of Schizophrenia. *Archives of General Psychiatry* 51:456–468, 1994.

157. National Institute of Mental Health. Genetics of mental disorders: Report of the National Institute of Mental Health's Genetics Work-Group. National Institute of Mental Health: Rockville, 1998.

158. I.V. Warner, M. Weissman, L. Mufson, and P. Wickramaratne. Grandparents, Parents, and Grandchildren at High Risk for Depression: A Three-Generation Study. *Journal of American Academy of Child Adolescent Psychiatry* Mar;38(3): 289–296, 1999.

159. S.B. Roberts, C.J. MacLean, M.C. Neale, L.J. Eaves, and K.S. Kendler. Replication of Linkage Studies of Complex Traits: An Examination of Variation in Location Estimates. *American Journal of Human Genetics* 65:876–884, 1999.

160. S. Hyman. The genetics of mental illness: Implications for practice. *Bulletin of the World Health Organization* 78(4):455–463, 2000.

161. K.S. Kendler, C.O. Gardner, and C.A. Prescott. Clinical Characteristics of Major Depression That Predict Risk of Depression in Relatives. *Archives of General Psychiatry,* Apr;56:323–327, 1999.

162. J. Cooper and N. Sartorius, eds. *Mental Disorders in China, Results of the National Epidemiological Survey in 12 Areas.* Gaskell Royal College of Psychiatrists: London, 1996.

163. L. Dennerstein. Psychosocial and mental health aspects of women's health. *World Health Statistics Quarterly* 46(4):234–236, 1993.

164. J. Broadhead and M. Abas. Life events and difficulties and the onset of depression among women in a low-income urban setting in Zimbabwe. *Psychology Medicine* 28:29–38, 1998.

165. J.I. Davar, D.J. Brull, S. Bulugahipitiya, J.G. Coghlan, D.P. Lipkin, and T.R. Evans. Prognostic value of negative dobutamine stress echo in women with intermediate

probability of coronary artery disease. *American Journal of Cardiology* Jan1;83(1):100–102, A8, 1999.

166. M. Weissman and M. Olfson. Depression in Women: Implications for Health Care Research. *Science* Aug 11(269):799–801, 1995.

167. A.E. Becker. Postpartum illnes in Fiji: A sociosomatic perspective. *Psychosomatic Medicine* 60:431–438, 1998.

168. T.D. Wade and D.S. Kendler. The Relationship between Social Support and Major Depression Cross-Sectional, Longitudinal, and Genetic Perspectives. *The Journal of Nervous and Mental Disease* May;188(5), 2000.

169. M.M. Weissman, P.J. Leaf, C.E. Holzer, J.K. Myers, and G.L. Tischler. The epidemiology of depression: An update on sex differences in rates. *Journal of Affective Disorders* 7, 179–188, 1984.

170. M. Shiva and A. Mukhopadhyay, eds. State of India's Health. New Delhi: Voluntary Health Association of India. *Women and Health* 1:265–302, 1992.

171. V. Skultans. Women and afflection in Maharashtra: A hydraulic model of health and illness. *Culture, Medicine and Psychiatry* Sep 15(3)321–359, 1991.

172. K. Uvnas-Moberg, E. Bjorkstrand, V. Hillegaart, and S. Ahlenius. Oxytocin as a possible mediator of SSRI-induced antidepressant effects. *Psychopharmacology* (Berlin) Feb;142(1):95–101, 1999.

173. V. Hendrick, L.L. Altshuler, and R. Suri. Hormonal changes in the postpartum and implications for postpartum depression. *Psychosomatics* Mar-Apr;39(2):93–101, 1998.

174. P.J. Lucassen, F.J. Tilders, A. Salehi, and D.F. Swaab. Neuropeptides vasopressin (AVP), oxytocin (OXT) and corticotropin-releasing hormone (CRH) in the human hypothalamus: Activity changes in aging, Alzheimer's disease and depression. *Aging* (Milano) 9(4):48–50, 1997.

175. S. Carranza-Lira and M.L. Valentino-Figueroa. Estrogen therapy for depression in postmenopausal women. *International Journal of Gynaecology and Obstetrics* Apr;65(1):35-38, 1999.

176. F. Benazzi. Female depression before and after menopause. *Psychotherapy and Psychosomatics* Sep-Oct;69(5):280–283, 2000.

177. H.D. Desai and M.W. Jann. Major depression in women: A review of the literature. *Journal of American Pharmacology Association* (Washington) Jul-Aug;40(4):525–537, 2000.

178. S. Nhiwatiwa, V. Patel, and W. Acuda. Predicting postnatal mental disorder with a screening questionnaire: A prospective cohort study from Zimbabwe. *Journal of Epidemiology and Community Health* Apr;52(4):262–266, 1998.

179. E. da S. Coutinho, N. de Almeida Filho, J. de J. Mari, and L.C. Rodrigues. Gender and minor psychiatric morbidity: Results of a case-control study in a developing country. *International Journal of Psychiatric Medicine* 29(2):197–208, 1999.

180. P.J. Cooper, M. Tomlinson, L. Swartz, M. Woolgar, L. Murray, and C. Molteno. Post-partum depression and the mother-infant relationship in a South African peri-urban settlement. *British Journal of Psychiatry* Dec;175:554–558, 1999.

181. R. Gubash and M.T. Abou-Saleh. Postpartum illness in Arab culture: Prevalence and psychosocial correlates. *British Journal of Psychiatry* Jul;171:65–68, 1997.

182. L.A. Rohde, E. Busnello, A. Wolf, A. Zomer, F. Shansis, S. Martins, et al. Maternity blues in Brazilian women. *Acta Psychiatrica Scandinavica* Mar;95(3):231–235, 1997.

183. C.H. Chen. Etiology of postpartum depression—A review. *Kao Hsiung I Hsueh Ko Hsueh Tsa Chih* Jan;11(1):1–7, 1995.

184. R.E. Kendell, J.C. Chalmers, and C. Platz. Epidemiology of puerperal psychoses. *British Journal of Psychiatry* 150:662, 1987.

185. M.E. Thase and R.H. Howland. Biological processes in depression: An updated review and integration. In: *Handbook of Depression,* 2nd edition. Beckham, E.E. and Leber, W.R., eds., Guilford: New York, 1995.

186. A.J. Rush, R.S. Stewart, D.L. Garver, and D.A. Waller. Neurobiological bases for psychiatric disorders. In: *Comprehensive Neurology* 2nd edition, Rosenberb, R.N. and Pleasure, D.E., eds. John Wiley and Sons: New York, pp555–603, 1998.

187. S. Checkley, ed. *Biological models of depression and response to antidepressant treatments.* In: *The Management of Depression,* Checkley, S., ed. Blackwell Science: Oxford, pp.42–69, 1998.

188. C.B. Nemeroff. New vistas in neuropeptide research in neuropsychiatry: Focus on corticotrophin-releasing factor. *Neuropsychopharmacology* 6: 69–75, 1992.

189. C.B. Nemeroff. Psychopharmacology of affective disorders in the 21st century. *Biological Psychiatry* 44: 517–525, 1998.

190. W.W. Zung, W.E. Broadhead, and M.E. Roth. Prevalence of depressive symptoms in primary care. *Journal of Family Practice* 4:337–344, 1993.

191. S.R. Kisley and G.P. Goldberg. Physical and psychiatric comorbidity in general practice. *British Journal of Psychiatry* 169: 236–242, 1996.

192. N. Sartorius, T.B. Ustun, Y. Lecrubier, and H.U. Wittchen. Depression comorbid with anxiety: Results from the WHO study on psychological disorders in primary health care. *British Journal of Psychiatry.* June(30)38–43, 1996.

193. M.F. Bonin, D.R. McCreary, and S.W. Sadava. Problem drinking behavior in two community-based samples of adults: Influence of gender, coping, loneliness, and depression. *Psychology and Addictive Behavior* Jun;14(2):151–161, 2000.

194. O.A. Abiodun. Alcohol-related problems in primary care patients in Nigeria. *Acta Psychiatrica Scandinavica* Apr;93(4):235–239, 1996.

195. C.A. Prescott, S.H. Aggen, and K.S. Kendler. Sex-Specific Genetic Influences on the Comorbidity of Alcoholism and Major Depression in a Population-Based Sample of U.S. Twins. *Archives of General Psychiatry* Aug;57:803–811, 2000.

196. D. Snow and C. Anderson. Exploring the factors influencing relapse and recovery among drug and alcohol addicted women. *Journal of Psychosocial Nursing in Mental Health Services* Jul;38(7):8–19, 2000.

197. L. Spak, F. Spak, and P. Allebeck. Alcoholism and depression in a Swedish female population: Co-morbidity and risk factors. *Acta Psychiatrica Scandinavica* Jul;102(1):44–51, 2000.

198. S.W. Perry, L.B. Jacobsberg, B. Fishman, A. Francis, J. Bobo, and B.K. Jacobsberg. Psychiatric diagnosis before serological testing for the Human Immunodeficiency Virus. *American Journal of Psychiatry* 147:89–93, 1990.

199. E.H. Kua. Psychiaric referrals of elderly patients in a general hospital. *Annals of Academic Medicine.* Jan 16(1):115–117, 1987.

200. M. Ganguli, S. Dube, J.M. Johnston, R. Pandav, V. Chandra, and H.H. Dodge. Depressive symptoms, cognitive impairment and functional impairment in a rural elderly population in India: A Hindi version of the geriatric depression scale (GDS-H). *International Journal of Geriatric Psychiatry* Oct; 14(10):807–820, 1999.

201. M. Cvjetkovic-Bosnjak, A. Knezevic, and B. Soldatovic-Stajic. Depression in older persons. *Medicinski Pregled* Mar-Apr;53(3–4)-184–186, 2000.
202. J.E. Wells, J.A. Bushell, A.R. Hornblow, P.R. Joyce, and M.A. Oakley-Browne. Christchurch psychiatric epidemiology study part 1: Methodology and lifetime prevalence for specific psychiatric disorders. *Australian and New Zealand Journal of Psychiatry* 23, 315–326, 1989.
203. H.U. Wittchen, S. Zhao, R.C. Kessler, and W.W. Eaton. DSM-III-R generalized anxiety disorder in the National Comorbidity Survey. *Archives of General Psychiatry* May;51(5):355–364, 1994.
204. M. Eddleston, M.H. Rezvi Sheriff, and K. Hawton. Deliberate Self-Harm in Sri Lanka: An overlooked tragedy in the developing world. *British Medical Journal* 137:133–135, 1998.
205. J.A. Bartlett, A. Andreoli, T. Pascual, and S.E. Keller. Recent benzodiazepine use in depressed patients: A confound of psychoimmunologic studies? *Brain, Behavior and Immunity* Dec;10(4):380–386, 1996.
206. A.F. Jorm. Does old age reduce the risk of anxiety and depression? A review of epidemiological studies across the adult life span. *Psychological Medicine* 30, 11–22, 2000.
207. E. Cemerinski, R.G. Robinson, and J.T. Kosier. Improved recovery in activities of daily living associated with remission of poststroke depression. *Stroke* Jan;32(1):113–117, 2001.
208. H. Brodaty. Think of depression—Atypical presentations in the elderly. *Australian Family Physician* Jul 22(7)1195–1203, 1993.
209. J. Scott, D. Eccleston, and R. Boys. Can we predict the persistence of depression? *British Journal of Psychiatry* Nov;161:633–637, 1992.
210. M.M. Weissman, S. Wolk, R.B. Goldstein, D. Moreau, P. Adams, S. Greenwald, et al. Depressed Adolescents Grown Up. *Journal of the American Medical Association* May 12;281(18):1707–1713, 1999.
211. M.M. Weissman, S. Wolk, P. Wickramaratne, R.B. Goldstein, P. Adams, S. Greenwald, et al. Children with Prepubertal-Onset Major Depresive disorder and Anxiety Grown up. *Archives of General Psychiatry* Sep;56:794–801, 1999.
212. M.B. Keller, P.W. Lavori, T.I. Mueller, J. Endicott, W. Coryell, R.M. Hirschfeld, et al. Time to recovery, chronicity, and levels of psychopathology in major depression. A 5-year prospective follow-up of 431 subjects. *Archives General Psychiatry* Oct;49(10):809–816, 1992.
213. M. Piccinelli and G. Wilkinson. Outcome of depression in psychiatric settings. *British Journal of Psychiatry* March 164(3)297–304, 1994.
214. J. Scott, W.A. Barker, and D. Eccleston. The Newcastle Chronic Depression Study. Patient characteristics and factors associated with chronicity. *British Journal of Psychiatry* Jan;152:28–33, 1988.
215. G.B. Cassano, L. Musetti, G Perugi, A. Soriani, V. Mignani, D.M. McNair, et al. A proposed new approach to the clinical sub-classification of depressive illness. *Pharmacopsychiatry* Jan 21(1):19–23, 1988.
216. A. Marneros, A. Deister, and A. Rhode. Stability of diagnosis in affective, schizoaffective and schizophrenic disorders. Cross sectional versus longitudinal diagnosis. *European Archives Psychiatry and Clinical Neurosciences* 241(3):187–192, 1991.

217. J. Angst and M. Preisig. Outcome of a clinical cohort of unipolar, bipolar and schizoaffective patients. Results of a prospective study from 1959–1985. *Archives of Neurological Psychiatry* 146(1):17–23, 1995.

218. R.S. Murthy, K. Kuruvilla, A. Verghese, and B.M. Pulimood. Psychiatric illness at general hospital medical clinic. *Journal of the Indian Medical Association.* Jan 1;66(1):6–8, 1976.

219. C. Shamsundar, R.L. Kapur, U.K. Sundaram, S. Pai, and G.N. Nagarathna. Involvement of the GPs in urban mental health care. *Journal of the Indian Medical Association,* 72:310–313, 1978.

220. S. Gautam, R.L. Kapur, and C. Shamasundar. Psychiatric morbidity and referral in General practice. *Indian Journal of Psychiatry* 22:295–297, 1980.

221. M.I. Isaac, R.L. Kapur, C.R. Chandrasekhar, M. Kapur, and R. Parthasarathy. Mental health delivery in rural primary health care—Development and evaluation of a pilot training programme. *Indian Journal of Psychiatry* 24:131–132, 1982.

222. C. Shamsundar, U.K. Sundaram, S. Kalyanasundaram, S. Pai, and R.L. Kapur. Training of GPs in mental health—Two year experience. *Indian Journal of Psychological Medicine,* 3:85–89, 1980.

223. C. Shamsundar, R.L. Kapur, M.K. Isaac, and U.K. Sundaram. Orientation course in psychiatry for GPs. *Indian Journal of Psychiatry* 25:298, 1983.

224. N.N. Wig and R.S. Murthy. *Manual of mental health for primary care physicians.* Indian Council of Medical Research: New Delhi, 1981.

225. M.K. Isaac, C.R. Chandrasekhar, and R.S. Murthy. Mental Health care by primary care doctors. National Institute of Mental Health and NeuroSciences: Bangalore, 1994.

226. T.G. Sriram, K. Kishore, S. Moily, C.R. Chandrashekar, M.K. Isaac, and R.S. Murthy. Minor psychiatric disturbances in primary health care: A study of their prevalence and characteristics using a simple case detection technique. *Indian Journal of Psychiatry* 3:212–226, 1987.

227. R.S. Murthy. Economics of mental health care in developing countries. In: *International review of psychiatry,* Lieh Mak, F. and Nadelson, C.C. eds. American Psychiatric Press: Washington, D.C.; 2:43–62, 1996.

228. A. Mohit. Mental health in the Eastern Mediterranean Region of the World Health Organization with a view of the future trends. *East Mediterranean Health Journal* Mar;5(2):231–240, 1999.

229. S. Davoid. Comprehensive report on integration of mental health into primary health care systems (in the Farsi language, limited circulation) Ministry of Health and Medical Education, Tehran, Iran, 1992.

230. N.N. Wig. WHO and mental health—A view from developing countries. *Bulletin of the World Health Organization* 78(4):502–503, 2000.

231. WHO/EMRO. Intercountry Meeting on development of mental health indicators, Alexandria, Dec, 1999. D. Shahmohammadi. Personal communication to Dr. Ahmad Mohit, Regional Advisor, Mental Health, WHO/EMRO, May 30, 2000.

232. D.G. Jacobs. National Depression Screening Day: Educating the public, reaching those in need of treatment, and broadening professional understanding. *Harvard Review of Psychiatry* Sept.–Oct. 3(3):156–159, 1995.

233. R.G. Priest, R. Gimbrett, M. Roberts, and J. Steinhart. Reversible and selective inhibitors of monoamine oxidase A in mental and other disorders. *Acta Psychiatrica Scandinavica* 386:40–43, 1995.

234. R.G. Priest, E.S. Paykel, and D. Hart. Progress in defeating depression. *Psychiatric Bulletin,* 19:491–495, 1995.
235. N. Rettersol. National Plan for Suicide Prevention in Norway. *Italian Journal of Suicidology.* 5:19–24, 1995.
236. E.S. Paykel, D. Hart, and R.G. Priest. Changes in public attitudes to depression during the defeat depression campaign. *British Journal of Psychiatry* Dec 173:519–522, 1998.
237. V. Patel and R. Thara. *Preventive programmes in low income countries.* Sage: New Delhi, 2000.
238. V. Eapen, L.I. al-Gazali, S. Bin-Othman, M.T. Abou-Saleh, K.A. el-Nasser, R. Ramzy, et al. School Mental Health Screening: A Model for Developing Countries. *Journal of Tropical Pediatrics* Feb;45:53–55, 1999.
239. M. Mubbashar. School mental health program in Pakistan. In: *Preventing Mental Illness—Mental Health Promotion in Primary Care.* Jenkins, R. and Ustun, T.B., eds. Wiley: Chicester, 1998.
240. A. Rahman, M.H. Mubbashar, R. Gater, and D. Goldberg. Randomized trial of impact of school mental health program in rural Rawalpindi, Pakistan. *Lancet* 352:1022–1025, 1998.
241. M. Olfson, J. Gorman, and H. Pardes. Investing in mental health research. *Journal of Nervous and Mental Disease* 183, 421–424, 1995.
242. S. J. Taylor, D. Kingdon, and R. Jenkins. How are nations trying to prevent suicide? An analysis of national suicide prevention strategies. *Acta Psychiatrica Scandinavica* 95:457–463, 1996.
243. W. Rutz, L. Von Knorring, and J. Walinder. Frequency of suicide on Gotland after systematic post-graduate education of general practitioners. *Acta Psychiatrica Scandinavica.* 80:151–154, 1989.
244. K. Michel, C. Frey, K. Wyss, and L. Valach. An exercise in improving suicide reporting in print media. *Crisis* 21(2):71–79, 2000.
245. B. Ahrens, M. Linden, H. Zaske, and H. Berzewski. Suicidal behavior—Symptom or disorder? *Comprehensive Psychiatry* Mar–Apr;41(2 Supplement1):116–121, 2000.
246. A. Varnik. Suicide in the former republics of the USSR. *Psychiatric Fennica* 29:150–162, 1998.
247. Department of Health. *Safer Services: National Confidential Inquiry into Suicide and Homicide by People with Mental Illness.* (Appleby, L., Director). Department of Health: London, 1999.
248. M. Upanne. A model for the description and interpretation of suicide prevention. *Suicide Life Threatening Behavior* 29(3):241–255, Autumn 1999.
249. L. Maruilli-Koenig, ed. *National Strategies for the Prevention of Suicide.* Information Support Unit of the United Nations Department for Policy Coordination and Sustainable Development. Kiosk Online Oct./Nov. 2(5), 1996.
250. R. Joffe, S. Sokolov, D. Streiner. Anti-depressant treatment of depression: A meta-analysis. *Canadian Journal of Psychiatry* Dec 41(10): 613–616, 1996.
251. C. Brown and H.C. Schulberg. The efficacy of psychosocial treatments in primary care: A review of randomized clinical trials. *General Hospital Psychiatry* Nov 17(6): 414–424, 1995.

252. M. Abas, J.C. Broadhead, P. Mbape, and G. Khumalo-Sakatukwa. Defeating depression in the developing world: A Zimbabwean model. *British Journal of Psychiatry* Mar;164(3):293–296, 1994.

253. M. Hollifield, W. Katon, and N. Morojele. Anxiety and depression in an outpatient clinic in Lesotho, Africa. *International Journal of Psychiatric Medicine* 24(2):179–188, 1994.

254. O.A. Abiodun. A study of mental morbidity among primary care patients in Nigeria. *Comprehensive Psychiatry* 34:10–13, 1993.

255. C. Wright, M.K. Nepal, and W.D.A. Bruce-Jones. Mental health patients in primary care services in Nepal. *Asia-Pacific Journal of Public Health* 3:224–230, 1989.

256. M. Joukamaa, V. Lehtinen, and H. Karlsson. The ability of general practitioners to detect mental disorders in primary health care. *Acta Psychiatrica Scandinavica* 91:52–56, 1995.

257. P.P. Sales. Primary mental health care in Nicaragua five years later. *Social Science Medicine* 37:1585–1586, 1993.

258. W. Katon. Will improving detection of depression in primary care lead to improved depressive outcomes? *General Hospital Psychiatry* 17:1–2, 1995.

259. A. Kigamwa. Psychiatry morbidity and referral rate among medical in-patients at the Kenyatta National Hospital. *East African Medical Journal* May;68(5):383–388, 1991.

260. G. Simon. Long term prognosis of depression in primary care. *Bulletin of the World Health Organization* 78(4):439–445, 2000.

261. W. Katon, M. Von Korff, E. Lin, T. Bush, and J. Ormel. Adequacy and duration of antidepressant treatment in primary care. *Medical Care* 30:67–76, 1992.

262. O. Spigset. Adverse reactions of selective serotonin reuptake inhibitors: Report from a spontaneous reporting system. *Drug Safety* March 20(3):277–287, 1999.

263. G. Isacsson, G. Boethius, S. Henriksson, J.K. Jones, and U. Bergman. Selective serotonin reuptake inhibitors have broadened the utilzation of antidepressant treatment in accordance with recommendations. Finding from a Swedish prescription database. *Journal of Affective Disorders* Apr;53(1):15–22, 1999.

264. E. Frank, D.J. Kupfer, J. M. Perel, C. Cornes, D.B. Jarrett, A.G. Mallinger, et al. Three-year outcomes for maintenance therapies in recurrent depression *Archives of General Psychiatry* Dec;47(12);1093–1099,1990.

265. P. Liu. Clinical psychopharmacology in China: The last decade. *Psychiatry Clinical Neurosciences* Dec;52 Supplement:S190–192, 1998.

266. I.M. Anderson. Selective sertonin reuptake inhibitors versus trycyclic antidepressants: A meta-analysis of efficacy and tolerability. *Journal of Affective Disorders* 58:19–36, 2000.

267. C.M. Pare. The present status of monoamine oxidase inhibitors. *British Journal of Psychiatry* Jun;146:576–584, 1985.

268. F. Quitkin, J.W. Stewart, P.J. McGrath, E. Tricamo, J.G. Rabkin, K. Ocepek-Welikson, E. Nunes, W. Harrison, and D.F. Klein. Columbia atypical depression. A subgroup of depressives with better response to MAOI than to tricyclic antidepressants or placebo. *British Journal of Psychology* Sep 21:30–34, 1993.

269. M.H. Lader. The Efficacy of antidepressant medication In: *The Management of Depression*, Checkley, S., ed. Blackwell: London, pp.188–211, 1998.

270. G. Singh and R. Sharma . Anxiety and Depressive Neurosis: Their response to anxiolytic and antidepressant treatment. *Indian Journal of Psychiatry* 29:49–56, 1987.

271. F. Song, N. Freemantle, T.A. Sheldon, A. House, P. Watson, A. Long, et al. Selective serotonin reuptake inhibitors: Meta-analysis of efficacy and acceptability. *British Medical Journal* Mar 13;306(6879):683–687, 1993.

272. E. Trindade and D. Menon. Selective serotonin reuptake inhibitors (SSRIs) for major depression. Part 1: Evaluation of the clinical literature. Canadian Coordinating Office for Health Technology Assessment (Report 3E): Ottawa, 1997.

273. R.J. Boerner and H.J. Moller. The importance of new antidepressants in the treatment of anxiety/depressive disorders. *Pharmacopsychiatry* Jul;32(4):119–126, 1999.

274. J.P. Lepine, J. Goger, C. Blashko, C. Probst, M.F. Moles, J. Kosolowski, et al. A double-blinded study of the efficacy and safety of sertraline and clomipramine in outpatients with severe major depression. *International Clinical Psychopharmacology* Sep;15(5):263–271, 2000.

275. S.M. Razali and C.T. Hasanah. Cost-effectiveness of cyclic antidepressants in developing countries. *Australian New Zealand Journal of Psychiatry* Apr;33:283–284, 1999.

276. M. Hotopf, G. Levis, and C. Normand. Are SSRIs a cost-effective alternative to tricyclic? *British Journal of Psychiatry* 168:404–409, 1996.

277. P.G. Janicak, J.M.Davis, S.H. Preskorn and F.J. Ayd. *Principles and Practice of Psychopharmacotherapy*, 2nd edition. Williams & Wilkins: Baltimore, MD, 1997.

278. G.L. Birbeck. Barriers to care for patients with neurologic disease in rural Zambia. *Archives of Neurology* March 57(3):414–417, 2000.

279. J.F. Gumnick and C.B. Nemeroff. Problems with currently available antidepressants. *Journal of Clinical Psychiatry* 10(Supplement 61):5–15, 2000.

280. M. Fava. New approaches to the treatment of refractory depression. *Journal of Clinical Psychiatry* 61(1):26–32, 2000.

281. A.I. Scott. Contemporary practice of electroconvulsive therapy. *British Journal of Hospital Medicine* Apr 6–19;51(7):334–338, 1994.

282. H. Folkerts. Electroconvulsive therapy of depressive disorders. *Therapeutische Umschau* Feb;57(2):90–94, 2000.

283. A.I. Scott. Does ECT alter brain structure? *American Journal of Psychiatry* Sep;152(9):1403, 1995.

284. Royal College of Psychiatrists. *The ECT Handbook*. Royal College of Psychiatrists: London, 1995 (Council report CR39).

285. A.S. Hale. ABC of mental health: Depression. *British Medical Journal* 315:43–46, 1997.

286. G. Goodwin. Mood Disorder. In: *Companion to Psychiatric Studies,* 6th Edition. Johnstone, E., Freeman, C.P.L., and Zealby, A.K., eds. Churchill Livingstone: Kent, U.K., 1998.

287. R. Desjarlais, L. Eisenberg, B. Good, and A. Kleinman. World Mental Health. Problems and Priorities in Low-income Countries. Oxford University Press: New York, 1995.

288. O.A. Abiodun. The role of psychosocial factors in the causation, course and outcome of physical disorders: A review. *Eastern African Medical Journal* Jan;71(1):55–59, 1994.

289. A.E. Zretsky, Z.V. Segal, and M. Gemar. Cognitive therapy for bipolar depression: A pilot study. *Canadian Journal of Psychiatry* Jun;44(5):491–494, 1999.

290. I.D. Glick, T. Suppes, C. DeBattista, R.J. Hu, and S. Marder. Psychopharmacologic treatment strategies for depression, bipolar disorder, and schizophrenia. *Annals of Internal Medicine* Jan2;134(1):47–60, 2001.

291. D.L. Evans, J. Staab, H. Ward, J. Leserman, D.O. Perkins, R.N. Golden, J.M. Petitto. Depression in the medically ill: Management considerations. *Depression and Anxiety* 4(4):199–208, 1996–1997.

292. S.W. Perry and J. Markowitz. Psychiatric interventions for AIDS-spectrum disorders. *Hospital Community Psychiatry* Oct;37(10):1001–1006, 1986.

293. A. Bergant, T. Nguyen, R. Moser, and H. Ulmer. Prevalence of depressive disorders in early puerperium. *Gynakol Geburtshilfliche Rundsch* 38(4):232–237, 1998.

294. D.S. Gruen. A group psychotherapy approach to postpartum depression. *International Journal of Group Psychotherapy* Apr;43(2):191–203, 1993.

295. A.T. Beck, M.Kovacs, and A. Weissman. Assessment of suicidal intention: The scale for suicide ideation. *Journal of Consulting Clinical Psychiatry* April 47(2):343–352, 1979.

296. P.C. Kendall and S.M. Panichelli-Mindel. Cognitive-behavorial treatments. *Journal of Abnormal Child Psychology* Feb 23(1):107–124, 1995.

297. L. Mynors-Wallis, I. Davies, A. Gray, F. Barour, and D. Gath. A randomized controlled trial and cost analysis of problem-solving treatment for emotional disorders given by community nurses in primary care. *British Journal of Psychiatry* Feb;170:113–119, 1997.

298. J.E. Barrett, J.W. Williams Jr., T.E. Oxman, W. Katon, E. Frank, M.T. Hegel et al. The treatment effectiveness project. A comparison of the effectiveness of paroxetine, problem-solving therapy, and placebo in the treatment of minor depression and dysthymia in primary care patients: Background and research plan. *General Hospital Psychiatry* Jul-Aug;21(4):260–273, 1999.

299. C. Dorwick, G. Dunn, J.L. Ayuso-Mateos, O.S. Dalgard, H. Page, V. Lehtinen, et al. Problem solving treatment and group psychoeducation for depression: Multicentre randomized controlled trial. Outcomes of Depression International Network (ODIN) Group. *British Medical Journal* Dec 9;321(7274):1450–1454, 2000.

300. D.J. Miklowitz and M.J. Goldstein. Behavorial family treatment for patients with Bipolar affective disorder. *Behavior Modification* Oct 14(4):457–489, 1990.

301. T. Kendrick. Primary care options to prevent mental illness. *Annals of Medicine* Dec;31(6):359–363, 1999.

302. N. Nalini, V. Kumaraiah, and D. Subbakrishna. Cognitive behaviour therapy in the treatment of neurotic depression. *National Institute of Mental Health and Neurosciences* 14, 31–35, 1996.

303. A. Sumathipale, R. Hanwella, S. Hwege and A. Mann. Randomised controlled trial of cognitive behaviour therapy for respected consultations for medically unexplained symptoms: A feasibility study in Sri Lanka. *Psychological Medicine* 30:749–758, 2000.

304. D. Dudek and A. Zieba. Development and application of cognitive therapy in affective disorders. [Article in Polish] *Psychiatrica Polska* 34(1):81–88, 2000.

305. S.X. Li and M.R. Phillips. Witch doctors and mental illness in mainland China: A preliminary study. *American Journal of Psychiatry* Feb;147(2):221–224, 1990.

306. A.P. Reeler. Pathways to psychiatric care in Harare, Zimbabwe. *The Central African Journal of Medicine* 38(1): 1–7, 1992

307. S. Bondestam, J. Garssen, and A.I. Abdulwakil. Prevalence and treatment of mental disorders and epilepsy in Zanzibar. *Acta Psychiatrica Scandinavica* Apr;81(4):327–331, 1990.

308. O. Gureje, R.A. Acha, and O.A. Odejide. Pathways to psychiatric care in Ibadin, Nigeria. *Tropical and Geographical Medicine* 47(3):125–129, 1995.

309. B. Bloch. Treatment of psychiatric patients in Tanzania. *Acta Psychiatrica Scandinavica* 364(83):122–126, 1991.

310. S.W. Acuda. Mental health problems in Kenya today: A review of research. *East African Medical Journal* Jan 60(1):11–14, 1983.

311. F. Schulsinger and A. Jablensky. The national mental health programme in the United Republic of Tanzania: A report from WHO and DANIDA. *Acta Psychiatrica Scandinavica* 83(364):1–132, 1991.

312. K.H. Heggenhougen and L. Gilson. Perceptions of efficacy and the use of traditional medicine, with examples from Tanzania. *Curare* 20:5–13, 1997.

313. S.F. Kaaya and M.T. Leshabari. Depressive illness and primary health care in sub-Saharan Africa: With special reference to Tanzania. *Central African Journal of Medicine*, 1999.

314. T.B. Ustun. The global burden of mental disorders. *American Journal of Public Health* Sep:89(9):1315–1318, 1999.

315. W. Gulbinat, R. Manderscheid, A. Beigel, and J.A. Costa e Silva. A multinational strategy on mental health policy and care. A WHO collaborative initiative and consultative program. In: *Handbook of Mental Health Economics and Health Policy. Schizophrenia.* Mosacarelli, M., Rupp, A., and Sartorius, N., eds. John Wiley & Sons: Chicester, 1996.

316. R.S. Murthy. Economics of mental health care in developing countries. In: *International Review of Psychiatry.* Lieh Mak, F. and Nadelson, C.C., eds. American Psychiatric Press: Washington, D.C., 2:43–62, 1996.

317. D. Chisholm. Challenges for the international application of mental health economics. *Epidemiology and Psychiatric Sociology.* Jan–March 8(1):11–15, 1999.

318. A. Shah and R. Jenkins. Mental health economic studies from developing countries reviewed in the context of those from developed countries. *Acta Psychiatrica Scandinavica* 100:1–18, 1999.

319. I. Blue and T. Harpham. The World Bank World Development Report 1993: Investing in Health. Reveals the burden of common mental disorders, but ignores its implications. *British Journal of Psychiatry* July 165(2):9–12, 1994.

320. R.S. Murthy. Conversion factor instability in international comparisons of health care expenditure: Some econometric comments. *Journal of Health Economics* Aug;11(2):183–187, 1992.

321. P. Cowley and J.R. Wyatt. Schizophrenia and manic-depressive illness. In: *Disease control priorities in developing countries.* Jamison, D.T., Mosley, W.H., Measham, A.R., and Bobadilla, J.L., eds. Oxford University Press: Oxford, pp.661–670, 1993.

322. W. Xiong, M.R. Phillips, R. Wang, Q. Dai, J. Kleinman, and A. Kleinman. Family-based intervention for schizophrenic patients in China: A randomised controlled trial. *British Journal of Psychiatry* 165:239–247, 1995.

323. Q. Wang, Y.Gong, K. Niu. Q. Wang., Y. Gong, and K. Niu. The Yantai model of community care for rural psychiatric patients. *British Journal of Psychiatry* 1994;165(Suppl24):107–113

324. M.K. Isaac and R.L. Kapur. A cost-effective analysis of three different methods of psychiatric case finding in the general population. *British Journal of Psychiatry* 137:540–546, 1980.

325. L.S. Gillis, A. Koch, and M. Joyi. The value and cost-effectiveness of a home-visiting programme for psychiatric patients. *South African Medical Journal* 77:309–310, 1989.

326. M. Knapp, J. Beecham, A. Fenyo, and A. Hallam. Community mental health care for former hospital in-patients. Predicting costs from needs and diagnoses. *British Journal of Psychiatry* 27:10–18, April 1995.

327. W. Hargreaves, M. Shumway, T. Hu, and B. Cuffel. *Cost Outcome Methods for Mental Health*. Academic Press: London, 1997.

328. A. Creese. Global trends in health care reform. *World Health Forum* 15(4):317–322, 1994.

329. L. Kumaranayake and C. Watts. Cost-effectiveness estimates of the Mwanza sexually transmitted diseases intervention. *Lancet* Mar 28;351(99107):989–990, 1998.

330. D. Chisholm, K. Sekar, K. Kishore Kumar, K. Saeed, S. James, M. Mubbahar, et al. Integration of mental health care into primary care: Demonstration cost-outcome study in India and Pakistan. *British Journal of Psychiatry* 176:581–588, 2000.

331. R. Sturm and K. Wells. Health insurance may be improving-but not for individuals with mental illness. *Health Services Research* April:35(1 pt 2):253–262, 2000.

332. D.J. Katzelnick, K.A. Kobak, J.H. Greist, J.W. Jefferson, and H.J. Henk. Effect of primary care treatment of depression on service use by patients with high medical expenditures. *Psychiatric Services* 48(10):59–64, Jan 1997.

333. D. Goldberg, G. Jackson, R. Gater, M. Campbell, and N. Jennett. The treatment of common mental disorders by a community team based in primary care: A cost-effectiveness study. *Psychological Medicine* May;26(3):487–492, 1996.

334. L.V. Rubenstein, M. Jackson-Triche, J. Unutzer, J. Miranda, K. Minnium, M.L. Pearson, et al. Evidence-based care for depression in managed primary care practices. *Health Affirmation* Sep–Oct;18(5):89–105, 1999.

335. J.R. Lave, R.G. Frank, H.C. Schulber, and M S Kamlet. Cost-effectiveness of treatments for major depression in primary care practice. *Archives of General Psychiatry* July;55(7):645–651, 1998.

336. W. Katon. Treatment trials in real world settings. Methodological issues and measurement of disability and costs. *General Hospital of Psychiatry* Jul–Aug.:21(4):237–238, 1999.

337. R.C. Kessler, C. Barber, H.G. Birnbaum, R.G. Frank, P.E. Greenberg, R.M. Rose, G.E. Simon, and P. Wang. Depression in the workplace: effects on short-term disability. Health Affairs (Millwood) 18(5):163–171, Sep–Oct 1999.

338. K.B. Wells and C.D. Sherbourne. Functioning and utility for the current health of patients with depression or chronic medical conditions in managed, primary care practices. *Archives of General Psychiatry* Oct;56(10):897–904, 1999.

339. R. Frank, J. Glazer, and T. McGurie. *Measuring Distortion from Adverse Selection in Managed Health Care*. Boston University: Boston, 1999.

340. G.P. Kilonzo and N. Simmons. Development of mental health services in Tanzania: A reappraisal for the future. *Social Science and Medicine* 47(4):419–428, Aug 1998.

341. R Alarcon and S. Aguilar-Gaxiola. Mental health policy developments in Latin America. *Bulletin of the World Health Organization* 78:483–490, 2000.

342. O. Gureje and A. Alem. Mental health policy development in Africa. *Bulletin of the World Health Organization* 78:475–482, 2000.
343. M. Shepherd. Mental health as an integrant of primary medical care. *Journal of the Royal College of General Practitioners* 30:657–664, 1980.
344. B.J. Burns, D.A. Regier, and A.M. Jacobson. Factors relating to the use of mental health services in a neighborhood health center. *Public Health Report* 93(3):232–239, May-Jun 1978.
345. R. Jenkins. Developments in the primary care of mental illness—A forward look. *International Review of Psychiatry* 4:237–242, 1992.
346. J. Scott, T. Jennings, S. Standart, R. Ward, and D. Goldberg. The impact of training in problem-based interviewing on the detection and management of pyschological problems presenting in primary care. *British Journal of General Practice* Jun;49:441–445, 1999.
347. M. Fulop. Residency training. *Annals of Internal Medicine* Jun;106(6):915, 1987.
348. S. Morley and S.B. Barton. Specificity of reference patterns in depressive thinking: Agency and object for self-representation. *Journal of Abnormal Psychology* Nov;108(4):655–66, 1999.
349. A.H. Mann, R. Blizard, J. Murray, J.A. Smith, N. Botega, E. MacDonald, et al. An evaluation of practice nurses working with general practitioners to treat people with depression. *British Journal of General Practice* 48:875–879, 1998.
350. O.A. Abiodun. Knowledge and attitude concerning mental health of primary health care workers in Nigeria. *International Journal of Social Psychiatry* 37(2):113–120, Summer 1991.
351. C.A. Orchard and R. Karmaliani. Community development specialists in nursing for developing countries. *Image Journal of Nursing School* 31(3):295–299, 1999.
352. G.E. Simon, E.H.B. Lin, W. Katon, K. Saunders, M. Von Korff, E. Walker, et al. Outcomes of "inadequate" antidepressant treatment. *Journal of General Internal Medicine* 10:663–670, 1995.
353. E.H.B. Lin and W.J. Katon. Beyond the diagnosis of depression. *General Hospital Psychiatry* 20:207–208, 1998.

**Summary of Findings:
Stroke in Developing Countries**

- Stroke ranked as the third leading cause of death in 1990 in developing countries and was responsible for about 2.4 percent of disability-adjusted life years (DALYs) worldwide. Projections for 2020 place stroke fifth among the causes of disease burden for developing countries.

- Prevalence and incidence rates for stroke vary dramatically among populations and may be influenced by economic, behavioral, and genetic factors, among others. Comparative epidemiological studies of stroke based on common definitions, methods, and modes of data presentation are needed to increase understanding of this disease.

- Because of the high risk for death, long-term disability, and recurrence after a first stroke, prevention is key to reducing the public health impacts of cerebrovascular disease. And prevention is feasible, given the remarkable reduction in stroke mortality achieved in several developed countries.

- Low-cost community health education programs that promote exercise, healthy diets, and smoking cessation may significantly reduce risk of stroke in developing countries.

- Several low-cost treatments for hypertension, diabetes, and other conditions are likely to reduce significantly the incidence and severity of stroke and stroke-related vascular disease in developing countries.

- Primary health care workers, nurses, and physicians play an important role in detecting, diagnosing, and treating hypertension and other conditions that increase stroke risk, and in ensuring compliance with treatment. Key resources such as stroke units in major hospitals, rehabilitation facilities, and post-stroke community support programs may serve a minority of patients, but promote the development and introduction of appropriate, cost-effective methods and technology for stroke prevention, treatment, and rehabilitation.

10

Stroke

DEFINITION

A stroke occurs when blood vessels in the brain rupture or become occluded. Deficits resulting from stroke are usually maximal at onset (rather than steadily worsening, like the symptoms of a brain tumor), last more than 24 hours, and coincide with injury to the brain's vasculature as demonstrated by neurological and neuroimagining examination. Typical symptoms include muscular weakness, loss of sensation, problems with vision, and impaired speech. Depending on the location and severity of neuronal damage, additional symptoms, including loss of consciousness, may occur.

There are two main types of stroke: hemorrhagic and thrombotic (also known as ischemic). A hemorrhagic stroke may be caused by a ruptured cerebral blood vessel, a ruptured intracranial aneurysm, or an arterio-venous malformation leading to an intracerebral hemorrhage in or near the brain. (In this report, we do not address hemorrhage from arterial aneurysms and arterio-venous malformations, as their epidemiology differs significantly from that of other types of stroke). A thrombotic stroke results from the occlusion of one or more cerebral blood vessels. A thrombus may form directly on a diseased small vessel, or a large-vessel atherosclerotic plaque may embolize and block a smaller cerebral artery.[1]

A temporary interruption of the blood supply to a region of the brain, called a transient ischemic attack (TIA), usually results from narrowing of the carotid arteries due to plaque accumulation (carotid stenosis). Patients with TIAs experience a sudden onset of stroke symptoms and a focal loss of brain function lasting less than 24 hours. Studies from the United States and Europe indicate that within 2 to 5 years of their first TIA, between 8 and 33 percent of patients go on to have a full stroke.[2]

SCOPE OF THE PROBLEM

Mortality

Stroke is a leading cause of disability and mortality throughout the world.[3,4] According to the World Health Organization (WHO), stroke kills approximately 4.6 million people (9 percent of all deaths) each year, and ranks as the second most common cause of mortality worldwide. The 1996 *Global Burden of Disease* study revealed that cardiac and cerebral vascular diseases have surpassed infectious and parasitic diseases to become the leading causes of death in the developing world, India and sub-Saharan Africa excepted.[5] In the People's Republic of China (PRC) alone, more than 1 million people die from stroke each year—three times the number of those who die from ischemic heart disease in that country.[6]

Among men and women aged 30–69, cardiac and cerebral vascular diseases cause three times as many deaths worldwide as infectious and parasitic diseases.[3] This age group generally comprises the most economically productive members of the workforce, a situation that serves to amplify the toll of death and disability associated with stroke and related disorders.[2,7] In South Africa, for example, stroke accounts for between 8 and 10 percent of all reported deaths and 7.5 percent of deaths among people of prime working age, 25 to 64 years old.[8]

Table 10-1 lists several additional reports describing stroke mortality in diverse populations. While the wide range of mortality rates shown may to some extent reflect population differences in exposure to risk factors for stroke (as discussed further below), the variation probably results as well from methodological differences among studies.[9] For example, in sub-Saharan Africa, most data on stroke mortality have been hospital-based, although the majority of stroke deaths in that region are thought to occur at home.[10] Box 10-1 describes an attempt to take this situation into account and produce more accurate measures of stroke mortality in urban and rural Tanzania.

Some studies in developing countries have found significant geographic [11] and ethnic [12,13] variations in stroke mortality within the same nation.[14,15] Other researchers, however, point out that such results need to be interpreted with caution as no standards exist for classifying ethnic groups.[16] Comparative data for more than 30 countries from 1950 to 1990 show increasing mortality from stroke in Eastern Europe, contrasting with declines seen in the United States; Europe; and Argentina, Chile, Uruguay, and Venezuela.[17]

Social and Economic Costs

In addition to causing early death, stroke results in significant nonfatal illness and disability. In the 1996 *Global Burden of Disease* study, stroke ranked as the sixth leading cause of lost years of healthy life and was responsible for about 2.4 percent of disability-adjusted life years (DALYs) worldwide.[5] Projections for 2020 place cerebrovascular disease—a more general term that describes any abnormality

BOX 10-1 Stroke Mortality in Urban and Rural Tanzania

Measuring stroke mortality in sub-Saharan Africa presents numerous problems. General mortality rates in this region are not well known because of the lack of reliable death certification systems, and few data are available on cerebrovascular disease or its risk factors. Community-based research in developed countries indicates that many people die of a first stroke before reaching a hospital, a scenario that appears even likelier to occur in Africa. A recent study by Walker and co-workers attempted to circumvent these problems through the use of key informants and so-called verbal autopsies in three contrasting regions of Tanzania, with a total population of more than 300,000. The three surveillance areas were urban Dar-es-Salaam; Hai district, a relatively prosperous rural area; and Morogoro district, an impoverished rural area.

Over a 3-year period, key informants provided mortality information for an annual or semiannual census. For each reported death, clinical officers identified the cause through the use of a standard questionnaire presented to family members of the deceased; the results were coded by physicians and further validated through a variety of measures. The study determined age-specific stroke mortality rates for men and women in the three areas, compared with 1993 rates for England and Wales. Stroke mortality rates for each of the Tanzanian communities were higher than rates in England and Wales for all age bands up to 65 years. The total number of adults dying from stroke in Tanzania is low in comparison with similar figures from other developing countries, however, since only about 6 percent of the Tanzanian population is older than 65. It appears likely that as increasing numbers of people in sub-Saharan Africa survive to old age, there will be a significant increase in mortality due to stroke.

Source: [10]

TABLE 10-1 Stroke Mortality: Selected Studies

Country	Population	Method	Rates (per 100,000)
China (PRC) [18]	Urban and rural (29 provinces, 5,800,000)	Door-to-door survey with follow-up neurological examination	77 (crude) 81 (age-adjusted)
China (PRC) [6]	Rural (Inner Mong olia)	Door-to-door survey with follow-up neurological examination	45 (age-standardized)
China (PRC) [6]	Rural (Tibet)	Door-to-door survey with follow-up neurological examination	370 (age-standardized)
Mexico [19]	Urban and rural; multiple sites in Mexico	Population-based; epid e-miological surveillance data from hospital records and surveys	25 (crude)
Philippines [20]	Urban and rural	Vital statistics records from ministry of health, 1963-76	32
Singapore [21]	Urban and rural	Population-based; annual death registries, 1970–1994	50–60 (crude) 59 (age-standardized)
South Africa [22]	Rural; 35 years and older (932 deaths)	Community-based study; census, death records, and verbal auto psies	127 (over 35 years) 80 (35 to 64 years) 338 (over 64 years)
Tanzania [10]	Three regions (urban poor and prosperous rural); 307,820 popul a-tion (181,888 aged 15 or older)	Death and hospital records confirmed with verbal autopsies	95–420 for men, 55–317 for women (age-adjusted; 15 years and older); 35–65 for men, 27–88 for women (age-adjusted; 15–64 years)
Venezuela [23]	All ages	Ministry of health records	30
Vietnam [24]	Three regions (Ho Chi Minh City and two rural areas) with a total population of 52, 649	Door-to-Door survey with follow up examination	131 (age-adjusted)

of the brain resulting from blood vessel pathologies—fifth among the causes of disease burden as measured in DALYs for developing countries, and fourth worldwide.[25]

The extensive and intensive care frequently required by stroke victims places disproportionate demands on limited resources for health care in many developing countries.[26] For example, in one Zambian bush hospital during a 6-month period, stroke patients comprised less than 5 percent of total admissions but consumed 14 percent of all intensive care unit bed days.[27]

When a person dies or becomes disabled as a result of stroke, the negative repercussions of that event extend beyond the victim's family to the community, the nation, and the global economy. The death of an adult family member can have a devastating impact on the household. Caring for a family member disabled by stroke can harm the caregiver's own health, productivity, and ability to earn money.[28] The resulting losses in production, earnings, investment, and consumption affect local, regional, national, and global economies. Among many developed-country populations, 0.2 percent suffer a stroke each year. Of those afflicted, one-third remain permanently disabled, and one-third make a reasonable recovery. The two-thirds who do not die form a large pool (about 1 percent of the population) of stroke survivors, of whom at least half are disabled, making stroke the most important single cause of severe disability among people living in their homes.[29] Unfortunately, such studies have not attempted to assess or document the social and economic costs of stroke in developing countries, where more than two-thirds of all strokes are thought to occur.[9]

The social and economic costs of stroke in developing countries are expected to persist—and probably increase—over the next two decades.[30] The following factors are most frequently cited to explain this trend [31]:

• Reductions in infant and childhood mortality, allowing greater proportions of people in developing countries to survive beyond age 64, when 75 percent of all strokes occur.[2,9,30]

• The growing adoption of behaviors and lifestyles known to elevate stroke risk, such as tobacco use and high saturated fat intake, that can lead to hypertension, obesity, and diabetes (see the discussion of risk factors below). For example, current predictions indicate that by 2020, 12 percent of all deaths and 9 percent of all DALYs will be attributable to tobacco alone; the vast majority of this increased burden is projected to arise in developing countries.[32,33]

• Although evidence from industrialized countries demonstrates that stroke and other vascular disorders can be significantly reduced through interventions at the individual, community, and national levels, this knowledge and experience have yet to be applied systematically among the populations of developing countries.[34,35]

• There is a lack of awareness of cost-effective options for reducing the impact of stroke, as well as concern in some quarters that such investments may detract from efforts to control communicable diseases and to promote maternal, child, and reproductive health.[30]

Along with the above factors, which influenced the rise of stroke and other cardiovascular and cerebrovascular diseases in developed countries and are now becoming prominent in the developing world, there appear to be additional factors specific to developing populations that could exacerbate the pending epidemic of these diseases. For example, researchers have documented relatively high rates of obesity, hypertension, glucose intolerance, and ischemic heart disease—all risk factors for stroke—among adults whose growth was stunted during childhood. Among populations where food has been historically scarce, "thrifty genes" appear to predispose bearers to obesity and diabetes when food is plentiful.[30]

The seriousness of the threat posed by cerebro- and cardiovascular disease must be clearly demonstrated to the governments of developing countries. Stroke deserves particular attention as a preventable and treatable illness with profound medical, economic, and social consequences. Confronting the epidemic of stroke that threatens developing countries will require a better understanding of the origins of the disease, prediction of its magnitude, and timely implementation of preventive and case-management strategies.[30]

PREVALENCE AND INCIDENCE

Prevalence and incidence rates for stroke vary dramatically from one population to another. The reasons for this heterogeneity are not completely understood and are currently being explored in several large-scale epidemiological studies. Three broad sets of factors have been proposed as likely explanations for differences in the prevalence and incidence of stroke [2]:

• The stage of economic development, which appears to play a role not only in the prevalence and incidence figures for a given geographic region, but also in the specific type of stroke present.

• Differences in behavior and lifestyle that expose populations to varying types and degrees of risk factors, such as smoking, physical inactivity, obesity, ethanol use and abuse, and high sodium and saturated fat intake.

• Differences in hereditary predisposition to cerebral and cardiovascular diseases. Although the results of research to determine specific genetic risk factors for stroke have been inconclusive, epidemiological data suggest the existence of significant differences in the cause, type, and prevalence of stroke among different ethnic populations.[36] Genetic studies in diverse populations could provide a new perspective on the basic pathogenic mechanisms underlying the vascular disease process.

Developing countries have recently begun to join the developed world in experiencing the so-called epidemiological transition of diseases. Control of infectious and parasitic diseases, along with improvements in nutrition, have lengthened the average life span in many parts of the world. As a result, the spectrum of disease is shifting away from communicable diseases and perinatal and nutritional disorders to predominantly noncommunicable diseases, most notably cardiovascular disease.[37,38] Early in the epidemiological transition, most strokes tend to be hemorrhagic. Hypertension is an important risk factor for this type of stroke, which often occurs in people with low blood cholesterol levels. As the transition progresses, thrombotic strokes account for an increasing fraction of mortality, and ultimately become the most prevalent stroke type.[2]

During the 1980s, WHO undertook a major international effort to monitor stroke prevalence and incidence in 10 countries of Asia and Europe: the Monitoring of Trends and Determinants in Cardiovascular Disease (MONICA) Project.[3,39] Unfortunately, neither Latin American nor African countries were studied. Despite this limitation, the MONICA Project, through the use of uniform and statistically valid procedures, provided comparisons across populations in areas as different as Novosibirsk in the Russian Federation and Fruili in Italy. In the ideal, community-based settings in which MONICA was conducted, overall stroke occurrence and mortality rates were found to be twice as high among men than women, and higher in Finland, Lithuania, the Russian Federation, and the PRC than in western and central Europe.

MONICA populations were defined as all residents of the study areas according to geographic and administrative boundaries. Stroke events were identified through standard protocols, and cases were coded according to the *International Classification of Diseases* (*ICD*). Death certificates provided the major source of data on stroke mortality; hospitalized cases were identified from admission lists, discharge diagnoses, and other available medical record information. While considerable effort was made to ensure the quality of the data, researchers have noted some discrepancies, as well as a general need to interpret multinational comparisons of stroke statistics with caution.[4]

Prevalence

Table 10-2 shows the broad range of stroke prevalence reported in studies conducted throughout the developing and developed worlds. Similar variation in stroke prevalence has also been reported within single countries. In India, for example, neuroepidemiological data on stroke collected over the past 30 years have revealed prevalence rates as low as 44 in rural areas and as high as 842 per 100,000, among the urban Parsi community in Bombay.[40] Studies conducted across many regions of India indicate that stroke accounts for 2 percent of hospital registrations, 1.5 percent of medical registrations, and 9 to 30 percent of neurological admissions.[41–44]

Reliable studies of stroke prevalence would be particularly valuable in estimating the impact of the disease since, as noted above, many stroke patients survive with some disability for many years. However, most studies on stroke prevalence in developing countries have been based on hospital records, and thus describe only those patients—a minority in many low-income communities—who received hospital treament. Community-based research, while difficult to perform in developing countries, represents the best means of obtaining accurate estimates of stroke prevalence—information that could be used not only for health care planning, but also for clues to risk factors, preventive strategies, and treatments.[22,45] Two examples of the few existing studies of this type were conducted in the Hai district of Northern Tanzania [22] and the island of Kinmen in the Republic of China (Taiwan).[45] Although the focus of each study was quite different, both employed door-to-door surveys, followed by neurological examination to confirm diagnoses.

Incidence

As is the case with studies of stroke mortality and prevalence, reports of stroke incidence rates indicate wide variation throughout the developing world (see Table 10-3). Rates of 200 per 100,000 or higher have been reported in several Asian countries [6, 24,26] and in Russia,[47] while stroke appears to be nonexistant in Kitava, New Guinea.[48] Researchers have offered a variety of explanations for low stroke incidence, including young populations, lack of influence of Western diets, low diastolic blood pressure, and low cholesterol levels.[49,50] A substantial decrease in stroke mortality noted over recent years in the United States remains unexplained, but appears to be due to individual lifestyle modifications, as well as improvements in the general environment and in medical care.[51]

Several studies have revealed high rates of stroke incidence among young people in low-income countries as compared with the developed world. In India, for example, an analysis of the Stroke Registry established at NIMHANS showed that 20 percent of strokes occurred in people younger than age 40. Stroke among children, while comparatively rare relative to adults, may prove more common among developing populations prone to sickle cell anemia, an apparent risk factor for stroke,[52] as well as other conditions discussed below.

Incidence studies have also revealed variation in the occurrence of the two types of stroke among different populations in the developing world. In several West African countries, approximately two-thirds of all stroke cases are ischemic, and one-third are hemorrhagic.[53–56] In Iran, two-thirds of strokes were found to be ischemic in origin.[57] In the PRC, hemorrhagic stroke is as common as ischemic. Consistently, 30 percent of stroke cases are hemorrhagic in Singapore, Malaysia, Thailand, Indonesia, Hong Kong, the Philippines, Taiwan, and South Korea.[58,59]

Comparing stroke incidence in different countries and observing incidence trends in specific populations may increase our understanding of the disease. However, such comparisons cannot be made until studies of stroke incidence use the same definitions, methods, and mode of data presentation. While MONICA and other recent studies have begun to address this problem in some parts of the world, the profound lack of comparable incidence data for Africa, Asia, and South America largely excludes the developing world from such analyses.[60,61]

TABLE 10-2 Stroke Prevelance: Selected Studies

Country	Population	Method	Rate (per 100,000)
China (PRC) [18]	Urban and rural sites (5,800,000)	Door-to-door survey with follow-up neurological examination	260 (age-adjusted) 246 (crude)
Colombia [62]	Urban (13,588)	Door-to-door survey	559
Ecuador [63]	Rural (1,113)	Door-to-door survey; questionnaire; neurological screening examina tion	360
Ethiopia [64]	Rural (60,820)	Door-to-door survey	15 (disability due to stroke only)
India [40]	Urban; Parsis living in Bombay (14,010)	Detailed neuro-epidemiological study	842
India [65]	Rural; Kashmir	House-to-house census	143
Nigeria [66]	Rural (18,594)	Questionnaire; examination	58
Peru [67]	Rural (3,246)	Door-to-door survey	647
Saudi Arabia [68]	Hospital-based (500)	Review of records; diagn o-sis confirmed by com - puted tomography	186
Taiwan (ROC) [45]	3,915 residents of the islet of Kinmen, age 50 and over	Door-to door interview; neurological examination of all partici pants	2,450 (lifetime prevalence)
Tanzania [10]	Rural; Hai District 148,135 (82,152 age 15 and over)	House-to-house census, interview, examina tion	73 (127 age 15 and over)
Tunisia [69]	Urban (34,874)	Community-based survey; follow-up co ntrol survey	140
Vietnam [24]	Three regions (Ho Chi Minh City and two rural areas) with a total population of 52, 649	Door-to-door survey with follow-up neurological examination	608 (age-adjusted)

TABLE 10-3 Stroke Incidence: Selected Studies

Country	Population	Method	Rate (per 100,000)
China (PRC) [18]	5,800,000	Door-to-door survey with follow-up neurological examination	116 (standardized to world populations) 110 (crude)
Singapore [70]	Urban and rural (5,920)	Cohort study examining three previous cross-sectional surveys and longitudinal follow-up from national registry data	Chinese: 230 (male); 120 (female) Malay: 160 (male); 280 (female) Indian: 220 (male); 150 (female)
Iran [57]			44 (men) 59 (women)
Kuwait [49]	Urban	Hospital and primary care clinic registries with clinical evaluation	28 (crude) 145 (age-adjusted)
Libya [71]	Benghazi (52,000)		63
Nigeria [72]	Urban (Ibadan)	Hospital-based; stroke registry	74.8 (standardized to world population)
Papua New Guinea [50]	Kitava Island; traditional horticulturalists uninfluenced by Western diets (220)	Cardiovascular and neurological screening examinations	0
Russia [73]	Novosibirsk (150,000)	Population-based; stroke registry	232
Saudi Arabia [74]	545,000	Stroke registry (1989–93)	30 (crude); 126 (standardized to 1976 U.S. population)
Taiwan (ROC) [75]	3,915 residents of the islet of Kinmen, age 50 and over	Door-to door interview; neurological examination of all participants	527
Tunisia [76]	Tunis	Stroke registry	192 (age-adjusted, 45 years and older)
Vietnam [24]	Three regions (Ho Chi Minh City and two rural areas) with a total population of 52,649	Door-to-door survey with follow-up neurological examination	250 (age-adjusted)
Zimbabwe [77]	Urban (black residents of Harare; total population 887,768)	Prospective community-based	68 (standardized to world population); 30.7 (crude)

Recommendation 10-1. Data collection should be improved to provide accurate information about stroke mortality, morbidity, incidence, prevalence, and mechanisms in developing countries using culturally sensitive tools and diagnostic techniques. Pathological studies of stroke should be conducted to determine the relative prevalence of various stroke subtypes among several diverse representative populations in developing countries. This research would be greatly enhanced if conducted in collaboration with research centers in high-income countries utilizing other existing data and research mechanisms.

RISK FACTORS

The term "risk factor" was coined by investigators in the Framingham Heart Study, one of the largest, longest-running, and best-known epidemiological studies of its kind. Considerable data on risk factors for stroke have come from the 850 participants who have experienced a stroke since the U.S. study began in 1950.[78] While several of the predominant modifiable risk factors for stroke identified in the Framingham study—most notably hypertension, diabetes, and smoking—appear generalizable to many populations, data documenting the relative impact of these factors in developing countries are sparse. This represents fertile ground for future epidemiological studies, as does the possibility that new stroke risk factors of particular significance in developing countries might be identified (for example, infectious agents, nutritional factors, or developmental syndromes that rarely occur in developed countries).[30] At present, the risk factors described in this section represent the most promising targets for preventing and treating stroke in the developing world. Additional factors associated with stroke outcome are subsequently discussed.

Physiological

Hypertension

The foremost risk factor for stroke throughout the industrialized world, hypertension may play an even greater role in causing stroke in low-income communities. Epidemiological studies among populations of East Asia, including the PRC [79] and Africa [80,81], indicate that controlling elevated blood pressure in these populations could prevent proportionately more strokes than equivalent measures in Western populations.[44] The reasons for the apparently stronger influence of hypertension on strokes among East Asian and black African populations remain to be identified, but may include both genetic and environmental effects, as well as longer exposure to untreated conditions of hypertension. Both populations were found to suffer a far higher proportion of hemorrhagic strokes as compared with Western populations.

Hypertension increased the risk of stroke threefold among both men and women in every age group monitored in the Framingham study.[82] A statistical overview of prospective epidemiological studies of middle-aged individuals with no previous history of vascular disease, examining the relationship between diastolic blood pressure and stroke, showed a doubling of the risk of stroke for every 7.5 (mm Hg) rise in blood pressure.[83] Similarly, among East Asians, projections indicate that a population-wide reduction in diastolic blood pressure of 3mm Hg would reduce stroke mortality by one-third.[79] In the PRC, carefully conducted epidemiological studies revealed a north–south gradient in stroke mortality and incidence that was shown to be due mainly to differences in the prevalence of hypertension, which was higher in the northern provinces.[6] The highest prevalence of hypertension was 22.3 percent in the province of Tibet, and the lowest was 4.8 percent in the province of Qinghai. A 10 percent higher prevalence of hypertension was associated with a 2.8-fold higher incidence of stroke, even after adjustment for differences in prevalence of cigarette smoking and alcohol consumption.[6,46]

Hypertension is a major public health problem in African countries, where it may affect up to 10 percent of the population and contributes to coronary heart disease, as well as to hemorrhagic and thrombotic stroke. Studies from Nigeria, Ivory Coast, and Zimbabwe found hypertension to be the main risk factor for both ischemic and hemorrhagic stroke.[22,72,77] The condition frequently goes unrecognized, however, in part because many African health care providers lack reliable equipment for measuring blood pressure.[27]

The results of controlled clinical trials of treatments for hypertension in developed populations may inform research in the developing world. Clinical studies in developed populations indicate that blood pressures of less than 140/83 mm Hg are optimal for stroke prevention. Therefore, the goal of antihypertensive therapy should be to normalize rather than just reduce blood pressure.[84] Additionally, recent studies and resulting data from both developed and developing countries indicate that high systolic blood pressure is equally or more important, especially in older adults (over age 65), as a predictor for stroke.[85–90] Antihypertensive therapy for systolic hypertension will be important for reducing the risk of stroke in elderly populations. Antihypertensive therapy has been found to reduce the risk of stroke by about 42 percent in people younger than age 65 suffering from high blood pressure.[88] Unfortunately, studies of patients who received antihypertenstion medication through urban clinics in both South Africa [89] and Saudi Arabia [91] indicate that many patients who receive the medication use it incorrectly, and few recognize that uncontrolled hypertension can lead to stroke.

Diabetes

Several studies in developed countries—notably the Framingham study [82] and the Honolulu Heart Study [92]—have documented diabetes as a risk factor for stroke. The Framingham study found a 10 percent increase in risk for having a stroke among males with diabetes; this proportion rose to over 20 percent when the patient was also hypertensive.[82] In Africa, studies from Senegal, Ivory Coast, Tunisia, and Nigeria link diabetes mellitus with stroke in 2–27 percent of cases.[56,72,93] A community-based study in rural and urban areas of Tanzania revealed that stroke accounted for approximately one-third of all deaths among those with diabetes. The researchers also discovered that, although the prevalence of diabetes in Tanzania was low in comparison with developed countries, mortality rates attributed to diabetes were on a par with those in the United States.[94] This result suggests that untreated diabetes, like untreated hypertension, represents a major contributor to stroke mortality in the developing world. Moreover, the number of adults with diabetes is projected to rise from 135 million in 1995 to 300 million in 2025, with 75 percent of those affected being expected to reside in developing countries.[2] If this increased prevalence of diabetes is not met with a comcomitant increase in access to medication, many of those affected will be at significantly increased risk for stroke.

Cardiac Disease

Cardiac disease has been shown to be a major predisposing factor for stroke among elderly people in developed countries, and is expected to rise in prominence in developing countries as increasing numbers of people reach old age. Most participants in the Framingham study who suffered stroke were found to have such comorbid conditions as congestive heart failure, coronary artery disease, or atrial fibrillation; the last condition appeared most significant among elderly populations, where it was found to account for approximately 30 percent of all strokes.[95]

In developing countries, cardiac diseases are also recognized risk factors for stroke; however, there are variations in the type of cardiac disease and the affected age groups. [96] Though not common in developed countries, rheumatic heart disease (and causal rheumatic fever) is especially predominant in sub-Saharan Africa and rural India, affecting mainly those aged 5–15. Rheumatic heart disease is frequently a risk factor for stroke in both children and adults who suffer the chronic and deteriorating affects of that disease.[97–100] A recent study of hospitalized black South African stroke patients (mean age 55 for men, 60 for women) found coronary artery disease to be much more prevalent than had previously been reported in similar groups, as well as in the general nonstroke black population. Such patients, the researchers concluded, may have a risk for coronary artery disease similar to that of white South Africans.[101] The difference in findings between this South African study and other studies conducted in Africa may be explained by two factors: (1) a lack of accurate data due to the absence of adequate data collection tools and proper diagnosis, and (2) increasing rates of coronary artery disease due to the demographic transition occurring in many African countries.[102,103] The prevalence of coronary artery disease in India and China continues to increase.[104–107]

Elevated Serum Cholesterol

Although elevated serum cholesterol is a well-documented risk factor for ischemic heart disease, which in turn is a risk factor for thrombotic stroke, several studies in developed countries have failed to demonstrate a relationship between cholesterol levels and stroke risk. The Honolulu Heart Study indicated that elevated serum cholesterol predicts a higher stroke rate when stroke is assessed 15 years after the cholesterol measurement.[108] Interestingly, clinical studies indicate that statins, cholesterol-lowering agents, reduce stroke risk by 30 percent, although this result may be due to other effects of these drugs, such as reduction of smooth muscle proliferation, reduction of inflammation, and restoration of impaired endothelial function.[109,110]

Few researchers have examined the relationship between stroke and serum cholesterol in developing countries. Among East Asians, elevated cholesterol appears to be a far less potent risk factor for stroke than hypertension. In these populations, elevated serum cholesterol appears to influence primarily stroke type, rather than occurrence.[79] Such a relationship might also be expected to occur in populations that experience relatively high rates of hemorrhagic stroke.

Elevated Serum Homocysteine

A recent study found that elevated serum homocysteine (15.4 mmol/liter or more) is associated with a fourfold increase in stroke risk among men.[111] Several recent studies indicate that elevated serum homocysteine is a risk factor for stroke in both adults and children.[112–115] Studies indicate that a deficiency of B-complex vitamins is attributable to elevated serum homocysteine.[111,116–119] How chronic, low-grade, or severe malnutrition and/or hypovitaminosis relate to the homocysteine/stroke issue is not known presently, but has significant implications for both children and adults in developing countries. Findings on this relationship would indicate the potential for preventing stroke by treatment with vitamins B6, B12, and folic acid.[111,120,121] More data are needed from developing countries to establish the likely causal relationships among vitamin deficiency, elevated levels of serum homocysteine, and the occurrence of stroke in these settings.

HIV/AIDS

Several clinical and autopsy studies have suggested an increase in stroke among those with HIV/AIDS. These studies, however, were conducted in populations with confounding factors, such as drug abuse and coexistent opportunistic infection.[122–126] A retrospective case-controlled study of young (below age 50) black African stroke patients in the KwaZulu Natal Province of South Africa found a higher rate of large-vessel stroke in patients who had HIV.[127] A recent study in Thailand has also shown stroke in children to be an indicator of undiagnosed HIV infection.[128]

Postpartum Cerebral Venous Thrombosis

Studies in both developed and developing countries indicate that postpartum cerebral venous thrombosis (CVT) is a risk factor for stroke.[129–132] In developed countries, postpartum (or puerperium) CVT accounts for 5 to 20 percent of all cases of CVT, but the figure in developing countries is estimated to be as high as 60 percent.[131–133] In developing countries, several risk factors, including low nutritional status, anemia, and dehydration resulting from the cultural practice of restraining fluids during the first days after delivery, are thought to account for this trend.[43,133] Postpartum CVT occurs frequently among the poorest Indian women; nearly 30 percent of those affected die from the disorder.[43,134] The administration of properly dosed anticoagulants immediately following the occurrence of CVT-induced stroke can reduce mortality to less than 20 percent and often reverses most of the initial disabling conditions (motor, vision, speech impairment).[129,130]

Risk Factors for Stroke in Children

As noted earlier, stroke in children is uncommon worldwide, but may occur at higher levels in some developing communities as a result of the presence of several known and suspected risk factors, including sickle cell disease, congenital heart disease, intracranial infections, and metabolic disorders.[43,52,135–137] Nearly one-third of the strokes suffered by a group of 35 Cameroonian children between 5 months and 15 years of age were attributable to sickle-cell disease; other identified risk factors included heart disease, cerebral malaria, and meningitis.[138]

Behavioral

Cigarette Smoking

Findings on the effect of cigarette smoking as a contributor to stroke have been variable in some populations. However, many studies have found an association between cigarette smoking and stroke risk, either directly or through smoking-related increases in blood pressure.[139–143] In the Framingham study, heavy smokers (> 40 cigarettes/day) were found to have a relatively high risk of stroke—twice that of light smokers (< 10 cigarettes/day). Participants (both men and women of all ages) who quit smoking, however, appeared to revert to risk levels near those of nonsmokers within 2 to 4 years.[141]

Cigarette smoking may prove an especially important risk factor for stroke in developing countries,[142] where nearly three-quarters of the more than 1 billion people who use tobacco regularly currently reside.[143] Moreover, the annual tobacco-related death toll in developing countries is predicted to triple by 2030, resulting in a yearly loss of 10 billion lives.[34] Epidemiologists already estimate that the rate of smoking among blacks in South Africa, for example, has doubled over the past 10 years, contributing to an increased risk of stroke in that population.[89]

Diet

Dietary change represents an important component of the epidemiological transition [30]. Increased consumption of foods high in saturated fat, cholesterol, and salt in developing populations is expected to produce concomitant increases in hypertension, obesity, and diabetes, all of which contribute to stroke risk.[144]

Alcohol Abuse

Alcohol has been reported to have a dose-dependent effect on the risk of hemorrhagic stroke.[145–148] Some studies have indicated that low to moderate levels of alcohol consumption may actually offer some protection against ischemic stroke,[147,149] while others [150,151] have found no such benefit. A prospective study of Chinese men aged 45 to 64 found an association between the consumption of small amounts of alcohol and lower overall mortality, including death from ischemic heart disease, but no beneficial effect of alcohol on death due to stroke; a study of elderly Taiwanese reached a similar conclusion.[152,153] The differing results of these studies may be influenced by genetic predisposition among different ethnic groups, indicating a need for more research on the relationship between moderate alcohol consumption and risk for ischemic stroke.

Physical Inactivity

The evidence is not conclusive on the role played by exercise in preventing stroke. Previous studies have found either no or a positive effect of exercise.[154–156] In the Framingham study, physical activity was found to be negatively correlated with stroke risk among men. Studies have shown that those who maintained moderate or high levels of exercise had a lower stroke risk than those who were inactive.[157, 158] Insofar as even moderate levels of exercise contribute to maintaining normal weight, controlling diabetes, and improving cardiovascular health, it can be surmised to serve as a preventive against other risk factors.[159, 160]

The remarkable reduction in stroke mortality achieved in several Western countries since 1970 suggests that population-wide efforts to educate people about causes and risk factors for stroke and other cardio- and cerebrovascular diseases are effective in reducing the impact of these disorders.[51] The concept of stroke as a serious condition may be highlighted at the public level using terms such as "brain attack," applied in the same context as heart attack. One such campaign was recently carried out in India (March 2000) as part of Brain

Awareness Week. The campaign was conducted by neurologists and featured a special education program in neurosciences for public audiences, as well as high school and college students. Presentations given on stroke introduced the concept of brain attack to emphasize the significant risk posed by stroke to overall health and functioning.[161] Indian medical professionals and government officials, as well as those from other developing countries, have begun to recognize that the evidence on stroke clearly indicates an impending public health disaster. Therefore, as a first step toward blunting the effects of these trends, the committee makes the following recommendation.

> **Recommendation 10-2. Public education strategies to raise awareness of stroke and of environmental and behavioral risk factors for the disease should be designed and implemented in developing countries by national public health agencies and community-level health care services. These strategies should be accompanied by urgent primary health care initiatives (see Recommendations 10-8 and 10-9) focused on the early detection and treatment of hypertension, diabetes, and other known risk factors for stroke.**

Although the available scientific evidence suggests that most of the risk factors for stroke identified for industrialized countries are also applicable to developing countries, the special genetic and environmental conditions prevalent in Africa, Asia, and Latin America call for specific case-control studies on risk factors for stroke among these populations. The scientific knowledge gained from these studies could be applicable to African-, Hispanic-, and Asian-American populations that at present are at higher risk of stroke morbidity and mortality in the United States.[95,162] The Countrywide Integrated Noncommunicable Diseases Intervention (CINDI) Program and Conjunto de Acciones para la Reduccion Multifactorial de las Enfermedades No Transmisibles (CARMEN) protocols could serve as a basis for conducting such studies in African, Asian, and Latin American countries.

> **Recommendation 10-3. Case-control studies should be designed and conducted to assess risk factors for stroke in Africa, Asia, and Latin America. To make the findings of this research widely available and inform efforts for ethnic populations worldwide, developing countries should become involved in existing international networks, such as the MONICA and CARMEN strategies sponsored by WHO and the Pan-American Health Organization (PAHO), respectively.**

Factors Affecting Course and Outcome

Extensive studies of stroke outcome have been limited largely to the developed world, but may be somewhat generalizable to developing populations as well. Overall, these studies indicate that stroke outcome depends primarily on the type of stroke and the presence of comorbid conditions.[36,113,145] Stroke outcomes are commonly described using the terminology of the National Institutes of Health (NIH) Stroke Scale.[163,164]

Stroke worsening occurs most frequently following large-vessel strokes. Early worsening must be distinguished from conditions such as cerebral edema, mass effect, hemorrhagic transformation, and metabolic disturbances.[164]

Stroke recurrence most frequently follows large-vessel and atherosclerotic strokes. The risk of recurrence has been found to be one to four percent in the first 30 days after a stroke, increasing to between 8 and 25 percent at 1 year (depending on stroke subtype and comorbidity), and climbing to 20 to 45 percent at 5 years.[165] Additional predictors of recurrence include elevated blood glucose, hypertension, age, coronary artery disease, atrial fibrillation, congestive heart failure, prior transient ischemic attacks, a low albumin/globulin ratio, and heavy alcohol consumption. Congestive heart failure also appears to be a strong predictor of stroke recurrence, and has been associated with about a 26 percent risk of recurrence at 3 years. Hyperglycemia is associated with about a 17 percent risk of 3-year recurrence.[164,165]

Functional disability is an approximate measure of a stroke's effect on a patient's daily activities. One simple scale, developed in France, classifies patients into four groups: Class 1, no sequelae, with the patient being able to return to previous work activities; Class 2, functional sequeleae, where the patient is autonomous but slightly impaired; Class 3, important sequelae, denoting severe impairment; and Class 4, bedridden.[166]

Quality of life reflects a combination of a patient's clinical status with social and psychological aspects of health. After a stroke, patients in developed countries are frequently unable to return to work, unwilling or unable to continue their rehabilitation once discharged from the hospital, and clinically depressed.[167] Many experience sexual dysfunction and stressful relationships and demonstrate abnormal social behavior.

Morbidity due to stroke is usually assessed as 30-day case fatality, which is greatest after intracerebral hemorrhage (48–82 percent) and lowest after ischemic infarct (8–15 percent). About 8 percent of patients experiencing ischemic strokes die within 30 days, about 21 percent within 1 year, 31 percent within 3 years, and 44 percent within 5 years. Approximately half of early deaths are attributable to the stroke itself, whereas recurrent stroke and cardiac disease have a greater impact on long-term mortality.[165] Large-volume strokes, decreased level of consciousness, and major basilar or hemispheric infarcts are associated with the highest case fatality, whereas patients with lacunar syndromes have the highest survival rates. Cardioembolic stroke is associated with about 15 percent of 30-day mortality, but with the worst long-term mortality.[166] Other predictors for long-term mortality due to stroke are age, cardiac disease, congestive heart failure, and elevated blood glucose.[167]

INTERVENTIONS

Prevention

Because of the high risk for death, long-term disability, and recurrence after a first stroke, prevention is key to reducing the public health impacts of cerebrovascular disease. Moreover, the relatively high costs and limited benefits of treatment and rehabilitation for stroke underscore the importance of efforts to prevent the disease in areas where health care resources are limited. Prevention strategies can be divided into three categories from the perspective of risk factors: (1) *primordial prevention* is directed toward the prevention of risk factors themselves; (2) *primary prevention* focuses on reducing the impact of existing risk factors; and (3) *secondary prevention* is directed toward early detection and management of existing clinical diseases (e.g., hypertension, diabetes, heart disease, and stroke itself).[2]

Primordial prevention tends to focus on entire populations. At this level, stroke prevention is best undertaken through a broad preventive health program for vascular disease that promotes a healthy lifestyle encompassing diet, exercise, and the avoidance of smoking and excess alcohol consumption.[8] Targeted campaigns may be directed at general, modifiable risk factors for cardio- and cerebrovascular disease, most notably smoking. Research indicates that community-wide education programs can result in a significant reduction in the prevalence of smoking and other cardiovascular risk factors and may be very cost-effective.[168] More specifically, in a randomized controlled trial, simple advice to give up smoking with a minimum of supportive counseling was found to reduce mortality from lung cancer and coronary heart disease, although the incidence of stroke was not analyzed separately.[169] Cost-effectiveness analyses demonstrate that tobacco-control campaigns cost US $20–70 per year of life saved.[2] Since smoking represents not only a significant modifiable risk factor for vascular disease, but also a growing drain on personal and public resources in developing countries, the committee makes the following recommendation.

Recommendation 10-4. Governments should develop, strengthen, and enforce legislation intended to reduce tobacco use. This could include tariffs or other programs designed to limit use of tobacco by raising its price, as well as legislation that protects nonsmokers from exposure to cigarette smoke in public places.

Primary prevention of stroke has been found effective in randomized trials in industrialized countries aimed at lowering stroke risk factors, such as high-fat, high-cholesterol, or high-sodium diets; hypertension; and cigarette smoking. As a first step toward undertaking similar efforts in developing countries, provisions must be made for the detection of conditions that represent risk factors for stroke at the level of primary care. This is particularly true of hypertension and diabetes, which frequently go undiagnosed in developing populations because of a lack of adequate medical services.[27]

Recommendation 10-5. Primary care providers in developing countries should be provided with the training and equipment necessary to conduct preventive monitoring of conditions that are known risk factors for stroke, including hypertension, diabetes, and coronary artery disease.

Secondary strategies for stroke prevention include treatment for conditions that are known risk factors for stroke, such as hypertension, diabetes, coronary artery disease, and TIAs, as well as measures to prevent stroke recurrence. Case-management strategies have been investigated extensively among patients with stroke. Recent projections from epidemiological data in the United States suggest that adequate control of hypertension, warfarin treatment for atrial fibrillation cases, and cessation of smoking could prevent more than half of the estimated 731,000 strokes that occur in the U.S. each year.[170] Other strategies that have been successful in industrialized countries involve sophisticated and expensive technologies, such as thrombolytic therapies, automated internal defibrillation, and cardiac surgery, that are unlikely to become available in developing countries in the near term.

On the other hand, several low-cost treatments for hypertension and other conditions are likely to significantly reduce the incidence and severity of stroke and stroke-related vascular disease in developing countries. These include low-dose thiazide, aspirin, and beta blockers (and, where costs permit, ACE inhibitors); sulfonylureas (with metformin if needed) for diabetes [171]; and low-cost statins for cholesterol control.[2] Indeed, it has been estimated that the relatively low-cost combination of aspirin and beta-blockers after acute myocardial infarction could prevent about 300,000 deaths due to ischemic heart disease and stroke in low- and middle-income countries in the year 2020 if coverage were increased from 30–40 percent to 85 percent of the patient population.[2,172] It will be important for health care personnel who administer and monitor antihypertensive drug treatments to be aware of the side effects of these drugs.

Hypertension deserves particular attention in developing countries because of its prominence as a risk factor for cardio- and cerebrovascular disease. Community-based hypertension control programs in rural Japan [173] and urban China [104] (see Box 10-2) have been shown to reduce stroke incidence, suggesting that similar programs would be both feasible and effective in many developing countries. Patient education should be a primary objective of such community-based programs, to ensure proper and continuous use of antihypertensive medication.[79,80] Sample guidelines for patient education at the primary care level, developed by the Hypertension Society of Southern Africa, appear in Box 10-3.

According to current guidelines, patients with a first cerebrovascular event due to cardioembolism should be treated with oral anticoagulants if there are no contraindications. Patients with atherothrombotic strokes should typically receive antiplatelet agents. For the best-studied agent, aspirin, the currently rec-

BOX 10-2 Stroke Prevention in Urban China

Stroke incidence has risen rapidly in the PRC over the past two decades, along with risk factors such as hypertension and smoking. Public understanding of healthy lifestyles appears to be poor; however, researchers have reason to believe that community-level efforts to reduce risk factors for stroke could be effective. Medical scientists from the Beijing Neurosurgical Institute, along with collaborators at the University of Washington, Seattle, established pilot intervention programs in seven Chinese cities to provide health education and treatment for hypertension, heart disease, and diabetes.

Beginning in May 1997, two geographically separated communities of approximately 10,000 people within each of the cities were selected as either intervention or control populations. Within each community, a cohort of 2,700 subjects age 35 or older and free of stroke were selected as subjects or controls for medical intervention. In the intervention community, subjects were treated for hypertension, diabetes, and heart disease as considered appropriate by their physicians, and a preventive education program was provided for all 10,000 residents.

After 3.5 years of intervention, the incidence rates for fatal and nonfatal stroke, as well as for ischemic and hemorrhagic stroke, were found to be significantly lower in the intervention cohort than in the control cohort. The sharp reduction in stroke incidence appeared to be due primarily to a blunting of the expected rise in hypertension as residents aged, as well as to earlier treatment of hypertension, especially borderline cases. Increased general health awareness and knowledge derived from health education may also have played a role in preventing some individuals from developing hypertension.

Source: [104]

ommended dose is 50–325 mg daily.[174] Other anticoagulant drugs require blood monitoring and standardization in dosing (which increases the overall cost of administration) to control adverse side effects, yet some may prove cost-effective in certain developing-country settings for the prevention of stroke recurrence or full stroke following a TIA. However, aspirin appears to be the more cost-effective option in many cases.[175]

Aspirin has been shown in clinical studies to reduce the relative risk of stroke or death by approximately 20 percent per year after a TIA or minor ischemic stroke.[168,176] This translates into an absolute benefit of 12 strokes prevented per 1000 patients treated for 1 year, at a cost of approximately one intracerebral hemorrhage. Recently, three other antiplatelet agents—ticlopidine, clopidogrel, and a combination of aspirin and extended-release dipyridamole—have been shown to be effective for stroke prevention. Ticlopidine and clopidogrel appear to be slightly more effective than aspirin in clinical trials, but they are also more

---

BOX 10-3   Education Guidelines for Patients with Hypertension

The following guidelines were developed by the Hypertension Society of Southern Africa, and endorsed by the Medical Association of South Africa and the Medical Research Council:

- Teach patients the distinction between having a risk factor (hypertension) and having a disease.
- Teach patients to understand hypertension and its consequences if not treated adequately.
- Inform patients of their blood pressure reading at every visit, and tell them whether it is controlled or otherwise.
- Teach patients to tell any medical practitioner they visit about their hypertension and what drugs they are taking, and encourage them to request a blood pressure measurement at each visit.
- Tell patients the name and dose of the drug(s) they are prescribed, the frequency of dosing, and the necessity of regular ongoing use. Ensure that patients know this at every visit.
- Provide reassurance as needed for patients with mild hypertension who have excess fear of stroke or other consequences of hypertension.

Source: [177]

---

expensive.[57,176] Cost comparisons, safety profiles, and availability will influence the choice of antiplatelet agent for patients in developing countries.

While drug combinations such as aspirin and beta-blockers may currently provide cost-effective prevention of stroke in emerging market economies, more expensive drugs, such as the cholesterol-lowering statins and ACE inhibitors, may not prove cost-effective for years to come. One means of increasing access to such useful but costly medications may be to negotiate pricing strategies and partnerships with pharmaceutical manufacturers (either individually or through collective agreements), which could supply a range of commonly prescribed medicines at reduced cost. For example, essential medicines for treating hypertension and hyperlipidemia could be offered in economical "vascular packages" that could be widely accessible.[2] Recognizing that the secondary prevention of hypertension, diabetes, and a variety of other comorbid conditions is key to stroke prevention, the committee makes the following recommendation.

> **Recommendation 10-6. Treatment, including essential medications, should be made available through primary care to all individuals with conditions such as hypertension, diabetes, and postpartum cerebral venous thrombosis that represent risk factors for stroke, as well as for those who have experienced TIAs. Medicines of proven cost-effectiveness should be used whenever possible; pricing strategies and partnerships should be undertaken to enable resource-limited developing countries to purchase costly essential medications.**

Treatment

Stroke is a particularly challenging condition to treat because of its sudden onset and the rapid tissue damage that ensues. Because of these limitations, the best option for managing stroke in developing countries is prevention, both of first stroke and of recurrence. A particularly thorny issue in the treatment of acute stroke is the need to diagnose stroke subtype, because existing treatments for ischemic stroke, such as aspirin, heparin, and recombinant tissueplasminogen activator (rtPA) (see below), can worsen the outcome of hemorrhagic stroke and vice versa.[8] Currently, the only reliable means of diagnosing stroke subtype is through the use of computed tomography (CT) brain scans, a rare option in developing countries.[15,178] Accurate, affordable clinical methods for diagnosing stroke subtype are thus urgently needed for use by the majority of the world's population.

The long search for a drug that can dissolve vascular obstruction and restore cerebral circulation following ischemic stroke appears to offer some promise with the success of rtPA in a clinical trial conducted by the National Institute of Neurological Disorders and Stroke. Patients suffering from an ischemic stroke who were treated with rtPA were significantly more likely to have minimal or no disability at 3 months after treatment than were those given placebos.[179] However, another large-scale study, conducted by the European Cooperative Acute Stroke Study (ECASS), did not show a significant benefit as compared with controls.[180] Although promising, not all countries have approved the use of rtPA, and further studies are necessary. For developing countries, there are additional limitations that may make this treatment option a lower priority, including (1) the need to begin treatment within 3 hours of stroke onset, which may limit use of rtPA where the technology is too distant and/or transportation is unavailable; (2) the limited availability of expensive CT scanning machines; (3) the limited availability and relatively high cost of rtPA; (4) the limited availability of special stroke teams with expertise in the use of the drug; (5) and the need to manage complications, especially the increased risk of hemorrhage.[181]

The above limitations apply to most of the available stroke treatment methods. These limitations point to areas in which additional resources for health spending would contribute to improvements in access to diagnostic tools, the availability of specialists who can interpret their results, and a better supply of cost-effective drug treatments for stroke.

Rehabilitation

The rehabilitation process has six major elements: (1) preventing, recognizing, and managing comorbid illnesses and medical complications; (2) providing training for maximum independence; (3) facilitating maximum psychosocial coping and adaptation by patient and family; (4) preventing secondary disability by promoting community reintegration, including resumption of home, family, recreational, and vocational activities; (5) enhancing quality of life in view of any residual disability; and (6) preventing recurrent stroke and other vascular conditions, such as myocardial infarction, that occur with increased frequency in patients with stroke.[182] Because depression and other mental disorders rank among the most prevalent and disabling consequences of strokes of all severity, mental health care represents an important component of stroke rehabilitation (see Chapter 10).[167,183,184]

No conclusive evidence demonstrates the cost-effectiveness of stroke rehabilitation in developed or developing countries. Where resources are limited, support for preventive efforts is a priority. However, if local communities have rehabilitation programs for other disabling conditions such as cerebral palsy or mental retardation, coordination and integration of stroke-related rehabilitation could prove to be cost-effective. (see Chapter 5 for detailed information about community-based rehabilitation). Research on home-based rehabilitation could also yield promising strategies for cost-effetive post-stroke care.

> **Recommendation 10-7. Existing community-based rehabilitation programs for developmental disabilities should explore cost-effective extension of care for stroke-related disabilities. Research on rehabilitation approaches in developing countries should examine home-based strategies and other potentially cost-effective means of supporting stroke patients and their families.**

Cost Analysis

Determination of the monetary costs of mortality, morbidity, disability, and handicap due to stroke is difficult, if not impossible, and many such studies performed to date have serious inadequacies. The principles of costing illness emphasize the importance of incorporating estimates of the direct costs to health services, social agencies, and patients, as well as the indirect costs to society and patients due to lost productivity and distress.[185] When prevention and treatment strategies involve drugs, their cost-effectiveness depends on the costs of these medications and their availability at the community level.

The costs of stroke have been studied in many countries, all developed. These studies have verified the huge economic impact of stroke, revealing that stroke-related costs account for 3–5 percent of the annual health care budget in some industrialized countries.[186,187] Because of the high rate of mortality associated with stroke and the equally high level of disability, prevention is the most cost-effective approach, although some forms of prevention—particularly medications such as cholesterol-lowering drugs—are unlikely to prove cost-effective in developing countries at this time (a sample cost analysis for various drug treatments for the prevention of stroke in the United States appears in Box 10-4). More promising strategies for developing countries lie in the promotion of behavioral changes (smoking cessation, fat- and sodium-reduced diets, lipid-lowering diets, physical activity, and weight reduction), as well as inexpensive drug interventions (lipid-lowering medications, aspirin, beta-blockers) that have been demonstrated to be highly cost-effective in developed countries.[168,175]

While several antihypertensive drugs appear likely to be cost-effective for preventing stroke even where health care resources are scarce, the initial investment required to purchase them may be prohibitive in some low-income settings. For many developing countries, the only cost-effective alternatives to drug therapy for lowering blood pressure are interventions such as sodium restriction, potasium supplementation, fish-oil supplementation, and a combination of these therapies with weight reduction and increased exercise over a longer period.[168] There is also evidence that a paramedical intervention program, including advice on diet, stress reduction, exercise, and smoking cessation, could result in net savings in drug costs among treated hypertensive patients: it is estimated that 25 percent of patients could cease drug therapy, and another 25 percent could reduce their drug requirements by half.[168,175] Dietary change may turn out to be the primary means of controlling hypertension in the developing world, where the cost of drug treatment for hypertension could amount to up to 5 percent of total health care costs.[168]

Where health care resources are limited, research is needed to ensure optimal allocation of funds and human capital to interventions for stroke. The Asia Pacific Consensus Forum on Stroke Management has pointed out the relevance of developing databases for use in assessing and evaluating (1) the needs of the community, (2) the accessibility of stroke care, (3) the effectiveness of acute stroke care, (4) the effectiveness of rehabilitation, (5) the adequacy of education programs, and (6) the key indicators of process and outcome.[58,90]

Recommendation 10-8. Research to assess local needs for stroke prevention, treatment, and rehabilitation should be conducted in developing countries to inform the planning and allocation of health care resources aimed at reducing the burden of illness associated with stroke. International support for such efforts should include the development of information technology and databases to aid research and multinational collaboration.

CAPACITY

This chapter has emphasized that prevention is key to reducing death and disability due to stroke. At the community level, health care workers and other paramedical personnel should provide basic education regarding stroke risk factors and promote a healthy diet, smoking cessation, and other lifestyle modifications, as well as regular checkups to test for hypertension and diabetes. Guidelines for accomplishing these tasks have been developed by WHO and PAHO [188]; training programs should be established to distribute such

---

BOX 10-4 Sample Cost Analysis of Medications for Stroke Prevention

The following figures estimate the benefit and cost of providing appropriate stroke-preventive drugs for 1 year to a population of 1 million people in the United States, who would otherwise be expected to experience 2,400 strokes. The total cost of such an initiative was estimated to be $2.6 million; however, the cost of treatment and rehabilitation for the strokes prevented was estimated to be $25 million. Thus, according to this scenario, an annual investment of $1 in stroke-preventing medicines would be expected to result in a savings of nearly $10.

Drug Type	Cost/Patient/Year (US$)	Strokes Prevented
Antihypertensive (bendrofluazide)	132	21
Anticoagulant (warfarin)	85	70
Anticholesterol (statin)	81	500
Antiplatelet (aspirin)	80	14

Source: [39]

---

information to health care workers. Primary health care workers, nurses, and physicians play an important role in detecting, diagnosing, and treating hypertension, hypercholesterolemia, and atrial fibrillation, and in ensuring compliance with treatment. Their training, too, should emphasize the importance of stroke prevention through both patient education and the management of conditions known to be risk factors for stroke.

Recommendation 10-9. Training guidelines for stroke prevention should be developed and established as part of basic education for both primary medical and paramedical personnel in developing countries. Medical school curricula for both general practitioners and neurological and psychiatric specialists should include training in the use of diagnostic tools and assessment methods that reflect the local and regional presentation of stroke in both primary care and secondary/tertiary care centers, as well as knowledge about local pathways to care for stroke.

Beyond primary care, key resources for stroke services include stroke units in major hospitals, rehabilitation facilities, and post-stroke community support programs.[189] While such amenities are likely to serve a small minority of stroke patients in a developing country, they can play an important role in the development and introduction of appropriate, cost-effective methods and technology for stroke prevention, treatment, and rehabilitation.[29,190] Facilities such as national and regional training and research centers proposed elsewhere in this report (see Chapter 4) should provide training and employment for greater numbers of neurologists, who could establish programs of secondary and tertiary stroke care.

Recommendation 10-10. Regional and national centers for training and research on brain disorders should include facilities and specialists for secondary and tertiary stroke care, research on locally appropriate interventions for stroke, and expert support for stroke-related training of primary health care workers.

REFERENCES

1. W. B. Saunders. *Dorland's Illustrated Medical Dictionary*. 25th edition. W.B. Saunders: Philadelphia, London, Toronto, 1974.
2. Institute of Medicine. *Control of Cardiovascular Diseases in Developing Countries*. Howson, C.P., Reddy, K.S., Ryan, T.J, and Bale, J.R., eds. National Academy Press: Washington, D.C., 1998.
3. WHO (World Health Organization). Stroke trends in the WHO MONICA Project. *Stroke* 28:500–506, 1997.
4. K. Asplund, R. Bonita, K. Kuulasmaa, A-M Rajakangas, V. Feigin, H. Schaedlich, et al. Multinational comparisons of stroke epidemiology. Evaluation of case ascertainment in the WHO MONICA study. *Stroke* 26:355–360, 1995.
5. C.J.L. Murray, and A.D. Lopez. The Global Burden of Disease: A comprehensive Assessment of Mortality and Disability from Diseases, Injuries, and Risk Factors in 1990 and Projected to 2020. Harvard University Press: Boston, 1996.
6. J. He, M.J. Klag, Z. Wu, and P.K. Whelton. Stroke in the People's Republic of China. I. Geographic variations in incidence and risk factors. *Stroke* 26:2222–2227, 1995.
7. M.B. Kahn, H.K. Patterson, J. Seltzer, M. Fitzpatrick, S. Smullens, R. Bell, et al. Early carotid endarterectomy in selected stroke patients. *Annals of Vascular Surgery*. September 3(5):463–467, 1999.
8. South African Medical Association—Neurological Association of South Africa Stroke Working Group. Stroke therapy clinical guidelines. *South African Medical Journal* 90:292–306, 2000.
9. R. Bonita, R. Beaglehole, and K. Asplund. The worldwide problem of stroke. *Current Opinion in Neurology* 7:5–10, 1994.
10. R.W. Walker, D.G.McLarty, H.M Kitange, D. Whiting, G. Masuke, D. M. Mtasiwa, et al. Stroke mortality in urban and rural Tanzania. Adult Morbidity and Mortality Project. *Lancet* May 13;355:1684–1687, 2000.
11. I. Lessa.Trends in relative mortality from cerebrovascular diseases in Brazilian state capitals, 1950–1988. *Bulletin of the Pan American Health Organization* 29:216–225, 1995.

12. N. Venketasubramanian. Interethnic differences in cerebrovascular disease mortality in Singapore. *Journal of Neuroimaging* 7:261, 1997.
13. C.H. Wyndham. Mortality from cardiovascular diseases in the various population groups in the Republic of South Africa. *South African Medical Journal* 56:1023–1030, 1979.
14. C. Sarti, D. Rastenyte, Z. Cepaitis and J. Tuomilehto. International trends in mortality from stroke, 1968–1994. *Stroke* 2000 Jul; 31(7):1588–1601.
15. T. Ingall, K. Asplund, M. Mahonen, and R. Bonita. A multinational comparison of subarachnoid hemorrhage epidemiology in the WHO MONICA stroke study. *Stroke* May; 31(5):1054–1061, 2000.
16. O. Fustinoni and J. Biller. Ethnicity and stroke: Beware of the fallacies. *Stroke*. May 31(5):1013–1015, 2000.
17. V.J. Kattapong, and T.M. Becker. Ethnic differences in mortality from cerebrovascular diseases among New Mexico's Hispanics, native Americans and non-Hispanic whites, 1958 through 1987. *Ethnic Diseases* 3: 75–82, 1993.
18. G. B. Xue, B. X. Yu, X. Z. Wang, G. Q. Wang, and Z. Y. Wang. Stroke in urban and rural areas of China. *China Medical Journal* Aug; 104(8):697–704, 1991.
19. M.J. Hoy-Gutierrez, E. Gonzalez-Figueroa, and P. Kuri-Morales. [Epidemiology of cerebrovascular disorders]. *Gaceta médica de México* [Spanish] Mar–Apr;132(2):223–230, 1996.
20. J. Tuomilehto, S. Morelos, J. Yason, S.V. Guzman, and H. Geizerova. Trends in cardiovascular diseases mortality in the Philippines. *International Journal of Epidemiology* Jun;13(2):168–176, 1984.
21. N. Venketasubramanian. Trends in cerebrovascular disease mortality in Singapore: 1970–1994. *International Journal of Epidemiology* Feb;27(1):15–19, 1998.
22. R. Walker. Hypertension and stroke in sub-saharan Africa. *Transactions of the Royal Society of Tropical Medicine and Hygiene* 88:609–611, 1994.
23. R. Hernández-Hernández, M. C. Armas-Padilla, M. J. Armas-Hernández, and M. Velasco. The prevalence of hypertension and the state of cardiovascular health in Venezuela and surrounding nations. *Ethnicity and Disease* Autumn;8(3):398–405, 1998.
24. L. van Thành, L. thi Lôc, N. thi Hùng, N. huu Hoàn, D. tien Xuàn, N. van Thành, P. minh Buu. Les accidents vasculaires cérébraux au Sud Viêtnam: Etude épidémiologique. *Review of Neurology* 155:137–140, 1999.
25. C.J.L. Murray and A.D. Lopez. Mortality by cause for eight regions of the world: global burden of disease study. *Lancet* 349:1269–1278, 1997.
26. G.D. Smith, C. Hart, D. Blane and D. Hole. Adverse socioeconomic conditions in childhood and cause specific adult mortality: Prospective observational study. *British Medical Journal* May 30;316(7145):1631–1635, 1998.
27. G.L. Birbeck. Barriers to care for patients with neurologic disease in rural Zambia. *Archives of Neurology*. Mar 57(3):414–417, 2000.
28. L.K.Wright, J.V.Hickey, K.C. Buckwater, S.A.Hendrix and T. Kelechi. Emotional and physical health of spouse caregivers of persons with Alzheimer's disease and stroke. *Journal of Advanced Nursing* Sep; 30(3):552–563, 1999.
29. G.J. Hankey. Stroke. How large a public health problem, and how can the neurologist help ? *Archives of Neurology* 56: 748–754, 1999.
30. T.A. Pearson. Cardiovascular disease in developing countries: Myths, realities, and opportunities. *Cardiovascular Drugs and Therapy* 13:95–104, 1999.

31. D.M. Reed. The paradox of high risk of stroke in populations with low risk of coronary heart disease. *American Journal of Epidemiology* 131:579–588, 1990.

32. R. Peto and A.D. Lopez. *Mortality from smoking in developed countries 1950–2000: Indirect estimates from national vital statistics.* Oxford University Press: Oxford, 1994.

33. R. Peto, A. D. Lopez, J. Boreham, M. Thun, C. Heath, and R. Doll. Mortality from smoking worldwide. *British Medical Bulletin* 53:12–25, 1996.

34. T.J. Thom. International mortality from heart disease: Rates and trends. *International Journal of Epidemiology.* Supplement 18:S20–S28, 1989.

35. M. Higgins and T.J. Thom. Trends in CHD in the United States. *International Journal of Epidemiology* 18:S58–S66, 1989.

36. O.H. Del Brutto, A. Mosquerra, X. Sanchez, J. Santos, and C.A. Noboa. Stroke subtypes among Hispanics living in Guayaquil, Ecuador. Results from the Luis Vernaza Hospital Stroke Registry. *Stroke* 24:1833–1836, 1993.

37. A.R. Omram. The epidemiological transition: A theory of the epidemiology of population change. *Milbank Memorial Fund Quarterly* 49:509–538, 1971.

38. S.J. Olshansky and A.B. Ault. The fourth stage of the epidemiologic transition: The age of delayed degenerative diseases. *Milbank Memorial Fund Quarterly* 64:355–391, 1986.

39. P. Thorvaldsen, K. Asplund, K. Kuulasmaa, A.M. Rajakangas, and M. Schroll. Stroke incidence, case fatality, and mortality in the WHO MONICA project. World Health Organization Monitoring Trends and Determinants in Cardiovascular Disease. *Stroke* 26:361–367, 1995.

40. N.E. Bharucha, E. P. Bharucha, A. E. Bharucha, A. V. Bhise, and B. S. Schoenberg. Prevalence of stroke in the Parsi community of Bombay. *Stroke* Jan;19(1):60–62, 1988.

41. A.K. Banerjee. Pathology of Cerebrovascular Disease. *Neurology India* Dec 48;305–307, 2000.

42. Epidemiological study on subarachnoid haemorrhage in India. Indian Council of Medical Research, New Delhi, 1987.

43. A.K. Banerjee, M. Varma, R.K. Vasista and J.S. Chopra. Cerebrovascular disease in north-west India: A study of necropsy material. *Journal of Neurology, Neurosurgery, and Psychiatry* Apr;52(4):512–515, 1989.

44. R.B. Singh, I.L. Suh, V.P. Singh, S. Chaithiraphan, P. Laothavorn, R.G. Sy, et al. Hypertension and stroke in Asia: Prevalence, control and strategies in developing countries for prevention. *Journal of Human Hypertension* Oct–Nov;14(10–11):749–763, 2000.

45. H.C. Liu, S.J. Wang, J.L. Fuh, C.Y. Liu, K.P. Lin, P.N. Wang, et al. The Kinmen Neurological Disorders Survey (KINDS): A study of a Chinese population. *Neuroepidemiology* 16(2):60–68, 1997.

46. J. He, M.J. Klag, Z. Wu, and P.K. Whelton. Stroke in the People's Republic of China II. Meta-analysis of hypertension and risk of stroke. *Stroke* 26:2228–2232, 1995.

47. V.L. Feign, D.O. Wiebers, J.P. Whisnant, and W.M. O'Fallon. Stroke incidence and 30–day case-fatality rates in Novosibirsk, Russia, 1982 through 1992. *Stroke* 26:924–929, 1995.

48. S. Lindeberg, E. Berntorp, P. Nilsson-Ehle, A. Terent, and B. Vessby. Age relations of cardiovascular risk factors in a traditional Melanesian society: The Kitava Study. *American Journal of Clinical Nutrition* Oct;66(4):845–852, 1997.

49. N.U. Abdul-Ghaffar, M.R. el-Sonbatty, A.B.M.S. el-Dn, M.S. Abdul-Baky, A.A. Marafie, and A.M. al-Said. Stroke in Kuwait: A three year prospective study. *Neuroepidemiology* 16:40–47, 1997.

50. S. Lindeberg, P. Nilsson-Ehle, A. Terent, B. Vessby, and B. Schersten. Cardiovascular risk factors in a Melanesian population apparently free from stroke and ischemic heart disease: The Kitava study. *Journal of Internal Medicine* 236:331–340, 1994.

51. R.F. Gillum, and C.T. Sempos. The end of the long-term decline in stroke mortality in the United States? *Stroke* 28:1527–1529, 1997.

52. A. Al-Sulaiman, O. Bademost, H. Ismail and G. Magboll. Stroke in Saudi children. *Journal of Child Neurology* 14:295–298, 1999.

53. H. Collomb, J. Graveline, M. Diop, and A. Bourgeade. [Systemic elastorrhexis in a sicklemia patient]. *Bulletin de la Société médicale d'Afrique Noire de Langue Francaise* [French] 10(4):597–602, 1965.

54. T.O. Dada, F. A. Johnson, A.B. Araba and S.A. Adegbite. Cerebrovascular accidents in Nigerians—A review of 205 cases. *West African Medical Journal of Nigerian Practice* Jun; 18(3):95–108, 1969.

55. B.O. Osuntokun. O. Bademosi, O.O. Akinkugbe, A.B. Oyediran, and R. Carlisle. Incidence of stroke in an African City: Results from the Stroke Registry at Ibadan, Nigeria, 1973–1975. *Stroke* Mar-Apr;10(2):205–207,1979.

56. B.Kouassi. Presentation at the Workshop of the IOM Committee on Nervous System Disorders in Developing Countries, November 8–9, Washington, D.C., 1999.

57. M. Janghorbani, A. Hamzehee-Moghadam, and H. Kachoiee. Epidemiology of nonfatal stroke in southeastern Iran. *Iranian Journal of Medical Sciences* 21 (3 & 4): 135–140, 1996.

58. Asian acute stroke advisory panel (AASAP). Stroke epidemiological data of nine Asian countries. *Journal of the Medical Association of Thailand* 83:1–7, 2000.

59. N. Poungvarin. Stroke in the developing world. *Lancet* 352(III): 19–22, 1998.

60. C.L. M. Sudlow and C. P. Warlow. Comparing stroke incidence worldwide. What makes studies comparable? *Stroke* 27:550–558, 1996.

61. INTERHEALTH Sterring Committee. Demonstration projects for the integrated prevention and control of noncommunicable diseases (INTERHEALTH programme): Epidemiological background and rationale. *World Health Statistics Quarterly* 44(2):48–54, 1991.

62. C.S. Uribe, I. Jimenez, M. O. Mora, A. Arana, J. L. Sanchez, L. Zuluaga, et al. [Epidemiology of cerebrovascular diseases in Sabaneta, Colombia (1992–1997)] [article in Spanish]. *Review of Neurology* Jul; 25(143):1008–1012, 1997.

63. M. E. Cruz, B. S. Schoenberg, J. Ruales, P. Barberis, J. Proano, F. Bossano, F. Sevilla, and C. L. Bolis. Pilot study to detect neurologic disease in Ecuador among a population with high prevalence of endemic goiter. *Neuroepidemiology* 4(2);108–116, 1985.

64. R. Tekle-Haimanot, M. Abebe, A. Gebre-Mariam, L. Forsgren, J. Heijbel, G. Holmgren, and J. Ekstedt. Community-based study of neurological disorders in rural central Ethiopia. *Neuroepidemiology* 9(5):263–277, 1990.

65. S. Razdan, R. L. Koul, A. Motto, and S. Koul. Cerbrovascular disease in rural Kashmir, India. *Stroke* Dec;20(12):1691–1693, 1989.

66. B.O. Osuntokun, A. O. Adeuja, B. S. Schoenberg, O. Bademosi, V.A. Nottidge, A. Olumide, et al. Neurological disorders in Nigerian Africans: A community-based study. *Acta Neurologica Scandanivica* May–Jan; 28(3):13–21, 1987.

67. A.S. Jaillard, M. Hommel, and P. Mazetti. Prevalence of Stroke at High Altitude (3380 m) in Cuzco, a Town in Peru: A population-based study. *Stroke* 26(4):562–568, 1995.

68. S. al-Rajeh, A. Awada, G. Niazi, and E. Larbi. Stroke in a Saudi Arabian National Guard community. Analysis of 500 consecutive cases from a population-based hospital. *Stroke* Nov;24(11):1635–1639, 1993.

69. N. Attia Romdhane, M. Ben Hamida, A. Mrabet, A. Larnaout, S. Samoud, A. Ben Hamida, et al. Prevalence study of neurologic disorders in Kelibia (Tunisia). *Neuroepidemiology* 12(5):285–299, 1993.

70. D.M. Heng, J. Lee, S.K. Chew, B.Y. Tan, K. Hughes, and K.S. Chia. Incidence of ischaemic heart disease and stroke in Chinese, Malays and Indians in Singapore: Singapore Cardiovascular Cohort Study. *Annals of the Academy of Medicine, Singapore* Mar;29(2):231–236, 2000.

71. P.P. Ashok, K. Radhakrishnan, R. Sridharan, and M.A. el-Mangoush. Incidence and pattern of cerebrovascular diseases in Benghazi, Libya. *Journal of Neurology, Neurosurgery, and Psychiatry* May;49(5):519–523, 1986.

72. B.O. Osuntokun, O. Bademosi, O.O. Akinkugbe, A. B. Oyediran, and R. Carlisle. Incidence of stroke in an African City: Results from the Stroke Registry at Ibadan, Nigeria. *Stroke* Mar–Apr;10(2):205–207, 1979.

73. V.L. Feigin, D.O. Wiebers, J.P. Whisnant, and W.M. O'Fallon. Stroke incidence and 30-day case-fatality rates in Novosibirsk, Russia, 1982 through 1992. *Stroke* 26:924–929,1995.

74. S. al-Rajeh, E. B. Larbi, O. Bademosi, A. Awada, A. Yousef, H. al-Freihi, et al. Stroke register: Experience from the eastern province of Saudi Arabia. *Cerebrovascular Disease* Mar–Apr;8(2):86–89, 1998.

75. J.L. Fuh, S.J. Wang, H.C. Liu, and H.Y. Shyu. Incidence of stroke on Kinmen, Taiwan. *Neuroepidemiology* Sep-Oct;19(5):258–264, 2000.

76. A. Mrabet, N. Attia-Romdhane, M. Ben Hamida, N. Gharbi, H. Le Noan, R Hentati, et al. [Epidemiologic aspects of cerebrovascular accidents in Tunisia]. *Review of Neurology* (Paris) 146(4):297–301, 1990.

77. J. Matenga. Stroke incidence rates among black residents of Harare—A prospective community-based study. *South Africa Medical Journal* 87:606–609, 1997.

78. P.A. Wolf, and R.B. D'Agostino. Epidemiology of stroke. In: *Stroke: pathophysiology, diagnosis, and management.* Barnett, H.J.M., Mohr, J.P., Stein, B.M., and Yatsu, F.M., eds. Churchill Livingstone: Philadelphia, 1998.

79. Eastern Stroke and Coronary Heart Disease Collaborative Research Group. Blood pressure, cholesterol, and stroke in eastern Asia. *Lancet* 352:1801–1807, 1998.

80. R.W. Walker, D. G. McLarty, Hypertension and stroke in developing countries. *Lancet* Sep 16; 346(8977):778, 1995.

81. D.R. Lisk. Hypertension in Sierra Leone Stroke population. *East African Medical Journal* 5:284–287, 1993.

82. L.N. Joseph, C.S. Kase, A.S. Beiser, and P.A. Wolf. Mild blood pressure elevation and stroke: the Framigham Study. *Stroke* 29:277, 1998.

83. C. J. Bulpitt, A.J. Palmer, A.E. Fletcher, D.G. Beevers, E.C. Coles, J. G. Ledingham, et al. Optimal blood pressure control in treated hypertensive patients. Report from the Department of Health Hypertension Care Computing Project (DHCCP). *Circulation* 90:225–233, 1994.

84. R. L. Sacco, B. Boden-Albala, R. Gan, X. Chen, D. E. Kargman, S. Shea, et al. Stroke incidence among white, black and Hispanic residents of an urban community:

The Northern Manhattan Stroke Study. *American Journal of Epidemiology* Feb 1;147:259–268, 1998.

85. P. Giannuzzi and E. Eleuteri. Elevated systolic and diastolic blood pressure vs. isolated systolic hypertension. *Italian Heart Journal* Jun;1(2):93–99, 2000.

86. D. Levy. The role of systolic blood pressure in determing risk for cardiovascular disease. *Journal of Hypertension* Supplement Feb;17(1):S15–S18, 1999.

87. Ji-Guang Wang, J.A. Staessen, L. Gong, and L. Liu. Chinese Trial on Isolated Systolic Hypertension in the Elderly. *Archives of Internal Medicine* Jan 24:160; 211–220, 2000.

88. S. MacMahon and A. Rodgers. The epidemiological association between blood pressure and stroke: Implications for primary and secondary prevention. *Hypertension Research* 17 (I): 23–32, 1994.

89. L.A. Hale, V.U. Fritz, and C. J. Eales. Do stroke patients realize that consequence of hypertension stroke? *South African Medical Journal* 88:451–454, 1998.

90. Asia Pacific Consensus Forum on Stroke Management. *Stroke* 29: 1730–1736, 1998.

91. L. S. Al-Sowielem and A. G. Elzubier. Compliance and knowledge of hypertensive patients attending PHC centres in Al-Khobar, Saudi Arabia. *Eastern Mediterranean Health Journal* 4(2):301–307, 1998

92. C.M. Burchfiel, J.D. Curb, B.L. Rodriguez, RD Abbott, D. Chiu, and K. Yano. Glucose intolerance and 22–year stroke incidence: The Honolulu Heart Program. *Stroke* 25:951–957, 1994.

93. E.L. Goulli, H. Chelli, and M. Chelli. [Maternal morality at the Charles Nicolle Hospital Maternity Department in Tunis between 1972 and 1975. With the exclusion of abortions (author's trans)]. *Journal de Gynécologie, Obstétrique et Biologie de la Reproduction* May-Jun;7(4):779–784, 1978.

94. D. G. McLarty, N. Unwin, H. M. Kitange, and K.G. Alberti. Diabetes mellitus as a cause of death in sub-Saharan Africa: Results of a community-based study in Tanzania. *Diabetic Medicine* Nov 13(11):900–904, 1996.

95. T.R. Dawber, G.F. Meadors, and F.E.J. Moore. Epidemiologic approaches to heart disease: The Framingham Study. *American Journal of Public Health* 41:279–286, 1951.

96. R.W. Walker, D.G. McLarty, G. Masuki, H.M. Kitange, D. Whiting, A.F. Moshi, et al. Age specific prevalence of impairment and disability relating to hemiplegic stroke in the Hai district of northern Tanzania. *Journal of Neurological and Neurosurgical Psychiatry* 68:744–749, 2000.

97. A.M. Groves. Rheumatic fever and rheumatic heart disease: An overview. *Tropical Doctor* Jul; 29(3):129–132, 1999.

98. S.B. Bavdekar, R. Soloman, J.R. Kamat. Rheumatic fever in children. *Journal of the Indian Medical Association.* Dec; 97(12):489–492, 1999.

99. F.F. Bitar, R. A. Jawdi, G. S. Dbaibo, K.A. Yunis, W. Gharzeddine, and M. Obeid. Paediatric infective endocarditis: 19–year experience at a tertiary care hospital in a developing country. *Acta Paediatrica* Apr; 89(4):427–430, 2000.

100. J.L. Deen, T. Vos, S.R. Huttly and J. Tulloch. Injuries and noncommunicable diseases: Emerging health problems of children in developing countries. *Bulletin of the World Health Organization* 77(6):518–524, 1999.

101. J. Joubert, C. A. McLean, C. M. Reid, D. Davel, W. Pilloy, R. Delport, et al. Ischemic heart disease in black South African stroke patients. *Stroke* 31:1294–1298, 2000.

102. R.W. Walker and D.G. McLarty. Hypertension and stroke in developing countries. *Lancet* Sep 16; 346(8977):778, 1995.

103. R.Walker, N. Unwin, and K. G. Alberti. Hypertension treatment and control in Sub-saharan Africa. Burden of cerebrovascular disease will increase as more people survive to old age. *British Medical Journal*, Jul 4; 317 (7150): 76–77,1988.

104. X-H Fang, R.A. Kronman, Shi-Chuo Li, W.T. Longstreth Jr., X-M Cheng, W-Z Wang, et al. Prevention of stroke in urban China. *Stroke* 30:495–501, 1999.

105. G. Premalatha, S. Shanthirani, R. Deepa, J. Markovitz and V. Mohan. Prevalence and risk factors of peripheral vascular disease in a selected South Indian population: The Chennai Urban Population Study. *Diabetes Care* Sep; 23(9):1295–1300, 2000.

106. L. Rajmohan, R. Deepa, and V. Mohan. Risk factors for coronary artery disease in Indians: Emerging trends. *Indian Heart Journal* Mar–Apr; 52(2):221–225, 2000.

107. A. Joseph, V. R. Kutty and C.R. Soman. High risk for coronary heart disease in Thiruvananthapuram city: A study of serum lipids and other risk factors. *Indian Heart Journal* Jan–Feb; 52(1):29–35, 2000.

108. H. Iso, D.R.J. Jacobs, D. Wentworth, J. D. Neaton, and J. D. Cohen. Serum cholesterol levels and six-year mortality from stroke in 350,977 men screened for the multiple risk factor intervention trial. *New England Journal of Medicine* 320:904–910, 1989.

109. R.P. Byington, J.W. Jukema, J.T. Salonen, B. Pitt, A.V. Bruschke, H. Hoen, et al. Reduction in cardiovascular events during pravastatin therapy: Pooled analysis of clinical events of the Pravastatin Atherosclerosis Intervention Program. *Circulation* 92:2419–2425, 1995.

110. C.J. Vaughan, M.B. Murphy, and B.M. Byckley. Statins do more than just lower cholesterol. *Lancet* 348:1079–1082, 1996.

111. C.J. Boushey, S.A.A. Beresford, G.S. Omenn, and A.G. Motuslky. A quantitative asessment of plasma homocysteine as a risk factor for vascular disease. *Journal of the American Medical Association* 274:1049–1057, 1995.

112. S. Gheye, A.V. Lakshmi, T.P. Krishna and K. Krishnaswamy. Fibrinogen and homocysteine levels in coronary artery disease. *Indian Heart Journal* Sep–Oct; 51(5):499–502, 1999.

113. J.W. Eikelboom, G. J. Hankey, S.S.Anand, E. Lofthouse, N. Staples, and R.I. Baker. Association between high homocysteine and ischemic stroke due to large- and small-artery disease but not other etiologic subtypes of ischemic stroke. *Stroke* May; 31(5):1069–1075, 2000.

114. E. Cardo, E. Monros, C. Colome, R. Artuch, J. Campistol, M. Pineda, et al. Children with stroke: Polymorphism of the MTHFR gene, mild hyperhomocysteinemia, and vitamin status. *Journal of Child Neurology* May 15(5): 295–298, 2000.

115. S. J. Kittner, W.H. Giles, R. F. Macko, J. R. Hebel, M. S. Wozniak, R. J. Wityk, et al. Homocysteine and risk of cerebral infarctions in a biracial population: The stroke prevention in young women study. *Stroke* Aug; 30(8):1554–1560, 1999.

116. J.L. Anderson, J.B. Muhlestein, B.D. Horne, J.F. Carlquist, T.L. Blair, T.E. Madsen, et al. Plasma Homocysteine Predicts Mortality Independently of Traditional Risk Factors and C-Reactive Protein in Patients with Angiographically Defined Coronary Artery Diseases. *Circulation* Sep 12; 102(11):1227–1232, 2000.

117. L.J. Appel, E.R. Miller, III, S.H. Jee, R. Stolzenberg-Soloman, P.H. Lin, T. Erlinger, et al. Effect of dictary patterns of serum homocysteine: Results of randomized, controlled feeding study. *Circulation* Aug 22; 102(8):852–857, 2000.

118. M.C. McKinley. Nutritional aspects and possible pathological mechanisms of hyperhomocysteinaemia: An independent risk factor for vascular disease. *Proceedings of the Nutrition Society* May;59(2):221–237, 2000.

119. D. J. VanderJagt, K. Spelman, J. Ambe, P. Datta, W. Blackwell, M. Crossey, et al. Folate and vitamin B12 status of adolescent girls in northern Nigeria. *Journal of the National Medical Association* Jul;92(7):334–340, 2000.

120. S.E. Gariballa. Nutritional factors in stroke. *British Journal of Nutrition* Jul; 84(1):5–17, 2000.

121. G. Boysen and T. Truelsen. Prevention of recurrent stroke. *Neurology Science* Apr; 21(2):67–72, 2000.

122. M.D. Connor, G.A. Lammie, J.E. Bell, C.P. Warlow, P. Simmonds and R.D. Brettle. Cerebral infarction in adult AIDS patients: Observations from the Edinburgh HIV autopsy cohort. *Stroke* Sep; 31(9):2117–2126, 2000.

123. L. Pontrelli, S. Pavlakis and L.R. Krilov. Neurobehavioral manifestations and sequelae of HIV and other infections. *Child Adolescent Psychiatry Clinics of North America* Oct; 8(4):869–878, 1999.

124. O. Picard, L. Brunereau, B. Pelosse, D. Kerob, J. Cabane, and J.C. Imbert. Cerebral infarction associated with vasculitis due to varicella zoster virus in patients infected with the human immunodeficiency virus. *Biomedical Pharmacotherapy* 51(10):449–454, 1997.

125. A.R. Gillams, E. Allen, K. Hrieb, N. Venna, D. Craven, and A.P. Carter. Cerebral infarction in patients with AIDS. *American Journal of Neuroradiology* Sep; 18(80):1581–1585, 1997.

126. S.S. Shah, R.A. Zimmerman, L.B. Rorke, and L.G. Vezina. Cerebrovascular complications of HIV in children. *American Journal of Neuroradiology* Nov-Dec; 17(10):1913–1917, 1996.

127. M. Hoffmann, J. R. Berger, A. Nath, and M. Rayens. Cerebrovascular disease in young, HIV-infected black Africans in the KwaZulu Natal Province of South Africa. *Journal of Neurovirology* 6(3):229–236, 2000.

128. A. Visudtibhan, P. Visudhiphan, and S. Chiemchanya. Stroke and seizures as the presenting signs of pediatric HIV infection. *Pediatric Neurology* Jan; 20(1):53–56, 1999.

129. K. Srinivasan. Ischemic cerebrovascular disease in the young. Two common causes in India. *Stroke* Jul–Aug;15(4):733–735, 1984.

130. I. Ben Hamouda-M'Rad, A. Mrabet, and M. Ben Hamida. Cerebral venous thrombosis and arterial infarction in pregnancy and puerperium. A series of 60 cases. *Review of Neurology* Oct;151(10):563–568, 1995.

131. P. Francois, M. Fabre, E. Lioret, and M. Jan. Vascular cerebral thrombosis during pregnancy and post-partum. *Neurochirurgia* Apr;46(2):105–109, 2000.

132. C. Lamy, J. B. Hamon, J. Coste and J. L. Mas. Ischemic stroke in young women: Risk of recurrence during subsequent pregnancies. *French Study Group on Stroke in Pregnancy Neurology* Jul 25; 55(2):269–274, 2000.

133. K. Srinivasan. Cerebral venous and arterial thrombosis in pregnancy and puerperium. A study of 135 patients. *Angiology* Nov; 34(11):731–746, 1983.

134. C. Lamy, T. Sharshar, and J.L.Mas. Cerebrovascular diseases in pregnancy and puerperium. *Review of Neurology* Jun–Jul;152(6–7):422–440, 1996.

135. K. Kumar. Neurological complications of congenital heart disease. *Indian Journal of Pediatrics* Apr;67(4):287–291, 2000.

136. J.S. Chopra, S.K. Prabhakar, K.C. Das, et al. Stroke in young—A prospective study. In: *Progress in Stroke Research* (1), Greenberg, R.M., Clifford Rose, F., eds. Pitman: London. 217, 1979.

137. G. deVeber, E.S. Roach, A.R. Riela, and M. Wiznitzer. Stroke in children: recognition, treatment, and future directions. *Semin Pediatrics Neurology* Dec;7(4):309–317, 2000.

138. J.M. T. Obama, L. Dongmo, C. Nkemayim, J. Mbede, and P. Hagbe. Stroke in children in Yaounde, Cameroon. *Indian Pediatrics* 32:791–795, 1994.

139. C. Dollery and P.J. Brennan. The Medical Research Council Hypertension Trial: The smoking patient. *American Heart Journal* 115:276–281, 1988.

140. J. Tuomilehto, R. Bonita, A. Stewart, A. Nissinen, and J.T. Salonen. Hypertension, cigarette smoking and the decline in stroke incidence in eastern Finland. *Stroke* 22:7–11, 1991.

141. P.A. Wolf, R.B. D'Agostino, W. B. Kannel, R. Bonita, and A. J. Belanger. Cigarette smoking as a risk factor for stroke: The Framingham Study. *Journal of the American Medical Association* 259:1025–1029, 1988.

142. M.R. Pandey. Tobacco smoking and hypertension. *Journal of the Indian Medical Association* 97:367–369, 1999.

143. E. Baris, L.W. Brigden, J. Prindiville, V.L. da Costa e Silva, H. Chitanondh, and S. Chandiwana. Research priorities for tobacco control in developing countries: A regional approach to a global consultative process. *Tobacco Control* Jun;9(2):217–223, 2000.

144. R.M. Selmer, I.S. Kristiansen, A. Haglerod, S. Graff-Iversen, H.K.Larsen, H. E. Meyer, et al. Cost and health consequences of reducing the population intake of salt. *Journal of Epidemiology Community Health* Sep; 54(9):697–702, 2000.

145. H. Tanaka. Age specific incidence of stroke subtype in Shibata Japan: 1976–1978. *Stroke* Jan–Feb;13(1):10, 1982.

146. J. S. Gill, A. V. Zezulka, M. H. Shipley, S. K. Gill, and D.G.B. Beavers. Stroke and alcohol consumption. *New England Journal of Medicine* 315:1041–1046, 1986.

147. H. Haapaniemi, M. Hillbom, and S. Jubel. Lifestyle-associated risk factors for acute brain infarction among persons of working age. *Stroke* 28:26–30, 1997.

148. M.J. Stampfer, G.A. Colditz, W.C. Willett, F.E. Speizer, and C.H. Hennekens. A prospective study of moderate alcohol consumptions and the risk of coronary heart disease and stroke in women. *New England Journal of Medicine* 319:267–273, 1988.

149. H. Rodgers, P.D. Aitken, J.M. French, R.H. Curless, D. Bates, and O.F.W. James. Alcohol and stroke: A case control study of drinking habits past and present. *Stroke* 24:1473–1477, 1993.

150. G. Boysen, J. Nyboe, M. Appleyard, P. S. Sorensen, J. Boas, F. Somnier, et al. Stroke incidence and risk factors for stroke in Copenhagen, Denmark. *Stroke* 149:1413–1416, 1988.

151. P. B. Gorelick, M. B. Rodin, P. Langenberg, D. B. Hier, and J. Costigan. Weekly alcohol consumption, cigarette smoking, and the risk of ischemic stroke: Results of a case-control study at three urban medical centers in Chicago, Illinois. *Neurology* 39:339–343, 1989.

152. J.M. Yuan, R.K. Ross, Y.T. Gao, B. E. Henderson, and M.C. Yu. Follow-up study of moderate alcohol intake and mortality among middle-aged men in Shanghai, China. *British Medical Journal* 314:18–23, 1997.

153. T.K. Lee, Z.S. Huang, S.K. Ng, K.W. Chan, Y.S. Wang, H.W. Liu, et al. Impact of alcohol consumption and cigarette smoking on stroke among the elderly in Taiwan. *Stroke* 26:790–794, 1995.

154. R. Shinton and G. Sagar. Lifelong exercise and stroke. *British Medical Journal* 307:231–234, 1993.

155. J. T. Salonen, P. Puska, and J. Tuomilehto. Physical activity and risk of myocardial infarction, cerebral stroke and death: A longitudinal study in Eastern Finland. *American Journal of Epidemiology* 115:526–537, 1982.

156. B. Herman, A. C. M. Leyten, J. H. van Luijk, C. W. Frenken, A. A. Op de Coul, and B. P. Schulte. An evaluation of risk factors for stroke in Dutch community. *Stroke* 13:334–339, 1982.
157. D.K. Kiely, P.A. Wolf, L.A. Cupples, A.S. Beiser, and W.B. Kannel. Physical activity and stroke risk: The Framingham study. *American Journal of Epidemiology* 140:608–620, 1994.
158. M. Anate, A. W. Olatinwo, and A.P. Omesina. Obesity—An overview. *West African Journal of Medicine* Oct–Dec;17(4):248–254, 1998.
159. R. Boedhi-Darmojo, B. Setianto, B. Sutedjo, D. Kusmana, D. Andradi, F. Supari, et al. A study of baseline risk factors for coronary heart disease: results of population screening in a developing country. *Review of Epidemiology Sante Publique* 38(5–6):487–491, 1990.
160. M. C. Gulliford. Controlling non-insulin-dependent diabetes mellitus in developing countries. *International Journal of Epidemiology* 24(1): S53–S59, 1995.
161. M. Gourie-Devi, Director-Vice Chancellor, and Professor of Neurology, National Institute of Mental Health and Neurosciences, personal communication, 2000.
162. W.T. Longstreth, C. Bernick, A. Fitzpatrick, M. Cushman, L. Knepper, J. Lima, et al. Frequency and predictors of stroke death in 5,888 participants in the Cardiovascular Health Study. *Neurology* Feb 13;56(3):368–375, 2001.
163. T. Brott, J.R. Marlar, C.P. Olinger, H.P. Adams, T. Tomsick, W.G. Barsan, et al. Measurements of acute cerebral infarction: A clinical examination scale. *Stroke* 20: 864–870, 1989.
164. R.L. Sacco, P.A. Wolf, and P.B. Gorelick. Risk factors and their management for stroke prevention: Outlook for 1999 and beyond. *Neurology* 53(4)L/S15–S24, 1999.
165. R.L. Sacco, T. Shi, M.C. Zamanillow, and D. Kargman. Predictors of mortality and recurrence after hospitalized cerebral infarction in an urban community: The Northern Manhattan Stroke Study. *Neurology* 44:626–634, 1994.
166. B.C. Walters. Outcome science and stroke. *Clinical Neurosurgery* 45:128–134, 1999.
167. J.R. McGuire and R. L. Harvey. The prevention and mangement of complications after stroke. *Physical Medicine and Rehabilitation Clinics of North America* 10(4):857–873, 1999.
168. D. Dunbabin. Cost-effective interventions in stroke. *PharmacoEconomics* 2 (6):468–499, 1992.
169. G. Rose, and L. Colwell. Randomised controlled trial of smoking advice: Final (20 year) results. *Journal of Epidemiology and Community Health* 46:75–77, 1992.
170. J. Broderick, T. Brott, R. Kothari, R. Miller, J. Khoury, J. Pancioli, et al. The Greater Cincinnati/Northern Kentucky Stroke Study: Preliminary first-ever and total incidence rates of stroke among blacks. *Stroke* 29: 415–421, 1998.
171. R. Coleman, G. Gill, and D. Wilkinson. Noncommunicable disease management in resource-poor settings: A primary care model from South Africa. *Bulletin of the World Health Organization* 76(6):633–640, 1998.
172. R. Heller, R. O'Connell, L. Lim, A. Aggrawal, A. Nogueira, L.H. Alvares Salis, et al. Variation in in-patient stroke management in ten centres in different countries: The INCLEN multicentre stroke collaboration. *Journal of the Neurological Sciences* Aug 1;167(1):11–15, 1999.
173. H. Iso, T. Shimamotot, Y. Naito, S. Sato, A. Kitamura, M. Iid, et al. Effects of a long-term hypertension control program on stroke incidence and prevalence in rural community in northeastern Japan. *Stroke* 29:1510–1518, 1998.

174. International Stroke Trial Collaborative Group. The International Stroke Trial (IST): A randomised trial of aspirin, subcutaneous heparin, both or neither among 19,435 patients with acute ischaemic stroke. *Lancet* 349:1569–1581.

175. S. Ebrahim. Systematic review of cost-effectiveness research of stroke evaluation and treatment. *Stroke* Dec.30(12):2759–2760, 1999.

176. B. Jonsson and M. Johannesson. Cost benefit of treating hypertension. *Clinical and Experimental Hypertension* 21(5 & 6):987–997, 1999.

177. Hypertension Society of Southern Africa. Guidelines for the management of hypertension at primary care level. *South African Medical Journal* 85:1321–1325, 1995.

178. A. Bryer and L. de Villiers. Is CT scan essential in the diagnosis of stroke? *South African Medical Journal* Feb 90(2):110–112, 2000.

179. The National Institute of Neurological Disorders, and Stroke rt-PA Stroke Study Group. Tissue plasminogen activator for acute ischemic stroke. *New England Journal of Medicine* 333: 1581–1587, 1995.

180. W. Hacke, M. Kaste, C. Fieschi, D. Toni, E. Lesaffre, R. von Kummer, et al. Intravenous thrombolysis with recombinant tissue plasminogen activator for acute hemispheric stroke: The European Cooperative Acute Stroke Study (ECASS). *Journal of the American Medical Association* 274:1017–1025, 1995.

181. M.D. Hill, and V. Hachinski. Stroke treatment: Time is brain. *Lancet* 352 (III):10–14, 1998.

182. G.E. Gresham, D. Alexander, D.S. Bishop, C. Giuliani, G. Goldberg, A. Holland, et al. American Heart Association Prevention Conference. IV. Prevention and Rehabilitation of Stroke. Rehabilitation. *Stroke* 28: 1522–1526, 1997.

183. H. Ueki, K. Washino, T. Fukao, M. Inoue, N. Ogawa, and A. Takai. Mental health problems after stroke. *Psychiatry and Clinical Neurosciences* 53:621–627, 1999.

184. S.E. Starkstein, B.S. Cohen, P. Fedoroff, R.M. Parikh, T.R. Price, and R.G. Robinson. Relationship between anxiety disorders and depressive disorders in patients with cerebrovascular injury. *Archives of General Psychiatry* Mar; 47(3):246–251, 1990.

185. M. Kaste, R. Fogelholm, and A. Rissanen. Economic burden of stroke and the evaluation of new therapies. *Public Health* 112.103–112, 1998.

186. N. Zethraeus, T. Molin, P. Henriksson, and B. Jonsson. Costs of coronary heart disease and stroke: The case of Sweden. *Journal of Internal Medicine* 246:151–159, 1999.

187. G.J. Hankey and C.P. Warlow. Treatment and secondary prevention of stroke: Evidence, costs, and effects on individuals and populations. *Lancet* 354:1457–1463, 1999.

188. J. Chalmers, S. MacMahon, G. Mancia, J. Whitworth, L. Beilin, L Hansson, et al. World Health Organization-International Society of Hypertension Guidelines for the management of hypertension. Guidelines Sub-Committee of the World Health Organization. *Clinical and Experimental Hypertension* Jul–Aug;21(5-6):1009–1060, 1999.

189. N. Venketasubramanian. Trends in cerebrovascular disease mortality in Singapore: 1970–1994. *International Journal of Epidemiology* Feb;27(1):15–90, 1998.

190. R.F. Heller, P. Langhorne, and E. James. Improving stroke outcome: The benefits of increasing availability of technology. *Bulletin of the World Health Organization* 78(11):1337–1343, 2000.

Epilogue

Two symbolic events marked the start and the conclusion of the committee's work on this report. First, the study's inception followed closely the conclusion of the Decade of the Brain, which yielded tremendous new insights into the development and workings of the nervous system. Second, the final stage of the preparation of this report for publication coincided with the publication of the two versions[1] of the full sequence of the human genome, a landmark achievement that heralds a new era in our conceptualization of human biology and in our capacity to prevent and treat disease. Against this background of historic scientific breakthroughs, the enormous disparities between the developed and developing worlds in the understanding, prevention, and treatment of brain disorders become dramatically apparent. These disorders, which frequently lead to death and long-term disability, are undermining the development of low-income countries, despite the fact that many low-cost preventive and treatment interventions are known and feasible to implement. Brain disorders are highly prevalent in settings characterized by persistent poverty-driven conditions, such as malnutrition and AIDS, which also adversely affect the nervous system. The hidden epidemic of children's disabilities and the fact that 50 percent of the population in many developing countries is under 12 years of age add to the importance of placing brain disorders high on the agenda as a public health problem in all nations. This report seeks to provide evidence that it is in the self-

---

[1] F.S. Collins and V.A. McKusick. Implications of the Human Genome Project for Medical Science. *Journal of the American Medical Association* Feb7;285(5):540-544, 2001.

interest of all governments to make a commitment to addressing brain disorders, building on the investments in health care they have already made.

ESTABLISHING NATIONAL AND LOCAL PRIORITIES FOR ADDRESSING BRAIN DISORDERS

In developing countries, the design and implementation of programs must be tailored to each country's needs and resources. The specific health needs of at-risk groups, resource constraints, the cultural context, and the local capacity to implement and sustain an intervention must all be taken into account. Building on evidence derived from programs in a variety of settings, this report highlights the need for rigorous operational research in conjunction with the provision of care. Several strategies for reducing the burden of brain disorders in the developing world emerged as this report was being prepared. Each requires further research for effective implementation based on consideration of the local resources and the community's health priorities.

THE POTENTIAL FOR PREVENTION

Prevention is critical in reducing the impact of brain disorders and in many instances is more cost-effective than treatment. Once established, impairment caused by these disorders is often irreversible. However, many potentially disabling disorders are now preventable. Examples include iodine supplementation to prevent mental retardation due to iodine deficiency; immunization against polio; folic acid supplementation and food fortification to reduce the number of children born with neural tube defects; and control of cysticercosis to prevent epilepsy. Appropriate, affordable treatment for other disorders, such as providing antidepressants or anticonvulsants, can prevent a lifetime of disability.

It is therefore essential to overcome existing barriers in developing countries to recognition of the public health importance of brain disorders and the development of strategies and programs for their prevention and treatment. Multifaceted research is needed to address these gaps, develop new prevention strategies, and assess the cost-effectiveness and sustainability of preventive strategies in specific settings. Multidisciplinary research involving collaboration between the health and social sciences and aiming to understand and remove these barriers should be targeted for increased funding.

INCREASING THE CLINICAL AND RESEARCH PROFESSIONAL CAPACITY IN DEVELOPING COUNTRIES

For a variety of historical, social, and economic reasons, many developing countries have a severe shortage of trained professionals with expertise in the assessment, treatment, and rehabilitation of brain disorders. Increasing the clinical and research professional capacity in developing countries is key to developing sustainable local programs. The approaches to addressing these deficits highlighted in this report include the following:

• Capacity building through on-site education, exchange programs, and distance learning using modern information technology;
• Development of local networks that link centers with the requisite expertise to their surrounding community and creation of regional networks linking such centers through joint training programs, staff exchanges, and collaborative research; and
• Partnerships between lead institutions in high-income countries and such collaborative networks in low-income countries.

COLLABORATIVE RESEARCH INTO GLOBAL HEALTH PROBLEMS

The demographic, cultural, and genetic diversity of populations in many developing countries offers unique opportunities for collaborative research addressing health issues of universal significance. For example, studies of Huntington's disease among a genetically unique population in Venezuela resulted in the identification of the responsible gene, an advance that will eventually lead to effective treatment. Similarly, epidemiological and genetic studies in Africa targeting the genetic basis of hypertension, conducted to complement similar studies in the United States and Europe, offer significant advantages in addressing the problem of stroke that will benefit all populations. A further example is research into the genetic basis and environmental factors associated with the good prognosis for schizophrenia in a substantial proportion of patients in developing countries. Both genetic (e.g., protective alleles) and environmental (psychosocial as well as dietary) factors may be involved, and collaborative research into this phenomenon holds promise for understanding key aspects of the etiology, treatment, and ultimate prevention of this debilitating disorder.

ACCESS TO AND AFFORDABILITY OF ESSENTIAL PHARMACEUTICAL PRODUCTS

In both the short and long terms, the availability and affordability of pharmaceutical products hold the key to important solutions for the treatment of brain disorders in the developing world. In most developing countries, the lack of adequate drug production facilities and the high prices of imported drugs restrict the availability of essential medicines. The medications needed to treat the disorders detailed in this report are simply not available on any scale in most low-income countries. However, the mere fact that the number of potential consumers of pharmaceuticals in developing countries far exceeds those currently being treated should indicate to the major pharmaceutical and biotechnology companies that both major needs and major opportunities exist. Satisfactory ways can be found to reduce the disparities between the need and the severe economic limitations that deprive millions of people in developing countries of adequate treatment. Some options include the following:

- Strengthening the research and development capacity in developing countries for local manufacturing of essential generic drugs that are cost-effective in the treatment of brain disorders.
- Facilitating developing countries' access to, and ensuring the affordability of, newer central nervous system pharmaceuticals by linking price structure to per capita gross domestic product (GDP); utilizing subsidies from the World Bank, United Nations agencies, or other sources; and providing incentives for price reduction, such as extending the period of patent protection.

AN INVESTMENT IN FUTURE OPPORTUNITIES

There are many incentives for governments, research institutions, foundations, the World Bank, and nongovernmental organizations to make continued and sustained investments in ameliorating the impact of brain disorders in developing countries. While each of the disorders detailed in this report represents a highly significant problem, bipolar disorder, depression, developmental disabilities, epilepsy, schizophrenia, and stroke are just the tip of the iceberg. These and many other disorders have in common the fact that by severely affecting the ability of millions of people to function as productive members of their communities, they diminish the human and social capital of entire societies.

The contribution of good mental health and neurobehavioral functioning goes beyond the reduction of clinical symptoms and disability, improved workplace productivity, and the lost productivity of caregivers. There is evidence that individual and population-based interventions aimed at reducing brain disorders would enhance constructive social interaction and contribute to the building of social capital in a country. A particularly telling example is provided by recent research in Rwanda and Cambodia that demonstrated that an increase in individual attributes such as interpersonal communication, trust, and resilience is contributing to the rebuilding of the social fabric in the post-conflict development of these countries.

Brain disorders have a severe impact on the ability to earn, and they therefore contribute to the poverty cycle. It is important to consider both paid and unpaid work in this calculation, as both contribute to economic development. There is a gender differential, in virtually all countries with women carrying out the majority of unpaid work, but this differential is much more marked in developing as compared to developed countries. Since women tend to have a higher prevalence of common disorders such as depression but are less likely to access treatment for such disorders, the actual negative impact of this gender disparity on the national economy is likely to be much greater than could be inferred from GDP and employment statistics.

Brain disorders also have an impact on key international health development targets, such as infant and child mortality. Child health improves when mothers are treated for depression, including postpartum depression. Reduced incidence of depression has proven links with better adherence to important health programs, such as antenatal care, vaccination, prevention and treatment of infectious diseases, and rehydration therapy for infant diarrhea.

Prevention and treatment of brain disorders can contribute significantly to the fundamental mission of a nation's health care system. Investment in these efforts proportional to the impact of brain disorders offers promise for building healthier, more productive communities and more prosperous nations. The success of innovative programs of treatment and research, coupled with recent initiatives and commitments from the international community, has created a favorable climate for meeting the challenge of brain disorders in developing countries.

APPENDIX A

The Study Approach

This appendix describes important definitions and the process by which disorders examined in this report were selected, analyzed, and evaluated to develop the report:

- definition of brain disorders and selection of specific disorders;
- definition of developing country;
- early history of the study;
- charge to the committee;
- commissioned papers and technical input to the study;
- workshop and committee meetings; and
- other IOM reports on global health.

BRAIN DISORDERS AND SELECTION OF
SPECIFIC DISORDERS FOR SECTION II

For the purposes of this report, neurological, psychiatric, and developmental disorders in the aggregate are referred to as *brain disorders*. These disorders include the following conditions from the classification system of the *Global Burden of Disease* study: neuropsychiatric conditions (unipolar depression, bipolar disorder, schizophrenia, epilepsy, alcohol use, dementia and other degenerative and hereditary CNS disorders, Parkinson's disease, multiple sclerosis, drug use, posttraumatic stress disorder, obsessive-compulsive disorders, and panic disorder); self-inflicted injuries (included in the wider category of intentional injuries); cerebrovascular disease (included under cardiovascular disease); and the developmental disabilities given in Table 6-1 of this report, but not included in the global burden of disease classification.

Part I of the report discusses the challenges posed by brain disorders: the global burden they impose, the stigma and lost productivity associated with these conditions, the role of poverty and gender, the capacity of local health systems to care for these conditions, and the priorities for services, training, and research to lessen the burden of these disorders in the early years of the 21st century. Estimation of the global burden caused by the broad range of disorders is complicated by their not all being included in estimates of the global burden of disease, and for those that are included, their not having been classified, analyzed, and reported in a way that allows the individual disorders to be assembled simply and accurately. Rather they are drawn from the group of neuropsychiatric disorders, with the additions of self-inflicted illness, cerebrovascular disease or stroke, and additional estimations for developmental disabilities (not included in the *Global Burden of Disease Study*) based on prevalence data from developing countries.

Part II of the report focuses on six classes of disorders—developmental disabilities, epilepsy, schizophrenia, bipolar disorder, unipolar depression, and stroke—in order to consider specific opportunities for cost-effective interventions and priorities for research. In selecting these categories of disorders, sponsors of the report considered the following criteria:

- the magnitude and severity of the disorder, as measured by prevalence and disability;
- inclusion of disorders that affect different age groups from infancy to senescence; and
- the likelihood of identifying cost-effective interventions for a disorder.

The framework for studying each category of disorder includes an overview of the epidemiology, a review of knowledge supporting existing and potential interventions, and projections of the feasibility, cost, and expected impact of those interventions.

DEVELOPING COUNTRIES

This report uses the term *developing countries* to describe those countries with economies classified as middle- and low-income in the 1999/2000 *World Development Report* (World Bank, 1999). They have per capita incomes that average less than $9,361 (see Figure A-1). These are subdivided into low-income countries with average per capita incomes of $760 or less, lower middle-income countries with average per capita incomes of $761 to $3,030, and upper middle-income countries with average per capita incomes of $3,031 to $9,361. The different countries in these groupings are developing at their own rates and have different capacities and challenges in providing health care services to their populations. They tend to share a number of the following characteristics:

- *Low GDP per capita*: In most developing countries, a serious disparity exists between increasing population size and low industrial and agricultural productivity. This situation is often aggravated by heavy external indebtedness, restricted access to global markets, and insecure prices of exportable raw commodities.
- *Young populations*: The pyramidal age structure in most developing countries has a very broad base, due to the relative and absolute predominance of young people, and a narrow tip.
- *High infant mortality and low life expectancy*: Although both indicators have moderated over the last decade, the vital statistics of a majority of the developing countries still lag behind the so-called developed world. The HIV/AIDS epidemic in Sub-Saharan Africa and the breakdown of health infrastructures throughout Central and Eastern Europe are creating worsening rates in these regions.
- *Epidemiological transition*: While communicable diseases and malnutrition remain prime causes of morbidity in developing countries, the incidence of noncommunicable diseases such as heart disease, stroke, cancer, and diabetes is increasing, creating a double burden of disease.
- *Weak health care infrastructure*: A shortage of skilled health care workers plagues most developing countries, where the relatively few medical professionals tend to be concentrated in urban areas. Health expenditure per capita in developing countries is typically a fraction of that in the developed world.
- *Social unrest and violent conflict*: The subsequent disruption to and loss of infrastructure reduces the availability of health services. Additionally, the attention and funds for social services and healthcare are diverted to military and defense efforts.
- *Other features*: Many, but not all, developing countries also suffer the following disadvantages: low literacy rates, especially among women; predominantly traditional, rural forms of social organization; extreme climates; frequent natural catastrophes such as drought, floods, and famine; large-scale population displacement; and epidemic rates of HIV/AIDS.

386

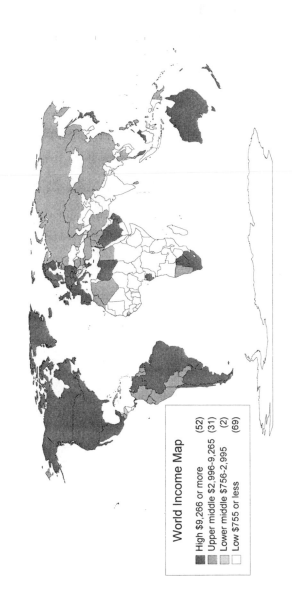

World Income Map

High $9,266 or more (52)
Upper middle $2,996-9,265 (31)
Lower middle $756-2,995 (2)
Low $755 or less (69)

Source: World Bank. World Development Report: Attacking Poverty 2000/2001. Oxford University Press, 1999.

EARLY HISTORY OF THE STUDY

In 1998 the Global Forum for Health Research* agreed to Dr. Donald Silberberg's request for support to develop a report on neurological and psychiatric disorders in low- and middle-income countries. Dr. Silberberg recommended that the study be undertaken by the Institute of Medicine's (IOM) Board on Global Health. It would provide an independent assessment of the magnitude of the health burden in developing countries due to these disorders, the risks for disorders, the health care currently provided, and gaps in that care. The study would then review for some specific disorders, such as developmental disabilities, epilepsy, schizophrenia, stroke and unipolar depression, affordable diagnostic assessment procedures, treatments, and rehabilitation for low-income populations. IOM's Board on Global Health discussed the study with the directors of four institutes of the National Institutes of Health (National Institute of Mental Health, National Institute of Neurological Disorders and Stroke, National Institute of Child Health and Human Development, and Fogarty International Center) and staff of the Centers for Disease Control and Prevention (CDC). The NIH and CDC directors proposed that the scope of the study be broadened to include bipolar disorder, and provided support for the expanded study. The Board on Global Health shaped the proposed study to be responsive to the needs and opportunities presented in its 1997 report, *America's Vital Interest in Global Health.*

CHARGE TO THE COMMITTEE

The committee will prepare a consensus report that defines the increasing burden caused by neurological, psychiatric, and developmental disorders, and identifies opportunities to effectively reduce that burden with cost-effective strategies for prevention, diagnosis, and treatment of several major conditions. It will also identify the areas for research, development, and capacity strengthening that would contribute most significantly to reducing the burden of these disorders.

The study will review the overall burden of disease caused by a range of disorders. It will then focus on the following disorders to identify strategies for prevention, low-cost treatment, priorities for research and development, and for capacity building to meet the needs of developing countries:

---

*The Global Forum for Health Research is a Swiss foundation, created in 1997 by the World Health Organization, the World Bank, bilateral cooperation agencies, international and national foundations, national and international nongovernmental organizations, and private sector companies to promote research to improve the health of poor people.

- developmental disabilities;
- unipolar depression;
- bipolar disorder;
- schizophrenia;
- epilepsy; and
- stroke.

COMMISSIONED PAPERS AND TECHNICAL INPUT
TO THE STUDY

The study covers diverse topics and diverse settings so the committee commissioned several papers on the broad range of topics to be covered in the report. These papers were as follows:

- "Health Services Research" by Vikram Patel;
- "Poverty, Gender, and Nervous System Disorders" by Vikram Patel;
- "The Role of Primary Care Providers and the Community" by Oyewusi Gureje;
- "Congenital Anomalies in Developing Countries" by Eduardo Castilla;
- "Disability in Sub-Saharan Africa: An Overview" by Gregory Powell;
- "Disability in Jamaica" by Marigold (Molly) Thorburn;
- "Disability in Bangladesh" by Nalia Khan; and
- "Bipolar Disorder in Developing Countries" by Kwame Julius McKenzie.

In addition, several experts were appointed as technical reviewers for specific chapters. They provided written reviews that were considered by the committee for the final drafting of the chapters.

- Chapter 2: Drs. Norman Satorius, Alex Cohen, and Joop de Jong;
- Chapter 3: Drs. Gretchen Birbeck, Joop de Jong, Matthew Menken, Vikram Patel, and Ellis D'Arrigo Busnello;
- Chapter 5: Drs. Robert Edgerton, Rune Simeonsson, and Molly Thorburn;
- Chapter 6: Drs. Gretchen Birbeck, Michel Dumas, Jerome Engel, Pierre-Marie Preux, Leonid Prilipko, J.W.A.S. Sander, and Robert Scott;
- Chapter 7: Dr. Oyewusi Gureje;
- Chapter 8: Dr. Kwame McKenzie;
- Chapter 9: Drs. Oyewusi Gureje and Jessie Mbwambo; and
- Chapter 10: Drs Jose Biller, William Harlan, Niphon Poungvarin, and Ralph Sacco.

WORKSHOP AND COMMITTEE MEETINGS

The committee held a workshop in Washington, D.C., on November 8–9, 1999, to hear the perspective of sponsors and presentations from other experts on the major areas of the study, and to identify or clarify issues that would be important for the study charge. This was a valuable opportunity to explore the thinking of additional experts and to identify with them sources of information on the range of topics and issues. The agenda for the workshop is given in Appendix C. The individuals and their presentation topics are listed below:

- Dr. Alex Cohen, "Mental Health of Indigenous People";
- Dr. Beugre Kouassi, "Epidemiology and Prevention of Epilepsy in Africa" and "Epidemiology and Prevention of Stroke in Africa";
- Dr. Thomas Langfitt, "Risk Factors and Outcomes for Children and Youth";
- Dr. Jessie Mbwambo, "Depression in Developing Countries";
- Dr. Vikram Patel, "Epidemiology of Common Mental Disorders in Developing Countries, with a Special Focus on Poverty and Female Gender as Risk Factors," and a "Health Systems Model of Approaching Mental Health Research and Program Implementation and the Overall Policy Implications of Cultural and Health System Diversity in Mental Health Care";
- Dr. Norman Sartorius, "The Global Burden of Disease";
- Dr. Peter Schantz, "Cysticercosis in Developing Countries"; and
- Dr. Harvey Whiteford, "Mental Health Economics."

Following the 2-day workshop, the committee met for deliberations twice in Washington D.C.: November 10, 1999, and May 9–10, 2000. Representatives of the committee's writing groups also met on March 29–30, 2000. Additionally, committee members along with IOM staff and consultants deliberated upon, contributed to, and reviewed the development of the report by e-mail, telephone, and mail between November 1999 and July 2000, then in September 2000 and January 2001 after revisions in response to external review.

OTHER IOM REPORTS ON GLOBAL HEALTH

This report on neurological and psychiatric disorders is one of a series of reports that address issues of global health and health policy:

- *Assessment of Future Scientific Needs for Live Variola Virus*, 1999;
- *Control of Cardiovascular Diseases in Developing Countries: Research, Development, and Institutional Strengthening*, 1998;
- *Prevention of Micronutrient Deficiencies: Tools for Policymakers and Public Health Workers*, 1998;
- *America's Vital Interest in Global Health*, 1997;
- *In Her Lifetime: Female Morbidity and Mortality in Sub-Saharan Africa*, 1996;

- *Vaccines Against Malaria: Hope in a Gathering Storm*, 1996;
- *Lead in the Americas: A Call for Action*, 1996;
- *The Children's Vaccine Initiative: Achieving the Vision*, 1993;
- *Emerging Infections: Microbial Threats to Health in the United States*, 1992; and
- *Malaria: Obstacles and Opportunities*, 1991.

Measurement Issues in Calculating the Global Burden of Disease

Official health statistics are the source of information for estimates of the global burden of disease. However, these statistics from developing countries are frequently incomplete, inaccurate, or out of date, and they rarely contain adequate information on neurological, psychiatric, or developmental disorders. At the same time these data provide the best starting point for understanding the magnitude of the burden of disease and for confronting the needs imposed by that burden.

In addition to mortality statistics, disability-adjusted life year (DALY) calculations require numerical inputs for the specific incidence of disease, the proportion of disease incidence leading to disability, the average age of disability onset, the duration of disability, and the distribution of disability across six levels of severity. Because such data are often unavailable, determinations of burden typically incorporate estimates for most of these values. The potential limitations and sources of errors in DALY estimates include:

- Disability-weights are presumed to be universal, but empirical studies are needed to validate these assumptions.
- Limitations in the data needed from countries to estimate the burden of disease. The cause of death age and gender are needed, but only about 30-40% of all deaths are captured by vital registration in most developing countries.
- The inability to quantify the contribution of risk factors in total burden of disease.
- The value choices that underlie the definition of the DALY are not universally accepted.

- The DALY does not reflect individuals' ability to cope with their functional limitations.
- Estimations may exclude some disabilities, which leads to an under-estimation of years lived with disability (e.g., childhood disabilities such as blindness or cognitive deficit), while some comorbidities might not be recognized (e.g., depression and substance abuse), leading to an over-estimation or double-counting.

Improving DALY measurements will require better data collection and analysis. Specific improvements might include:

- Validation of the methods to measure the time lived with disability of different severity;
- More accurate monitoring systems to be able to generate real estimates of mortality and disability by cause; and
- Projection methods that incorporate known levels and trends of major risk factors such as smoking and trends in other diseases.

The lack of data on psychiatric disorders in many countries has led to estimates based on methods that might not be transferable to assess the health status of the global poor. Further work is needed on standardizing assessment indicators to obtain a more realistic view of the burden of disease affecting developing countries.

Workshop Agenda

Nervous System Disorders in Developing Countries
Board on Global Health,
Institute of Medicine

Academy of Educational Development
Washington, D.C.

MONDAY, NOVEMBER 8
Open Meeting

9:00–9:30 a.m.   **Welcome and Opening Remarks**
Kenneth Shine
Judith Bale

Study Charge

Sponsors
Walter Gulbinat, Global Forum for Health Research
Darrel Regier, NIMH
Joana Rosario, NINDS
Mary Lou Oster-Granite, NICHD
Coleen Boyle, CDC

Introduction of Co-Chairs
Assen Jablensky
Richard Johnson

Opening Session

9:30–10:15   **Nervous System Disorders:**
Norman Sartorius, The Global Burden Disease

10:15–10:30   **Break**

Session I

Depression
Moderator: Rachel Jenkins

10:30–11:00   **Depression in Developing Countries**
Jessie Mbwambo

11:00–11:30   **Mental Health of Indigenous People**
Alex Cohen

11:30 a.m.–12:30 p.m.   **Small Working Group Discussion**
Srinivasa Murthy
Bedirhan Ustun
Sylvia Kaaya
Jessie Mbwambo
Alex Cohen
Darrel Regier

12:30–1:00   **Open Discussion**

1:00–2:00   **Lunch**

Session II

Developmental Disabilities
Moderator: Maureen Durkin

2:00–2:30   **Risk Factors and Outcomes for
Children and Youth**
Thomas Langfitt

2:30–3:30   **Small Working Group Discussion**
Julius Familusi
Donald Silberberg
Thomas Langfitt
Mary Lou Oster-Granite
Vikram Patel

3:30–3:45	**Break**

3:45–4:15	**Open Discussion**

4:15–5:00   **Epidemiology of Common Mental Disorders in Developing Countries, with a Special Focus on Poverty and Female Gender as Risk Factors**
Vikram Patel

5:00–5:15   **Closing Comments**
Norman Sartorius

TUESDAY, NOVEMBER 9

8:00–8:30   a.m.   **Breakfast**

Session III

Epilepsy
Moderator: M. Gourie-Devi

8:30–9:00   **Cysticercosis**
Peter Schantz

9:00–9:30   **Epidemiology and Prevention of Epilepsy in Africa**
Beugre Kouassi

9:30–10:30   **Small Working Group Discussion**
Marcelo Cruz
Donald Silberberg
Peter Schantz
Beugre Kouassi

10:30–10:45   **Break**

10:45–11:15   **Open Discussion**

Session IV

Schizophrenia
Moderator: Assen Jablensky

11:15–12:00 noon   **Health Systems Model of Approaching Mental Health Research and Program Implementation**

and the Overall Policy Implications of Cultural and Health System Diversity in Mental Health Care.
Vikram Patel

12:00–1:00 p.m.   **Lunch Presentation: Mental Health Economics**
Thomas McGuire
Harvey Whiteford

1:00–2:00   **Small Working Group Discussion**
Srinivasa Murthy
Vikram Patel
Bedirhan Ustun
Jessie Mbwambo
Darrel Regier

2:00 –2:30   **Open Discussion**

Session V

Stroke
Moderator: Marcelo Cruz

2:30–3:00   **Epidemiology and Prevention of Stroke in Africa**
Beugre Kouassi

3:00–4:00   **Discussion**
M. Gourie-Devi
Donald Silberberg
Richard Johnson
Beugre Kouassi

4:00–4:15   **Break**

4:15–4:45   Open Discussion

Closing Session

4:45–5:30   **Closing Discussion**
Co-Chairs

APPENDIX D

Economic Analysis

GUIDELINES FOR ECONOMIC ANALYSIS OF COMMUNITY MENTAL HEALTH CARE PROGRAMS IN LOW-INCOME COUNTRIES

From: *Integration of Mental Health Care into Primary Care: Demonstration Cost-Outcome Study in India and Pakistan*
D. Chisholm, K. Sekar, K.K. Kumar, K. Saced, S. James, M. Mubbashar, and R.S. Murthy
Reprinted with permission from the Royal College of Psychiatrists
© 2000

The guidelines have been drawn up in order to provide an overview of issues, principles and procedures related to the economic analysis of mental health care programs in low-income countries; are aimed at mental health workers who have an interest in incorporating an economic perspective into their evaluative research activities; are largely based on the principles and methods used in the United States and United Kingdom, but also reflect an additional set of features associated with the implementation of these methods in the context of low-income countries; and do not attempt to be comprehensive, and it is recommended that a local health economist or closest equivalent is consulted in their application.

THE RATIONALE FOR AN ECONOMIC PERSPECTIVE

The increasing recognition of mental health as a significant public health issue globally has led to additional demands for resources that are already stretched. There is therefore a requirement to demonstrate that investment of resources into mental health care and prevention is needed and worthwhile. This translates into generating evidence on affordable and cost-effective mental health care and prevention strategies. Economic evaluation provides a methodology that allows policy makers, managers and clinicians to make choices between differing treatments, settings and illnesses in order to facilitate the judicious use of scarce resources. The current lack of mental health economic evaluative studies in low-income countries is a significant stumbling block to the investment of resources in mental health by governments and international agencies.

PRINCIPLES OF ECONOMIC ANALYSIS

Key to the understanding of an economic approach towards mental disorder is the notion of resource scarcity, since this necessarily prompts the requirement to make choices between different courses of possible action or investment. Making a choice implies in turn the sacrifice or foregoing of the alternative action or investment. The economic approach therefore attempts to value the worth of a particular resource, decision or strategy with reference to its "opportunity cost," namely the value attached to the next best alternative. To give an example, the opportunity cost of an acute psychiatric bed is derived with reference to the alternative use with which those resources could be put to, such as within another medical speciality, outside medicine completely, or investment into an interest-bearing savings account. A further important principle of economic analysis is that it takes a broad, societal perspective, such that account is taken of costs falling to all relevant parties; for example, allowance should be made for inputs of unpaid volunteers/family carers as well as formal care inputs.

PLANNING AND DESIGNING AN ECONOMIC STUDY

For an appropriate economic evaluation of a mental health care intervention, program or strategy, a number of study design features need to be considered. Since economic evaluations often take place alongside clinical evaluations or trials, the *design of the study* will typically need to be agreed to in conjunction with other evaluators. The most desirable design requirements for the economic evaluation of a mental health care intervention revolve around the presence of a control group (against which to draw comparisons with the intervention group), and the prospective follow-up of these two groups over time (one year would be sufficient for most studies). This "experimental" study design is the "gold standard" of clinical and economic evaluation, since it is able to demonstrate most clearly that changes in selected measures are attributable to the intervention, as opposed to other possible explanatory factors ("confounding" variables). Where it is not possible or practicable to carry out an experimental study, an observational study design can be used; this design may have better external validity—preserving the context in which care is provided—but shifts the focus of the analysis towards identifying associations between the intervention and changes in costs or outcomes (as opposed to attributing a causal relationship). A further desirable is recruitment of a sufficient sample of patients and/or centers to show statistically significant changes between groups (at least 100–200 subjects per group is probably required); the sample size necessary to show a significant economic difference may be greater than that necessary to show a clinical difference between study groups.

Alongside decisions regarding the most appropriate study design, consideration must also be given to the *mode of economic evaluation* (i.e., the manner in which costs and outcomes data are to be combined). The simplest of cost evaluations is commonly referred to as cost-minimization analysis, but this is only appropriate if it is known that outcomes are identical (very unlikely), in which case the task is merely to establish the least cost method of achieving these outcomes. A much more common mode of economic evaluation in the field of mental health care is cost-effectiveness analysis, which assesses not only the costs but also the outcome of an intervention, expressed in terms of cost per reduction in symptom level, cost per life saved, etc. Where there is more than a single measure of outcome being investigated, as is often the case in psychiatry and related fields (see "Outcomes" below), it is more correct to label this type of study as a cost-consequences analysis. This mode of evaluation is likely to represent the default choice in most contexts, and has the advantage of presenting an array of outcome findings to decision-makers. A further mode of evaluation is cost-utility analysis, which has considerable appeal for decision-makers since it generates equivalent and therefore comparable study data ("utilities," expressed by a combined index of the mortality and quality of life or disability effects of an intervention), upon which priorities can then be based. However, there are technical difficulties in using this approach, and where it has been used in psychiatry, it has not performed very well to date. The final option is cost-benefit analysis, which refers to a form of evaluation in which all costs and outcomes are valued in monetary units, thereby allowing assessment of whether a particular course of action is worthwhile, based on a simple decision rule that benefits must exceed costs. This approach is difficult to undertake because of the requirement to quantify outcomes in monetary terms, and consequently is found very rarely in mental health care evaluation.

One other key decision to make at the design stage of the study is the scope or *perspective of the evaluation*. This refers to the viewpoint from which the analysis is being taken, which, in ascending order of comprehensiveness, might be that of a particular agency or government department (e.g., ministry of health), the statutory/formal sector as a whole (e.g., including social services), or a societal perspective which assesses the impact of the intervention on all agencies, including patients themselves as well as their carers or households. The choice of viewpoint, which will influence what costs and outcomes are to be measured, should be determined according to whether the intervention under study is expected to exert a differential impact on these various agencies/sectors.

In summary, it is possible to list a number of stages which typically comprise the conduct of an economic evaluation, all of which need to be considered and carried out in order to obtain a valid and reliable set of findings:

- definition of the alternative interventions to be evaluated (design);
- identification of the costs and outcomes to be included in the study (scope);
- quantification of these identified costs and outcomes (valuation);
- comparison of costs and outcomes (analysis);
- revision of findings in the light of risk, uncertainty and sensitivity (qualification); and
- examination of distributional effects (equity implications).

DATA COLLECTION

Resource Utilization

The collection of service utilization data at the level of the individual patient enables the generation of detailed information on the consumption of a wide range of resources. Opportunity cost estimates can be applied subsequently to these data in order to calculate the overall economic costs associated with an individual's care, or at a more aggregated level, a particular intervention or strategy. An initial stage in the recording of resource utilization data is the identification of relevant components of potential service receipt by users, such as contacts with primary care physicians and other health workers, community-based private or voluntary sector providers and hospital inpatient and outpatient care (both psychiatric and general). Services to include will differ with respect to a number of evaluative concerns, including the scope, objectives and setting of the study, as well as the particular service needs of the client group(s). For example, users with more severe or enduring mental disorders, such as persons with a diagnosis of schizophrenia, often need a wider range of service supports than people with common mental disorders such as depression and anxiety (e.g., day care services and residential care). For economic analyses carried out alongside clinical evaluations (the expected norm in this context), the most convenient means of data collection is often via an interviewer-administered service receipt schedule, which can record service use over defined retrospective periods at the various assessment points of the study. It is also important to ensure that data is available or collected on the socio-demographic and socio-economic characteristics of the individuals, including lost opportunities to work (this latter category may be an important economic outcome).

Resource Costs

For each item of resource utilization, a unit cost estimate is required, such as a cost per inpatient day, or cost per contact with a primary care worker. It will be necessary to compute these estimates using a range of data sources, including national/local government statistics, health authority figures and specific facility or organization revenue accounts. The broad perspective to be employed in the costing of services is an economic one, such that in principle service costs are derived by reference to their marginal long-term opportunity costs. In practice, derivation of costs in this way is difficult. It is therefore common to use short-term average costs as a proxy for long-run marginal costs. The main categories of cost that need to be quantified for each service are:

- Salaries/wages of staff employed in the direct care and management of patients. Salary costs can be obtained from local or national pay scales. The ideal salary value to use is a weighted average of all grades on a pay scale. Supplementary (fringe) benefits, bonuses and allowances should be included. Also include employer contributions to local/national taxes, pension or health insurance schemes, etc., which can be given as a percentage add-o to the salary/wage.

- Facility operating costs where the service is provided (cleaning, catering, consumables, water, electricity etc.). This covers the costs associated with running the establishment where the professional is employed, for example, a rural health center. This can be worked out by dividing pro rata the total running costs of the establishment (excluding capital costs or rent) by the total number of "full-time equivalent" staff. For government facilities, these costs can usually be obtained from the finance or planning departments of local or federal government.

- Any overhead costs relating to the service (personnel, finance, etc.). Costs associated with service management and administration, such as finance and personnel functions, are often difficult to identify with accuracy, and it may only be possible to establish a percentage add-on to known revenue (operating) costs.

- The capital costs of the facility where the service is provided (land, buildings, etc.). The (opportunity) cost of capital is calculated as the annuity (the constant stream of payments arising from interest, taken to be the best alternative use for the capital) which will deplete the lump sum value over the lifetime of the capital. The lump sum value can be obtained from government contracts for similar buildings. The lifetime of land and buildings is best set at 20 years, and the lifetime of equipment (including furniture and vehicles) can be set at 5 years. The other determining feature of the annuity factor is the prevailing discount rate for public and/or private capital assets (this should be available through local government offices). For example, using the 5% discount rate, a hospital worth $500,000 would have an annual capital cost of $40,122.

In order to reach a unit cost of contact time, the aggregate of these cost components needs to be divided by the typical availability of the service or the working time of the professional (for example, 35 hours per week, with 4 weeks holiday per year and 1 week sickness leave allowance).

It should be emphasized that economic or opportunity costs are *not* the same as market prices, charges, fees or per diems. Profit motives, varying accounting and reimbursement practices mean that the use of per diems and hospital charges may not represent a good proxy of opportunity cost. For example, a private, for-profit company may charge a fee above what it actually costs to provide care. Where used, this should be clearly stated and, if possible, adjusted to reflect the real economic cost.

Outcomes

There is an important distinction to be made between indicators of intermediate outcomes and final outcomes. The former category, which can also be referred to as process indicators, should not ideally be the focus of the analysis, since positive changes in, for example, attendance or detection rates may not in fact result in improved patient welfare or mental health. Thus, while process indicators are undoubtedly an important source of differentiation between study samples at the institutional level, their use as indicators of improved patient welfare needs to be treated with caution. Final outcomes, on the other hand, are concerned with detecting changes in the physical, psychological or social well-being of individuals, and commonly revolve around the measurement of symptoms, functioning and disability, quality of life and service satisfaction.

Local Service Structures

The take up and subsequent effectiveness of services is determined to a significant extent by the access, availability and quality of mental health services. Without comparable and standardized descriptions of the structure and content of service systems, analysis of the role of organizational characteristics in evaluating costs and outcomes is severely compromised. It is therefore vital to have an understanding of the features that characterize each site's local service system. Data is needed at a local area level in two domains: sociodemography, to include the age, sex, education and employment profiles of the population; and primary and secondary health services, to include the structure, organization and financing of both general medical and mental health services, plus the availability of/access to these services to/by the population(s) under study.

DATA ANALYSIS AND PRESENTATION

Economic evaluation provides a means of comparing the costs and outcomes of a mental health care intervention or program together in an explicit framework. This in turn enables decision-makers to assess the extent to which the intervention or strategy offers a good use of (scarce) resources. An analysis of costs alone, or indeed of outcomes alone, does not provide such information.

In analytical terms, there are a number of scenarios that can be considered when assessing whether an intervention represents a worthwhile use of resources:

If statistical analyses of cost and outcome data show that the new intervention is both significantly less costly and more beneficial than the control group (usual care), then one can immediately conclude that the intervention is preferable. Likewise, usual care is the preferred choice when it is cheaper and more effective.

If the costs and outcomes are found to be equivalent, then either is acceptable. If only cost is equivalent, then the more effective intervention is preferable, and if only outcome is equivalent, then the cheaper intervention is preferable.

When the evidence shows that one of the two (or more) interventions is both more costly and more effective, it is necessary to assess whether the additional costs are worth the greater effectiveness. This can be established by calculating a cost-effectiveness ratio (the difference in cost over the difference in outcome between the experimental intervention and the control or comparison group). The ratio is positive when one of the groups both costs more and produces a superior outcome. For example, an intervention that costs an extra Rupees 1,000 over a year and produces an additional improvement of 5 points on a social functioning measure compared to usual care, would result in a positive ratio of Rupees 200, interpreted as the increased average cost necessary to gain an average of 1 point of improvement per year. The cost-effectiveness ratio is negative when the innovative intervention costs less but has superior outcomes (i.e., cost saving), or when the innovation costs more but produces worse outcomes (i.e., a bad investment).

In any of these circumstances, the usefulness of these estimates depends on the validity and credibility of the evidence about the sampled populations of the study, and this is never perfect. A key activity of the analysis stage of an economic evaluation is therefore to carry out a sensitivity analysis, which involves the introduction of alternative values to key study parameters (e.g., the cost per inpatient day, or the rate at which capital costs have been discounted) with a view to assessing whether overall conclusions are robust to these plausible changes to values or whether in fact results are very sensitive to such changes.

While the addition of economic analysis to mental health care evaluations introduces an extra dimension that offers a wider assessment of the implications of new or existing courses of action, it is important to mention some of the limitations of the approach. Many economic evaluations fall short of the ideal, whether that be in terms of sample size, or comprehensiveness of cost and outcome measurement. Conclusions based on a small trial with less than 50 subjects per arm can often only be tentative, while the failure to measure the indirect consequences associated with two alternative treatments (e.g., lost opportunities for work) may give rise to misleading results. There are also a number of ongoing methodological debates with respect to certain aspects of economic evaluation, such as the alternative techniques available for measuring health state preferences (essential for both cost–utility and cost–benefit analysis). In this context, it is worth noting that economic evaluation is no panacea for making difficult allocative and policy decisions; rather, it is one additional tool that together with clinical and social dimensions can facilitate explicit, evidence-based decision-making.

CONTACT POINT

If you have any queries regarding these guidelines, please contact:

Daniel Chisholm, Economist
Classification, Assessment and Surveys (CAS)
World Health Organization
1211 Geneva 27
Switzerland
e-mail: ChisholmD@who.int

FURTHER READING

Drummond MF, O'Brien B, Stoddart GL, Torrance GW (1997). Methods for the Economic Evaluation of Health Care Programmes. Second edition, Oxford Medical Publications, Oxford.

Hargreaves W, Shumway M, Hu T, and Cuffel B (1998). Cost-Outcome Methods for Mental Health. Academic Press.

Knapp MRJ (1995). The Economic Evaluation of Mental Health Care. Ashgate, Aldershot.

Shah A and Jenkins R (1999). Mental health economic studies from developing countries reviewed in the context of those from developed countries. Acta Psychiatrica Scandinavica, 100, 1–18.

MONEY MATTERS IN EPILEPSY

S.V. Thomas
Department of Neurology
Sree Chitra Institute for Medical Sciences and Technology
Trivadrum-695 011, India
Reprinted with permission from Neurology India
© December 2000

INTRODUCTION

Epilepsy is the most common neurological disorder in the world. There have been remarkable advancements in clinical epidemiology in the recent past. Many new anti-epileptic drugs (AED) have been marketed in this decade. Epilepsy surgery has established itself as a safe and effective option for intractable epilepsy. Cognitive, psychosocial and gender issues have gained more attention, with the result that quality of life has become the central focus of epilepsy care. Progress in epilepsy care has inevitably escalated its cost as well. Recently, there had been much debate on the economic aspects of newer modalities of treatment of epilepsy [1,2]. The International League Against Epilepsy (ILAE) Commission on economic aspects, in a recent report, has highlighted the need for thorough appraisal of the economic aspects of epilepsy [3]. Thorough economic appraisal of newer strategies in epilepsy care, be it newer AEDs or epilepsy surgery, would enable the clinician to make judicious decisions in patient care. Most clinicians have little exposure to health economics, as it is a relatively new discipline in health sciences. In the future, as third party payment of medical bills becomes more prevalent, there will be greater pressure for cost containment without compromising on quality of services. In this article, the broad principles of estimating the cost of epilepsy and standard techniques of making economic evaluation of treatment protocols are reviewed.

COST

In socioeconomic evaluation, costs are the resources expended to obtain a desired state of health. All resource exenditures (medical and non-medical services) incurred for the prevention, diagnosis, treatment and rehabilitation of a particular disease are included under cost (Table 1). Traditionally, resource expenditure is estimated under the direct and indirect cost. A third component of intangible cost compromised of the money equivalents for the social stigma, psychological stress and pain is also computed in some cases (Table 2).

TABLE 1 Resources That Are Frequently Expended in a Medical Encounter

1.	The physician's time;
2.	Activities of physician's ancillary staff;
3.	Use of medical office space;
4.	Laboratory services;
5.	Cost of medicines and its storage;
6.	Pharmacist's time;
7.	Patient's time away from work; and
8.	Cost of patient transportation to office.

Direct cost

Direct cost can be further divided into medical costs related to the prevention, diagnosis, treament and rehabilitation of epilepsy and non-medical costs related to travel expenditure, etc. Most of the out-of-pocket expenses for the patients and their families come under this category. However, the actual cost of these services is frequently much more than what a patient pays. In many instances, government or other agencies may be subsidising this component; e.g., in a government hospital, the services of the neurologists and other specialists may be provided free, and the charges for video EEG or MRI may be only the cost of consumables. Many institutions also provide some cross subsidy by which they reduce the charges for poor patients by compensating it from more well off patients. Hence, the final bill charged to the patient may be quite diffrent from the actual costs. The cost of services may be different in different parts of the country. The cost of infrastructure in a big city may be more than that for the same in a more modest setting. These factors also should be considered while computing the cost of epilepsy care. The direct cost of epilepsy is gathered in one of the three methods viz. (1) self reported treatment data from providers or patients, (2) medical charts or billing data obtained from the provider or patient, and (3) hypothetical model based on disease characteristics.

TABLE 2 Cost Benefit Evaluation of Epilepsy

Costs	Benefits
Direct Medical Cost	*Morbidity*
Outpatient services in patient services	Control of seizures
Fixed cost of utilities	Improvement in cognition
Variables cost (diagnostic tests, drugs, devices)	Morbidity due to adverse drug reaction
Home care services	Morbidity due to surgery if any
Ancillary services	
Volunteers	
Direct Non-Medical cost	*Mortality*
Care provided by family and friends	Lives saved
Transportation to and from hospitals	Lives lost due to adverse drug effects or surgery
Child care	
Housekeeping	
Social services	
Indirect Cost	*Psychosocial*
Time and productivity	Improvement in quality of life
Change in productivity	Quality adjusted life years
Income lost by family members	
Forgone leisure time	
Intangible Cost	*Economic*
Cost attributed to pain	Use of health resources
Suffering, social stigma, etc.	Increase in productivity
	Reduction in patient care expenditures

Indirect cost

Indirect cost commonly has three components (1) employment related—the lost earnings associated with reduced output when people withdraw from work due to morbidity or premature mortality; (2) productivity related—the reduced earnings from absence or reduced productivity due to morbidity for those who continue to work despite the illness; and (3) household related—the lost value of household production when people alter the time they devote to such work because of epilepsy. Calculation of indirect cost involves in-depth examination of the impact of the illness on the socioeconomic life of the patients and their families.

Intangible cost

This aspect of epilepsy care has not yet been adequately examined. The social stigma, pain and suffering that an individual suffers because of epilepsy constitutes intangible costs. In some studies they are expressed in unit terms or scales and in some studies an economic equivalent of this loss is expressed.

CONSEQUENCE (BENEFIT)

Consequences or benefits are the result of using a medical service or in economic terms, the outcome of using a particular resource. With regard to epilepsy, the positive consequences would include control of seizures, years of increased productivity and probably years of life saved (by avoiding death due to accidents) and improvement in social life. The negative consequences would include adverse effect of the drugs or the investigations carried out, and time expended in making repeated visits to clinic and pharmacies (Table 3).

PERSPECTIVE

Economic evaluation can be performed from different perspectives or viewpoints. Patient's perspective emphasizes the out-of-pocket expenditure to the

TABLE 3 Annual Per Person Cost of Epilepsy (modified from ref. 14)

Country, year	Population	Cost measures	Direct cost	Indirect cost
Australia, 1993	All epilepsies	Direct medical, some indirect age +5	US$2,751	US$3,381
Switzerland, 1993	Individuals on AED	Direct medical, non-medical, some indirect	US$9,400	US$5,130
UK, 1990	All active and inactive epilepsies	Direct medical, non-medical, some indirect	US$2,600	US$5,989
USA, 1994	Refractory adult epilepsy	Direct medical, some indirect	US$2,971	US$9,418
India, 1998	Active and inactive epilepsy	Direct medical, non-medical, some indirect	INR 5,070	INR 6,000

patient and his family. The costs borne by the provider or society at large are less important. Quality of life, time lost to work, etc. are also important from the patient's perspective. Provider's perspective evaluates costs from the service provider's (such as hospital) viewpoint. Third party payer's perspective examines cost evaluation from the insurance company or employer's viewpoint. Societal perspective examines the entire social and economic effect of the new treatment (e.g., epilepsy surgery) on all segments of the society. Such studies would examine the lifetime medical and surgical cost and consequences. Costs related to a wide array of services such as institutional care and home services need to be included in addition to hospital care, outpatient care, etc. Perspective is a key factor in defining the research question and evaluating the cost and consequence of any new program for epilepsy. The most comprehensive study examines the cost and benefits from the societal perspective.

COST OF ILLNESS STUDIES (COI)

This is a form of evaluation which computes the current economic impact of a disease including the costs and consequences of treating the disease. No comparison of treatment modalities is made. Traditionally there are two methods of estimating the cost of an illness. The commonly used approach is the human capital method that divides cost into direct and indirect components. An alternative approach to estimate the cost of illness is the willingness to pay method. This approach defines the cost of an illness in terms of what people would be willing to pay for a hypothetical permanent cure for the disease. The former approach is more frequently used. Most of the COI studies on epilepsy have been based on prevalence based estimates [4-7]. Such studies do not express the variation in the cost of management due to changes in the natural history of epilepsy. Longitudinal studies are ideal for estimating the cost of epilepsy over a period of time. Two such studies have been published recently [8,9].

The first comprehensive study on epilepsy in the USA was carried out in 1975 [10]. That study estimated the national cost of epilepsy at $3.6 billion for 2.1 million cases. On a per patient basis, the 1975 figure represents US $7,440 in 1995, $1,150 (15%) for direct treatment-related costs and $6,290 (85%) for indirect employment-related costs. Begley et al. estimated the cost of epilepsy based on its natural history [9]. They identified six prognostic groups of epilepsy. Based on epidemiological data and these models, they estimated the lifetime cost of epilepsy for a cohort of persons diagnosed in 1990 in the United States. The total lifetime cost in 1990 for all perons with onset of epilepsy in 1990 was estimated at $3.0 billion (direct cost accounting for 62%). The cost per patient ranged from $4,272 for persons with remission after initial diagnosis and treatment to $138,602 for persons with intractable seizures.

An exhaustive cost of illness study on epilepsy was carried out in the UK [11]. This is based on data from the National Epilepsy Society and National

General Practice Study Group for Epilepsy. A longitudinal cost profile of epilepsy was calculated, with an average initial direct cost of £611 (US$917) per patient per annum which decreased after eight years of follow-up to £169 (US$254) per patient per annum. The cost of newly diagnosed epilepsy in the first year of diagnosis in the UK was £18 million (US$27 million). The total annual cost of established epilepsy in the UK was estimated to be £1930 million (US$2,895 million), over 69% of which was due to indirect costs (unemployment and excess mortality). The cost of active epilepsy per patient was approximately £4167 (US$6,251), and of inactive epielpsy £1630 (US$2,445) per patient per annum. Recently, another study had been carried out in the UK based on the prevalence of epilepsy.[12] The per annum per patient direct cost of epilepsy was £1568. The largest single element of cost (58%) to the health service was the cost of inpatient episodes followed by drug cost (23%). There are well-conducted "cost of illness studies" from Switzerland, Australia and other western countries (Table 3).[13]

These studies indicate that epilepsy is an enormous economic burden to the society and the major component of the cost is the indirect cost constituted by lost productivity. With effective treatment, 70–80% of patients can go in for remission and can be effectively rehabilitated with positive economic gain.

SPECIAL PROBLEMS IN EVALUATING COST OF EPILEPSY

Several methodological issues that influence the economic appraisal of epilepsy should be kept in mind while interpreting data on cost of epilepsy studies [14]. It is important to ensure that all major components of cost are included in a given study. The definition of epilepsy also assumes importance when the cost is evaluated from the societal perspective. The commonly used definition of two or more unprovoked seizures has many limitations. Considerable cost may be involved in the evaluation of single seizures which would not be included if we follow this definition.

Epilepsy is a collection of syndromes that differ widely in terms of severity. The cost of mild epilepsy with rare seizures that do not interfere with normal life is quite different from severe epilepsy with very frequent seizures and considerable morbidity. Hospital based studies are likely to reflect the client characteristics and may accordingly bias the data. There may be other co-morbidities such as mental retardation or motor disability that may inflate the cost unless suitable adjustments are done. It is also important to differentiate between prevalence based studies and longitudinal studies.

GENERAL TOOLS OF ECONOMIC EVALUATION

The value of a procedure, e.g., epilepsy surgery, is equal to the sum of all costs subtracted from all consequences discounted over time at a particular discount rate.[15] There are four commonly used approaches of cost and benefits evaluations.

Cost Benefit Analysis

This is the most exhaustive approach in which real cost and consequences are expressed in monetary terms. In this regard, many of the resources and consequences have to be given somewhat arbitrary monetary value. For example, the anxiety that one may lose memory following the surgery is a cost and the peace of mind that seizures will not occur is a benefit which are difficult to translate into monetary units. By using monetary values on both sides of the economic appraisal equation, it is possible to estimate the net gain to the society from a particular treatment. In principle this is an excellent tool to make comparisons between different treatment protocols for the disorder and different disorders altogether. However, the monetary value assigned to many benefits is arbitrary to a large extent and may not be comparable.

Cost Effectiveness Analysis

In this approach, the benefits are not converted into monetary units but are evaluated as such. This approach is frequently adopted to compare different treatment protocols that apparently achieve the same outcome; e.g., the costs of medical and surgical treatment can be compared against the outcome of seizure frequency, measured as the number of seizures in unit period.

Cost Utility Analysis (CUA)

CUA is another approach that measures costs in monetary terms, but measures consequences in terms of their quality or utility. In CUA no attempt is made to measure health outcomes in monetary terms. Rather, CUA employs a common non-monetary tool to measure those consequences that are not amenable to economic expression. One of the recommended tools to measure the outcome is quality adjusted life years (QALY). Disability Adjusted Life Years (DALY) is another outcome measure that can be used instead of QALY. However, utility measures have a number of disadvantages including the bias against the elderly, the impossibility of generalizing quality of life across or within patient groups.

Cost Minimization Analysis (CMA)

CMA assumes that the outcomes of two treatment options are the same and a direct comparison of costs for two alternate treatment protocols can be made. For example, if the remission rates of different AEDs are the same, how do we minimize the cost by choosing the AEDs.

PHARMACO-ECONOMIC EVALUATION OF EPILEPSY

The increase in the cost of epilepsy care due to the use of newer AEDs has been the focus of interest recently. It is estimated to be approximately US$500 million a year in United States. Certain methodological issues need to be kept in mind while interpreting such data, e.g., the cost of newer AEDs (acquisition cost) may be many-fold more than conventional AEDs. However the overall cost of treating epilepsy with such drugs could be less because of savings from fewer hospital visits for seizures, or management of adverse drug reactions or increased productivity. Similarly, the one-time cost of presurgical evaluation and epilepsy surgery is many times more than that of medical treatment, but the lifetime cost would be less for patients who achieve complete remission by surgery.

COMPARISON OF NEWER AEDS AGAINST CONVENTIONAL AEDS

Comparative studies of monotherapy have been published for lamotrigine [17,18] and vigabatrin as compared to carbamazepine.[19,20] A cost minimization study was carried out by Shakespeare and Simeon in which carbamazepine and lamotrigine were compared as monotherapy for partial or generalized epilepsy.[21] They observed that cost of therapy with carbamazepine was about one third of lamotrigine (£179 vs. £522) even after the costs associated with the management of adverse events and therapeutic switching were considered. Markowitz et al. have used another model to examine the cost-effectiveness of lamotrigine as an add-on therapy for epilepsy [22]. In this model, they estimated the cost of treating patients with intractable epilepsy with conventional AED and the cost of presurgical evaluation and surgery as the base data. The difference in cost due to introduction of lamotrigine in the ensuing 10 years was projected. The results showed that in the first year the lamotrigine regime costs an additional US$83.90 per seizure free day, and US$16.30 per seizure free day gained in the 3rd to 10th year. In the second year lamotrigine costs less because fewer persons from the lamotrigine group underwent presurgical evaluation and surgery. Another recent study had examined the lifetime cost utility of lamotrigine as an add-on therapy.[23] They have observed that adjunctive lamotrigine would cost approximately US$41,000 per unit increase in quality adjusted life year.

The cost of medical treatment of epilepsy with Vigabatrin (VGB) was compared with the cost of evaluation and surgery for epilepsy in 52 patients with intractable epilepsy [24]. In this study, the direct costs associated with treatment with the conventional AED, VGB, epilepsy surgery evaluation (ESE) and epilepsy surgery were analyzed. Sixty percent of the 52 patients obtained a reduction in seizure frequency of 50% or more with VGB. Of the 21 operated patients, 57% became seizure free. Corresponding figures for VGB responders who did not go through ESE and VGB non-responders who were not operated on were 6% and 0%, respectively. The mean yearly costs (expressed as 1991 prices) of epilepsy-related health care including AED treatment were US$1,594, the year before starting VGB therapy, and US$2,959 in the first year of VGB treatment including a mean yearly cost of VGB of US$1,572. The mean total cost for ESE and surgery was US$46,778 (N = 21), while the mean cost of ESE in patients evaluated but not accepted for surgery (N = 14) was US$24,054. Considering the costs for ESE and surgery in the whole patient series, the mean total cost of rendering one patient seizure free with surgery was US$110,000. Surgery is the most effective treatment option in selected cases of severe partial epilepsy. If its costs are distributed over the patient's expected lifetime, the yearly cost is comparable to the present yearly cost of medication with VGB. They opined that, since many patients achieve satisfactory seizure control with VGB, and considering the risks of surgery, it is a rational policy to let patients try this drug (or another of the new generation of AED) before entering ESE.

ACQUISITION COST MAY NOT REFLECT THE OVERALL COST

Fosphenytoin is a new AED which can be administered intravenously or intramuscularly for status epilepticus. This drug is about 15 times more expensive than phenytoin, but was shown to have better efficacy and less adverse effects in controlled clinical trials. Two recent studies [25,26] have shown that the outcome cost (acquisition cost plus the cost of treating adverse drug reactions) is less for fosphenytoin (US$156.68) than phenytoin (US$543.47), although the former is 15 times more expensive (US$90.00 vs. US$6.70).

ECONOMIC ASPECTS OF EPILEPSY: SCENARIO IN DEVELOPING COUNTRIES

Ninety per cent of the world's 40 million people with epilepsy live in developing countries. The vast majority of them are not on regular treatment. These countries have meager facilities for advanced care for epilepsy. The capital investment in epilepsy care would involve import of substantial sophisticated equipments, and spares, as well as training of personnel to handle this equipments properly. There is fierce competition for resources from several corners and its allocation is often a political decision. Quantification of the benefits of treating epilepsy also has problems in such countries. Unemployment among the healthy population, the traditional social underexpectations from sick people, and the impact of joint families all need to be taken into consideration. Direct conversion of local currency to equivalent US dollars would also be misleading as the purchasing power and monetary value of local currency may not be adequately reflected in it. Interaction with anti-cysticercal drugs, anti malarial and anti tubercular drugs that are frequently prescribed for people residing in tropical countries add another dimension to this problem [27]. A recent study from Latin America has highlighted the need for detailed studies on economic aspects of epilepsy in developing countries [28]. Chandra has drawn attention to some of the difficulties in estimating the cost of epilepsy in his study from Indonesia [29].

COST OF EPILEPSY CARE IN INDIA

There is no published report on cost of epilepsy from India. In a previous study, we had examined the various services that are utilized in the care for epilepsy in Kerala State [30]. This study, carried out at a tertiary referral center for epilepsy, indicated that primary care services are underutilized by people with epilepsy. The mean delay in diagnosis of the condition is about nine months. A study from another tertiary referral center for epilepsy in North India has suggested that the cost of epilepsy care can be reduced and the quality of care improved by proper clinical evaluation and education of general physicians.[31] Another recent study had shown that the frequency of polytherapy with its associated higher cost can be reduced by intervention from a tertiary referral center [32]. A multicenter study involving one center each from eight states of India was carried out recently [33]. This is the first large scale study that has addressed the medical service utilization by patients with epilepsy. It had also examined some of the direct cost of epilepsy care in India. Patients included all age groups (mean age 23 years). Half of them had localization related epilepsy. The mean delay in diagnosis of the condition was 1.5 ± 4 years. The average number of hospital visits was three per year (range 1–30). The median of hospitalization because of epilepsy was one per year (range 1–18). About six percent of them were never on any AED. Polytherapy was reduced from 48% to 22% of patients after referral to an advanced epilepsy center. Nearly three-quarters of them (70.2%) have had at least one EEG, one-third (36.1%) had one or more CT scan, and only 8.5% of them had one MRI scan. The direct cost of treatment was over Rs. 5000/- (Table 4).

TABLE 4 Some of the Direct Costs of Treatment of Epilepsy in India per year [33].

Particulars	Rs.
Outpatient service	310
Investigations	1,560
AEDs	1,050
Hospitalizations	1,830
Travel	320
Total	5,070

The mean loss of workdays was about 58 days. The indirect cost related to loss of work may be to the tune of Rs. 6000/-. The out-of-pocket expenditure for anterior temporal lobectomy for intractable temporal lobe epilepsy in Kerala is approximately Rs. 46700/-.

These studies have brought out some interesting aspects of pharmaco-economics and selection of cases. Newer drugs and more expensive AEDs like lamotrigine, if administered without any selection criteria, would increase the cost of treatment many-fold over treatment with conventional drugs. However, these drugs may have a clear economic advantage in the case of intractable epilepsy. Similarly, the savings in terms of fewer hospital visits or admission, fewer adverse drug reactions that need intervention and better quality of life may overcome the higher acquisition cost of some of the newer drugs or surgical treatment. However, the cost of epilepsy care from the societal perspective would increase many-fold if the same treatment and investigations are administered to all patients. Economic evaluation of epilepsy care is a relatively newer branch. Scientists from the field of clinical epileptology, health economics and health administrators need to work together to appraise the subject satisfactorily. Further, economic evaluation of treatment of epilepsy and its consequences in our settings would enable the physicians to improve evidence-based practice as we enter the next millenium.

REFERENCES

1. Chadwick D.: Do new antiepileptic drugs justify their expense? *Arch Neurol* 1998; 55: 1140–1142.
2. Hachinski V.: New antiepileptic drugs: The cost of innovation. *Arch Neurol* 1998; 55: 1142.
3. Beran RG, Pachlatko C : Final report of the ILAE commission on economic aspects of epilepsy, 1994–1997. *Epilepsia* 1997; 38: 1359–1362.

4. Banks GK, Regan KJ, Beran RG: The prevalence and direct costs of epilepsy in Australia. In: Beran RG, Pachlatko C (eds.) Cost of Epilepsy: Proceedings of the 20th International Epilepsy Congress, Ciba Geigy Verlag, Baden, Germany, 1995; 39–48.

5. Beran RG, Banks GK: Indirect costs of epilepsy in Australia. In Beran RG, Pachlatko C (eds.) Cost of Epilepsy: Proceedings of the 20th International Epilepsy Congress, Ciba Geigy Verlag Baden, Germany 1995; 49–54.

6. Gessner U, Sagmeister M, Horisberger B: The cost of epilepsy in Switzerland. *Int J Health Sci* 1993; 4: 121–128.

7. Cockrell OC, Hart YM, Sanders JWAS et al.: The cost of epilepsy in United Kingdom: An estimation based on the results of two population-based-studies. *Epilepsy Res* 1994; 18: 249–260.

8. Cockerell OC: Pharmacoeconomic considerations in the drug treatment of epilepsy. *CNS Drugs* 1996; 6: 450–461.

9. Begley CE, Annegers JF, Lairson DR et al.: Cost of epilepsy in the United States: A model based on incidence and prognosis. *Epilepsia* 1994; 35: 1230–1243.

10. Commission for the control of epilepsy and its consequences. Economic cost of epilepsy. In: Plan for nationwide action on epilepsy, Vol. IV, DHEW Publication No. 78-279. NIH, Washington, D.C. 1978; 117–118.

11. Cockrell OC, Hart YM, Sanders JWAS et al.: The cost of epilepsy in United Kingdom: an estimation based on the results of two population-based studies. *Epilepsy Res* 1994; 18: 249–260.

12. Jacoby A, Buck D, Baker G et al.: Uptake and costs of care for epilepsy: findings from a UK regional study. *Epilepsia* 1998; 39: 776–786.

13. Gessner U, Sagmeister M, Horisberger B: The cost of epilepsy in Switzerland. *Int J Health Sci* 1993; 4: 121–128.

14. Begley CE, Annegers JF, Lairson DR et al.: Methodological issues in estimating the cost of epilepsy. *Epilepsy Res* 1999; 33: 39-55.

15. Luce BR, Elixhauser A: Standards for the socioeconomic evaluation of health care services. Springer Verlag, New York, 1990.

16. Cockerell OC: Pharmacoeconomic considerations in the drug treatment of epilepsy. *CNS Drugs* 1996; 6: 450–461.

17. Brodie MJ, Richens A, Yuen AW: Double blind comparison of lamotrigine and carbamazepine in newly diagnosed epilepsy. UK Lamotrigine/Carbamazepine Trial Group. *Lancet* 1995; 345: 476–479.

18. Reunanen M, Dam M, Yen AW: A randomized open multicentre comparative trial of lamotrigine and carbamazaepine as monotherapy in patients with newly diagnosed or recurrent epilepsy. *Epilepsy Res* 1996; 23: 149–155.

19. Chadwick D, Roi L, Kennedy KM : Vigabatrin (Sabril) as a first line monotherapy in newly diagnosed epilepsy. A double blind comparison with carbamazepine. (Abstract) *Epilepsia* 1996; 37: 6.

20. Kalviainen R, Aikia M, Saukkonen AM et al.: Vigabatrin vs carbamazepine monotherapy in patients with newly diagnosed epilepsy. *Arch Neurol* 1995; 52: 989–996.

21. Shakespeare A, Simeon G: Economic analysis of epilepsy treatment: A cost minimisation analysis comparing carbamazepine and lamotrigine in UK. *Seizure* 1998; 7: 119–125.

22. Markowitz MA, Mauskopf JA, Halpern MT: Cost effectiveness model of adjunctive lamotrigine for the treatment of epilepsy. *Neurology* 1998; 51: 1026–1033.

23. Messori A, Trippoli S, Becagli P et al : Adjunctive lamotrigine therapy in patients with refractory seizures: A lifetime cost-utility analysis. *Eur J Clin Pharmacol* 1998; 53: 421–427.
24. Malmgren K, Hedstrom A, Granquist R et al : Cost analysis of epilepsy surgery and of vigabatrin treatment in patients with refractory partial epilepsy. *Epilepsy Res* 1996; 25: 199–207.
25. Ramsay RE, Wilder BJ : Parenteral fosphenytoin: Efficacy and economic considerations. *Neurologist* 1998; 4: S30–S34.
26. Marchetti A, Magar R, Fischer J et al.: Pharmacoeconomic evaluation of intravenous fosphenytoin (Cerebyx) versus phenytoin (Dilantin) in hospital emergency departments. *Clin Ther* 1996; 18: 953–966.
27. Trevathan E, Medina MT: Antiepileptic drugs in developing countries. *Lancet* 1998; 351: 1210–1211.
28. De-Bittencourt PR : The social and economic reality vis-à-vis the availability and use of medical care for eplieptic patients in Latin America. *Epilepsies* 1998; 10: 135–142.
29. Chandra B : Economic aspects of epilepsy in Indonesia. In Beran RG, Pachlatko CH. Cost of Epilepsy. Ciba Geigy Verlag, Baden. 1995; 75–82.
30. Sanjeev V. Thomas, Ramankutty V, Aley Alexander: Management and Referral Patterns of Epilepsy in India. *Seizure* 1996; 5: 303–306.
31. Sawhney IMS, Lekhra OP, Shashi JS et al : Evaluation of epilepsy management in a developing country: A prospective study of 407 patients. *Acta Neurol Scand* 1996; 94: 19–23.
32. Radhakrishnan K, Pradeep, Nayak : Profile of antiepileptic pharmacotherapy in a tertiary referral center in South India: A pharmacoepidemiological and pharmacoeconomic study. *Epilepsia* 1999; 40: 179–185.
33. Thomas SV, Abraham PA, Alexander M et al : Utilization of services for epilepsy and its economic burden in India: A multicenter study. *Epilepsia* 1999; 40: (Suppl 2) 198.

APPENDIX E

Committee and Staff Biographies

ASSEN V. JABLENSKY, M.D., *(Co-chair)* is Professor and Head of the Department of Psychiatry and Behavioral Science, University of Western Australia in Perth. He is a co-chair for this committee. Dr. Jablensky has formerly served as the Senior Medical Officer for the Division of Mental Health at the World Health Organization, Geneva (1975–1986), where he was responsible for cross-cultural collaborative research into the epidemiology of schizophrenia and other mental disorders. He has served as the Director of the National Program of Neuroscience and Behavior Research and President of the Academy of Medicine in Sofia, Bulgaria. His recent research includes an examination of the interactions between genetic vulnerability and environmental risk factors in schizophrenia; and the role of prenatal exposures and obstetric complications in the causation of schizophrenia, bipolar disorder, and mental retardation. Dr. Jablensky's experience in developing countries and his contribution to the development and evaluation of national mental health programs in Tanzania, Bulgaria, and other countries is of particular importance to this study.

RICHARD T. JOHNSON, M.D., *(Co-chair)* is Professor of Neurology and Microbiology and Neuroscience at the Johns Hopkins University Medical School and the School of Hygiene and Public Health. He is a member of the Institute of Medicine and a co-chair of this committee. His most recent research has been concentrated on HIV-associated neurological disease and cytokines and cofactors in development of disease in the central nervous system. Dr. Johnson is the founding Director of the Neuroscience Institute of Singapore. He has been a visiting professor at the Universidad Peruana Cayetano, Lima, Peru; Imperial College of Health Sciences, Pahlavi Medical Center, Tehran, Iran; Mahidol University, Bangkok, Thailand; and Institut fur Virologie and Immunobiologie, Wurzburg, Germany. Dr. Johnson has served previously on IOM committees, research panels, and review committees.

WILLIAM E. BUNNEY, M.D., is Distinguished Professor and Chair of the Department of Psychiatry and Human Behavior at University of California, Irvine. Dr. Bunney is a member of the Institute of Medicine and is a member of this committee. He serves on the National Scientific Advisory Board of the National Alliance of Research in Schizophrenia and Depression (NARSAD), and the National Depressive and Manic-Depressive Association, and previously served on the extramural scientific advisory board at the National Institute for Mental Health. His major research interests involve clinical psychobiological studies of manic depressive illness, schizophrenia, and childhood mental illness. These include behavioral studies of the efficacy and mode of action of psychopharmacological agents, brain imaging studies, and investigation of brain circuitry abnormality which may be related to the major psychosis period. Dr. Bunney is the author of more than 360 scientific publications and the editor of seven books.

MARCELO CRUZ, M.D., is Professor of Neurology, Neurosciences Institute, Central University of Ecuador. He is a member of this committee. He has published on neuroepidemiology, epilepsy, parasitic diseases, and neurodevelopmental disabilities. His current research examines cerebral cysticercosis as the cause of epilepsy, hydrocephalus, and dementia, as well as the clinical description, the distribution, and means of prevention and control of this parasitic infection. Dr. Cruz is the former Minister of Public Health of Ecuador, and a World Bank consultant for health reform. He currently serves as president of the Ecuadorean Academy of Neurosciences, and is an Honorary Member of the American Academy of Neurology. He also belongs to the Latin American Society of Pediatric Neurology, the Pan American Society of Neuroepidemiology, and the Francophone Network on Research of the Nervous System.

MAUREEN DURKIN, PH.D., DR.P.H., is Associate Professor of Public Health (Epidemiology) at Columbia University's Mailman School of Public Health and Sergievsky Center, and Research Scientist at the New York State Psychiatric Institute's Epidemiology of Brain Disorders Unit. She is a member of the committee. Dr. Durkin has developed methodology for and directed comparative studies of the prevalence and causes of neurodevelopmental disabilities in developing countries. Her current research pertains to international policies relevant to public health and developmental disabilities, the epidemiology and prevention of pediatric neurotrauma, and long-term outcomes of premature birth. She has published widely on these topics, presented at national and international scientific meetings, and taught graduate-level courses. Dr. Durkin has served as an advisor to the World Health Organization and a consultant to numerous organizations including the United Nations Statistical Office and the National Institutes of Health.

JULIUS FAMILUSI, M.D., is the Chair of the Department of Pediatrics, University of Ibadan, Nigeria, and a Consultant Pediatric Neurologist of the University College Hospital. He is a member of this committee. Dr. Familusi has previously served as a Visiting Professor of Pediatrics and Neurology at SUNY-Albany, King Saud University, Saudi Arabia, and the University of Zimbabwe, Harare. His recent research includes a comparison of folate levels in convulsing and non-convulsing febrile children, and cerebellar disorders in childhood. Dr. Familusi has researched and published in the areas of pediatrics and pediatric neurology with special emphasis on viral and bacterial infections of the central nervous system, seizure disorders, neurotoxins, and hemoglobinopathies. Dr. Familusi is an Executive Board member of the International Child Neurology Association.

MANDAVILLE GOURIE-DEVI, M.B.B.S., M.D. (MED), D.M. (NEURO), is the Director–Vice Chancellor and Professor of Neurology at the National Institute of Mental Health and Neuro Sciences in Bangalore, India. She is a member of this committee. She is a fellow of the Indian Academy of Neurology, National Academy of Medical Sciences, and National Academy of Sciences in India. She was the President of the Neurological Society of India. Dr. Gourie-Devi's research focuses on the prevalence and pattern of neurological disorders in the Indian population (which includes the epidemiology of epilepsy), tuberculous meningitis, motor neuron disease, muscular dystrophy, leprosy, stroke, and Japanese encephalitis. She has authored the book, *Neuroepidemiology in Developing Countries*. Dr. Gourie-Devi is the founding editor of the *Annals of the Indian Academy of Neurology*.

DEAN JAMISON, PH.D., is the Director of the Program on International Health, Education and Environment at University of California, Los Angeles. Jamison serves as a liaison member to the committee from the IOM's Board on Global Health. He is the lead author of the World Bank's *1993 Development Report, Investing in Health*. Jamison has researched and published on health policy for low- and middle- income countries, cost-effectiveness analysis, and assessment of health research and development priorities. The Institute of Medicine elected him to membership in 1994.

RACHEL JENKINS, M.D., is the Director of the WHO Collaborating Centre and Professor at the Institute of Psychiatry in London, England. She is a member of the committee. She has published widely on the global burden of mental disorders, mental health policy, and planning using epidemiology and disability measurements, primary care, and epidemiology and outcome indicators. Dr. Jenkins was formerly Principal Medical Officer of the Mental Health Division at the British Department of Health. She developed the mental illness key area of England's Health of the Nation strategy, and the first national survey program of psychiatric morbidity in Great Britain. Dr. Jenkins has conducted research and mental health policy support in many developing countries.

SYLVIA KAAYA, M.D., is Head of the Department of Psychiatry at the Muhimbili University College of Health Sciences of the University of Dar es Salaam, Tanzania. She is a member of the committee. Dr. Kaaya is a senior lecturer in psychiatry. She has researched and published in the areas of adolescent and youth development and risk behaviors as well as depression in sub-Saharan Africa. Dr. Kaaya is a member of the International Scientific Advisory Committee of the Essential Health Interventions Project of the International Development Research Council, the Medical Association of Tanzania, and serves on the Executive Committee of the Tanzania Public Health Association.

ARTHUR KLEINMAN, M.D., is the Presley Professor of Anthropology and Psychiatry, Departments of Anthropology and Social Medicine at Harvard University. He is a member of the Institute of Medicine and a member of the committee. Dr. Kleinman has published widely on mental illness in developing countries, and most recently on the relationship between mental health and social health perspectives and Chinese communities undergoing change from local, national, and global forces. Dr. Kleinman is Chair of the World Health Organization Technical Advisory Committee for the Mental Health of Underserved Populations Action Program and a WHO Consultant for the Chinese Ministry of Health in Beijing.

THOMAS MCGUIRE, PH.D., is Professor of Economics at Boston University. He is a member of the Institute of Medicine and a member of the committee. Dr. McGuire's fields of expertise include health and mental health economics, industrial organization, and public health finance. His recent research work examining economics and mental health will contribute to the committee's evaluation of low-cost treatments and program development. Dr. McGuire has published on mental health and substance abuse coverage under health care reform; demand and supply-side cost sharing in health care; payment and financing of mental health services; and optimal market structures for health care. Dr. McGuire has served as co-chair of four National Institute of Mental Health-sponsored conferences on economics and mental health.

R. SRINIVASA MURTHY, M.B.B.S., M.D., is Dean and Professor of Psychiatry at the National Institute of Mental Health and Neuro Sciences in India.

He is a member of the committee. Dr. Murthy is a fellow in the Indian Psychiatric Society and the National Academy of Medical Sciences. He has researched and published on the epidemiology of schizophrenia and the application of community-based interventions in primary care settings to prevent mental illness and promote mental health. Dr. Murthy has consulted with governments of many developing countries on the development of national mental health programs and the training of providers. Dr. Murthy is currently the Chief Editor of the upcoming World Health Organization *World Health Report*, 2001.

DONALD SILBERBERG, M.D., is Professor of Neurology, Senior Associate Dean (Chair Emeritus) and Director of International Programs at the University of Pennsylvania School of Medicine. He is a member of the committee. Dr. Silberberg's research has focused on metabolic disorders affecting brain development, clinical and basic aspects of multiple sclerosis, and approaches to ameliorating neurological disease in developing countries. Dr. Silberberg serves as a consultant for the World Health Organization (currently Consultant for the Global Burden of Mental and Neurological Diseases project), Global Forum for Health Research, National Institutes of Health, and the World Bank.

BEDIRHAN USTUN, M.D., is the Coordinator of the Classification, Assessment and Surveys Unit at the World Health Organization. He is a member of the committee. Dr. Ustun conducted various international studies on diagnosis, classification, and management of mental disorders in primary care settings and developed structured intervention strategies. Dr. Ustun, in his role at WHO, has a broad public health view of nervous system disorders globally and direct access to worldwide data on the burden of disease and mental health programs.

STUDY STAFF

JUDITH BALE, PH.D. is Director of the Board on Global Health at the Institute of Medicine (IOM), and co-director of Neurological, Psychiatric, and Developmental Disorders in Developing Countries. She directed The Assessment of Future Scientific Needs for Live Variola Virus and co-edited Control of Cardiovascular Disease in Developing Countries. Before IOM, while in the National Academies' Office of International Affairs, she developed and directed collaborative research programs on health and agriculture in more than 30 developing countries. She directed studies on technology transfer in Pakistan; technological challenges for megacities; population growth and land use change in India, China, and the United States; and international nutrition. Dr. Bale serves as a reviewer for several journals and speaker on international health issues. Prior to joining the National Academies, her laboratory research was at the National Institute of Heart, Lung, and Blood, where she published on enzyme kinetics, structure, and mechanisms.

STACEY KNOBLER, is a program officer at the Institute of Medicine (IOM). She is the co-director of Neurological, Psychiatric, and Developmental Disabilities in Developing Countries and study director of the Board on Global Health's Forum on Emerging Infections. Ms. Knobler is actively involved in program research and development for the Board on Global Health. Previously, she has held positions as a Research Associate at the Brookings Institution, Foreign Policy Studies Program and as a Human Rights and Development Consultant for the Organization for Security and Cooperation in Europe in Vienna and Bosnia-Herzegovina. Ms. Knobler has also worked as a research and negotiations analyst in Israel and Palestine. Ms. Knobler is currently a member of the CBACI Senior Working Group for Health, Security, and U.S. Global Leadership. She has conducted research and co-authored published articles on biological and nuclear weapons control, foreign aid, health in developing countries, poverty and public assistance, human rights, and the Arab-Israeli peace process.

Glossary

Acquired Immunodeficiency Syndrome (AIDS): A syndrome that is a result of being infected with human immunodeficiency virus resulting in killing or impairing of the T4 cells—essential for immune system function. The result is an inability of the body to fight infections and certain cancer, and delayed development in infected children.

Asperger Syndrome: A pervasive developmental disorder characterized by an inability to understand how to interact socially. Other typical features of the syndrome include clumsy and uncoordinated motor movements, social impairment with extreme egocentricity, limited interests and/or unusual preoccupations, repetitive routines or nrituals, speech and language peculiarities, and nonverbal communication problems.

Atherothrombotic Stroke: Condition that results from the occlusion of one or more cerebral arteries leading to necrosis of the brain tissue dependent on the blood flow. This may lead to transient (reversible ischemic neurological deficit) or permanent loss of neurological function. Most frequently, it is due to embolization of the atherosclerotic plaque or the thrombus forming in it (i.e., breaking off of material in the aorta, carotid, or vertebral arteries with material floating downstream until it lodges in one of the smaller cerebral arteries).

Autism: A developmental disorder that is characterized by impaired development in communication, social interaction, and unusual and repetitive behavior.

Autism is classified as a Pervasive Developmental Disorder (PDD), which is part of a broad spectrum of developmental disorders affecting young children and adults.

Benzodiazepine: Among the best known and most widely prescribed drugs in the world, benzodiazepines are used mainly as tranquilizers for the control of symptoms due to anxiety or stress.

Bipolar Depression: A psychiatric disorder also known as manic-depressive illness involving dramatic mood swings from periods of excessive activity and rapid thought (manic phase) to periods of hopelessness and depression (depressive phase).

Cerebral Palsy: A term describing a group of chronic conditions affecting body movement and muscle coordination. It is a non-communicable, non-progressive disorder that is a result of injury to the motor areas of the brain that occurred during pregnancy, birth, or early childhood. The condition may present with a combination of different symptoms, including: spasticity (stiff and difficult movement), hypotonia (muscle weakness), ataxia (inability to coordinate voluntary movement, unsteadiness), dyskinesia (inability to coordinate smooth movements resulting in fragmented or jerky movements), or dystonia (involuntary muscle contractions and spasm).

Community-Based Rehabilitation (CBR): A strategy to use and build on resources of the community in order to equalize opportunities for impaired, disabled, and handicapped persons, their families, and the community.

Down's Syndrome (Trisomy 21): A chromosomal abnormality which manifests itself in a set of common physical and mental characteristics, including: extra fold over the eyes, floppy muscles, loose joints, mental retardation, hearing loss, and visual problems. This abnormality is due to the presence of an extra chromosome and has an increased incident related to maternal age.

Dyscalculia: A specific developmental disability affecting a person's ability to conceptualize and perform mathematics. Mild cases can often be compensated for with use of a calculator, but those with severe dyscalculia will need special education services.

Dyskinesia: The presence of involuntary movements, such as the choreaform movements seen in some cases of rheumatic fever or the characteristic movements of tardive dyskensia. Some forms of dyskensia are a side effect of using certain medications, particularly L-Dopa and, in the case of tardive dyskensia, the anti-psychotics.

Dystonia: A state of abnormal (either excessive or inadequate) muscle tone. There are many forms of dystonia. Dystonia disorders cause involuntary movements and prolonged muscle contraction, resulting in twisting body motions, tremor, and abnormal posture. These movements may involve the entire body, or only an isolated area.

Framingham Study: A landmark study begun in 1948 in which some 12,000 residents of the town of Framingham, Massachusetts, were enrolled in a study designed to gather medical data and, more recently, DNA samples. The participants in the Framingham study came in for regular medical exams and provided the information that researchers requested. This extraordinary longitudinal (long-term) study has yielded a vast set of data from which invaluable health information has been extracted.

Hemorrhagic Stroke: Neurological deficit caused by the bursting of an intra-cerebral artery. The disruption of brain tissue and increase in cranial pressure are often fatal and almost always disabling.

Human Immunodeficiency Virus (HIV): Virus responsible for attacking the T4 cells of the immune system resulting in the body's inability to ward off infection.

Hypotonia: Decreased tone of skeletal muscles; in a word, floppiness. Hypotonia is a common finding in cerebral palsy and other neuromuscular disorders. Untreated hypotonia can lead to hip dislocation and other problems.

Infectious Diseases: Any illness that is caused by a specific microorganism.

Intrauterine Growth Retardation: Poor fetal growth, usually due to a fetal defect or to failure of the placenta to provide adequate nutrients. Intrauterine growth retardation causes the fetus to be smaller than expected for the length of gestation. Intrauterine growth retardation may be due to a chromosomal defect, such as Down's syndrome.

Low Birth Weight (LBW): A baby weighing less than 2500 grams at birth.

Neonatal: Pertaining to the newborn period which, by convention, is the first four weeks after birth.

Neural Tube Defect: A developmental failure affecting the spinal cord or brain in an embryo. This defect leads to failure of the bony arch to fuse over the back of the spinal cord, thus causing spina bifida. The best known neural tube defects are anencephaly (absence of the cranial vault and absence of most or all of the cerebral hemispheres of the brain) and spina bifida (an opening in the vertebral column protecting the spinal cord), sometimes with a meningomyelocele (protrusion of the meningeal membranes that cover the spinal cord).

Neurocysticercosis (NCC): Cysts found in the brain (and other parts of the body) as a result of ingestion of the pork tapeworm, *Taenia solium*. The most common symptoms include seizures, headaches, confusion, lack of attention to surroundings, difficulty with balance, and hydrocephalus.

Nosocomial: Originating, taking place, or acquired in a hospital.

Onchocerciasis: Also known as river blindness, a disease caused by a parasitic worm (*Onchocerca volvulus*) which is transmitted to persons by biting blackflies (buffalo gnats) that breed in fast-flowing rivers. The adult worms can live for up to 15 years in nodules beneath the skin and in the muscles of infected persons, where they produce millions of worm embryos (microfilariae) that invade the skin and other tissues, including the eyes.

Otitis media: Infection and inflammation of the middle ear space and ear drum. Symptoms include earache, fever and in some cases, diminished hearing.

Perinatal: Pertaining to the period immediately before and after birth. The perinatal period is defined in diverse ways. Depending on the definition, it starts at the 20th to 28th week of gestation and ends 1 to 4 weeks after birth.

Phenylketonuria (PKU): A rare, inherited metabolic disease that causes mental retardation due to an absence of phenylalanine hydroxylase—the enzyme that converts phenylalanine to tyrosine. The build-up of phenylalanine is toxic but can be controlled by diet.

Posttraumatic Stress Disorder (PTSD): A psychiatric disorder associated with a traumatic event (war, rape, tragic accident, etc.) resulting in the patient reliving the event through nightmares and disturbing recollections during the day.

Psychosocial: Relating social conditions to mental health.

Risperidone: An antipsychotic medication that works on nerves throughout the body and brain by blocking several of the receptors on nerves (dopamine type 2, serotonin type 2, and alpha 2 adrenergic receptors). This alters the chemical messages which nerves transmit to each other.

Schizophrenia: Chronic and disabling disorder which typically has an onset in young adults (teens or early 20s) that may be the result of altered brain chemistry or brain structure. It is defined by characteristic but nonspecific disturbances in the form and content of thought, perception, emotion, sense of self, volition, social relationships, and psychomotor behavior.

Tay Sachs Disease: An inherited condition that is caused by an absence of the enzyme hexosaminidase A (Hex-A), resulting in the accumulation of the lipid GM2 ganglioside. This accummulation, primarily in neurons, progressively damages the cells and results in death of the child by age 3–4.

Unipolar Depression: A psychiatric disorder also known as major depressive illness that is clinically diagnosed when five or more symptoms (sad mood, loss of interest in activities that were once enjoyed, difficulty sleeping or oversleeping, physical slowing or agitation, energy loss, feeling of worthlessness, difficulty concentrating, and thoughts of death or suicide) are present for at least a two-week period and interfere with daily living.

EPIDEMIOLOGICAL TERMS

Disability-Adjusted Life Years (DALYs): A measurement for estimating the burden of disease by taking into account both mortality and non-fatal conditions by summing years of life lost and years lived with disability. The calculation is based on assumptions put forth by Murray and Lopez, *The Global Burden of Disease*, 1997.

Incidence: Ratio of the number of new cases of the disease occurring in a population during a specified time to the number of persons at risk for developing the disease during that period.

Prevalence: Ratio of the number of cases of a specific disease present in a population at a specific time to the number of persons in the population at the time specified.

Primary Prevention: Prevention of the development of disease in a person who does not have the disease.

Secondary Prevention: Prevention of recurrence of a disease in a person who has already been diagnosed with the disease.

Tertiary Prevention: Prevention of disability, poor quality of life, and death in persons with advanced stages of a disease.

Years Lived with Disability (YLD): The number of years lived with a disability or non-fatal health outcomes.

Years of Life Lost (YLL): The number of life years lost prior to a given age of expected survival, usually 65 years.

Definitions for this glossary were compiled from the following sources:

Dorland's Illustrated Medical Dictionary, 28th ed. Philadelphia: W.B. Saunders Co., 1994.

Medicine.Net. *Medical terms and glos*sary. Available at http://www.medicinenet.com, 2001.

Medline plus (date of last update March 18, 2000). Available at http://www.nlm.nih.gov/.

Acronyms

5-HT	5-Hydroxytryptamine (serotonin)
ACE	Angiotensen-Converting Enzyme
ADL	Activities of Daily Living
AED	Anti-Epileptic Drug
AIDS	Acquired Immunodeficiency Syndrome
APA	American Psychological Association
BDI	Beck Depression Inventory
CARMEN	Set of actions for the multifactorial reduction of noncommunicable diseases (Conjuncto de Acciones para la Reducion Multifactorial de las Enfermedades No Transmisibles)
CBR	Community-Based Rehabilitation
CDC	Centers for Disease Control and Prevention
CEDC	Children in Especially Difficult Circumstances
CEU	Clinical Epidemiology Unit
CINDI	Countrywide Integrated Noncommunicable Diseases Intervention Program
CIS-R	Clinical Interview Schedule-Revised
CMD	Common Mental Disorders
CMV	Cytomegalovirus
CNS	Central Nervous System
CP	Cerebral Palsy
CT	Computerized Tomography
CVT	Cerebral Venous Thrombosis

CWD	Children with Disability
DALYs	Disability-Adjusted Life Years
DIS	Diagnostic Interview Schedule
DNA	Deoxyribonucleic Acid
DSM-IV	*Diagnostic and Statistical Manual* (Fourth Edition)
DZ	Dizygote
ECA	Epidemiological Catchment Area
ECASS	European Cooperative Acute Stroke Study
ECLAMC	Latin American Collaborative Study of Congenital Malformations
ECT	Electro-Convulsive Therapy
EEG	Electroencephalogram
EITB	Enzyme-Linked Immunoelectro-Transfer Blot
ERR	Event-Related Potentials
ESAP	Economic Structural Adjustment Programs
FAS	Fetal Alcohol Syndrome
GABA	Gamma-Aminobutryic Acid
GBD	Global Burden of Disease
GCAE	Global Campaign Against Epilepsy
GDP	Gross Domestic Product
GP	General Practitioner
GTCS	Generalized Tonic-Clonic Seizures
HEA	Health Education Authority (U.K.)
HIV	Human Immunodeficiency Virus
HPA	Hypothalamic-Pituitary-Adrenal
HSR	Health Systems Research
IBE	International Bureau for Epilepsy
ICD-10	*International Statistical Classification of Disease* (Tenth Revision)
ICIDH	International Classification of Impairments, Disabilities and Handicaps
ICMR	Indian Council of Medical Research
ILAE	International League Against Epilepsy
ILO	International Labor Organization
IMF	International Monetary Fund
INCLEN	International Clinical Epidemiology Network
IOM	Institute of Medicine
IQ	Intelligence Quotient
IPSS	International Pilot Study of Schizophrenia
LBW	Low Birth Weight
LDL	Low-Density Lipoprotein
MAOI	Monoamine Oxidase Inhibitor
MMSE	Mini-Mental State Examination
MONICA	Multinational Monitoring of Trends and Determinants in Cardio-vascular Disease

MR	Mental Retardation
MRI	Magnetic Resonance Imaging
MRS	Magnetic Resonance Spectroscopy
MZ	Monozygote
NCC	Neurocysticercosis
NCS	National Co-Morbidity Survey
NGO	Nongovernmental Organization
NICHD	National Institute of Child Health and Human Development
NIH	National Institutes of Health (U.S.)
NIMH	National Institute of Mental Health (U.S.)
NIMHANS	National Institute of Mental Health and Neuro Sciences (India)
NMHP	National Mental Health Programme of India
NOMASS	Northern Manhattan Stroke Study
OMAR	Operations Monitoring and Analysis of Results
OPV	Oral Polio Vaccine
PAHO	Pan-American Health Organization
PAS	Periodic-Acid Schiff
PCB	Polychlorinated Biphenyl
PET	Positron Emission Tomography
PHC	Primary Health Care
PHCW	Primary Health Care Worker
PKU	Phenylketonuria
PND	Postnatal Depression
PRC	People's Republic of China
PRDP	Population Rate Difference Percentage
PSE	Present State Examination
PTSD	Posttraumatic Stress Disorder
QALY	Quality-Adjusted Life Years
RCS	Research Capability Strengthening
RITM	Research Institute for Tropical Medicine
RTPA	Recombinant Tissue Plasminogen Activator
SAARC	South Asian Assistance for Regional Cooperation
SBK	Shishu Bikash Kendro
SCAN	Schedules for Clinical Assessment in Neuropsychiatry
SMR	Standard Mortality Ratio
SPECT	Single Photon Emission Computed Tomography
SPI	Study of Perioperative Ischemia
SSRI	Selective Serotonin Reuptake Inhibitor
TCA	Tricyclic Antidepressants
TDR	The Special Program for Research and Training in Tropical Diseases
TIA	Transient Ischemic Attack
TQ	Ten-Question Method

TSH	Thyroid Stimulating Hormone
UK	United Kingdom
UN	United Nations
UNDP	United Nations Development Program
UNESCO	United Nations Educational, Scientific, and Cultural Organization
UNHCR	United Nations High Commissioner for Refugees
UNICEF	United Nations International Children's Emergency Fund
USAID	United States Agency for International Development
USD	United States Dollar
WHO	World Health Organization
YLD	Years Lived with Disability
YLL	Years of Life Lost
ZPHCA	Zimbabwe Parents of Handicapped Children Association